Pediatric Integrated Care

Editors

TAMI D. BENTON
GREGORY K. FRITZ
GARY R. MASLOW

CHILD AND ADOLESCENT PSYCHIATRIC CLINICS OF NORTH AMERICA

www.childpsych.theclinics.com

Consulting Editor
HARSH K. TRIVEDI

October 2017 • Volume 26 • Number 4

ELSEVIER

1600 John F. Kennedy Boulevard • Suite 1800 • Philadelphia, Pennsylvania, 19103-2899

http://www.theclinics.com

CHILD AND ADOLESCENT PSYCHIATRIC CLINICS OF NORTH AMERICA Volume 26, Number 4
October 2017 ISSN 1056–4993, ISBN-13: 978-0-323-54656-0

Editor: Lauren Boyle
Developmental Editor: Kristen Helm

Child and Adolescent Psychiatric Clinics of North America (ISSN 1056-4993) is published quarterly by Elsevier Inc., 360 Park Avenue South, New York, NY 10010-1710. Months of issue are January, April, July, and October. Business and Editorial Offices: 1600 John F. Kennedy Boulevard, Suite 1800, Philadelphia, PA 19103-2899. Periodicals postage paid at New York, NY and additional mailing offices. Subscription prices are $316.00 per year (US individuals), $566.00 per year (US institutions), $100.00 per year (US students), $367.00 per year (Canadian individuals), $688.00 per year (Canadian institutions), $200.00 per year (Canadian students), $439.00 per year (international individuals), $688.00 per year (international institutions), and $200.00 per year (international students). International air speed delivery is included in all *Clinics* subscription prices. All prices are subject to change without notice. **POSTMASTER:** Send address changes to *Child and Adolescent Psychiatric Clinics of North America*, Elsevier Health Sciences Division, Subscription Customer Service, 3251 Riverport Lane, Maryland Heights, MO 63043. **Customer Service: 1-800-654-2452 (U.S. and Canada); 314-447-8871 (outside U.S. and Canada). Fax: 314-447-8029. E-mail:** JournalsCustomer Service-usa@elsevier.com **(for print support) or** journalsonlinesupport-usa@elsevier.com **(for online support).**

Reprints. For copies of 100 or more of articles in this publication, please contact the Commercial Reprints Department, Elsevier Inc., 360 Park Avenue South, New York, New York 10010-1710 Tel.: 212-633-3874; Fax: 212-633-3820, E-mail: reprints@elsevier.com.

Child and Adolescent Psychiatric Clinics of North America is covered in *MEDLINE/PubMed (Index Medicus), ISI, SSCI, Research Alert, Social Search, Current Contents,* and *EMBASE/Excerpta Medica.*

Contributors

CONSULTING EDITOR

HARSH K. TRIVEDI, MD, MBA

President and Chief Executive Officer, Sheppard Pratt Health System, Clinical Professor and Vice Chair, Department of Psychiatry, University of Maryland School of Medicine, Baltimore, Maryland

EDITORS

TAMI D. BENTON, MD

Chair, Department of Child and Adolescent Psychiatry and Behavioral Sciences, Children's Hospital of Philadelphia, Associate Professor, Department of Psychiatry, Perelman School of Medicine, University of Pennsylvania, Philadelphia, Pennsylvania

GREGORY K. FRITZ, MD

Professor and Director, Division of Child and Adolescent Psychiatry, Vice Chair, Department of Psychiatry and Human Behavior, The Warren Alpert Medical School of Brown University, Academic Director, E.P. Bradley Hospital, Associate Chief and Director of Child Psychiatry, Rhode Island Hospital/Hasbro Children's Hospital, Bradley Hasbro Children's Research Center, Providence, Rhode Island

GARY R. MASLOW, MD, MPH

Assistant Professor, Department of Psychiatry and Behavioral Sciences, Program Training Director Child and Adolescent Psychiatry Fellowship, Co-Chief, Division of Child and Family Mental Health and Developmental Neurosciences, Department of Psychiatry and Behavioral Sciences, Assistant Professor of Pediatrics, Primary Care Pediatrician, Duke University School of Medicine, Durham, North Carolina

AUTHORS

JOAN ROSENBAUM ASARNOW, PhD

Professor of Psychiatry and Biobehavioral Sciences, Semel Institute for Neuroscience & Human Behavior, David Geffen School of Medicine at UCLA, Los Angeles, California

KALINA BABEVA, PhD

Postdoctoral Scholar, Department of Psychiatry and Biobehavioral Sciences, Semel Institute for Neuroscience & Human Behavior, David Geffen School of Medicine at UCLA, Los Angeles, California

ADRIENNE BANNY, PhD

Department of Psychiatry and Behavioral Sciences, Duke University School of Medicine, Durham, North Carolina

LEE S. BEERS, MD
Associate Professor of Pediatrics, Child Health Advocacy Institute, Children's National Health System, Washington, DC

TAMI D. BENTON, MD
Chair, Department of Child and Adolescent Psychiatry and Behavioral Sciences, Children's Hospital of Philadelphia, Associate Professor, Department of Psychiatry, Perelman School of Medicine, University of Pennsylvania, Philadelphia, Pennsylvania

MATTHEW G. BIEL, MD, MSc
Associate Professor, Clinical Psychiatry and Pediatrics, Department of Child and Adolescent Psychiatry, Georgetown University School of Medicine, Washington, DC

DIANE E. BLOOMFIELD, MD
Medical Director, Montefiore Family Care Center Pediatric Teams, Assistant Professor, Division of Academic General Pediatrics, The Children's Hospital at Montefiore, Albert Einstein College of Medicine, Bronx, New York

TIFFANY WEST BRANDT, PhD
Assistant Professor, Psychiatric Research Institute, University of Arkansas for Medical Sciences, Little Rock, Arkansas

RAHIL D. BRIGGS, PsyD
Associate Professor, Department of Pediatrics, Psychiatry and Behavioral Sciences, Director, Pediatric Behavioral Health Services, Montefiore Medical Group, Yonkers, New York

JONATHAN D. BROWN, PhD, MHS
Director of Health Policy Assessment, Mathematica Policy Research, Washington, DC

MELISSA BUCHHOLZ, PsyD
Department of Psychiatry, Pediatric Mental Health Institute, Children's Hospital Colorado, University of Colorado School of Medicine, Aurora, Colorado

MAYA BUNIK, MD, MPH
Department of Pediatrics, Children's Hospital Colorado, University of Colorado School of Medicine, Aurora, Colorado

BRIDGET BURNETT, PsyD
Department of Psychiatry, Pediatric Mental Health Institute, Children's Hospital Colorado, University of Colorado School of Medicine, Aurora, Colorado

JACQUELYN M. COLLURA, MD
Physician, NW Permanente, PC, Physicians and Surgeons, Portland, Oregon

SILVIE COLMAN, PhD
Health Economist, Network Performance Group, Montefiore Medical Center, Bronx, New York

DAVID R. DeMASO, MD
Professor of Child Psychiatry and Pediatrics, Harvard Medical School, Psychiatrist-in-Chief and Chair, Department of Psychiatry, Boston Children's Hospital, Boston, Massachusetts

DIANE DERMARDEROSIAN, MD
Pediatric Director, The Hasbro Children's Partial Hospital Program, Clinical Assistant
Professor of Pediatrics, The Warren Alpert Medical School of Brown University,
Providence, Rhode Island

MIGUELINA GERMÁN, PhD
Assistant Professor, Department of Pediatrics, Director of Quality and Research, Pediatric
Behavioral Health Integrated Program (BHIP), Montefiore Medical Center, Albert Einstein
College of Medicine, Bronx, New York

LISA L. GILES, MD
Director, Behavioral Health Consultation and Community Services, Primary Children's
Hospital, Associate Professor of Pediatrics and Psychiatry, Department of Pediatrics,
University of Utah School of Medicine, Salt Lake City, Utah

MARY MARGARET GLEASON, MD, FAAP
Associate Professor, Psychiatry and Behavioral Sciences, Department of Pediatrics,
Tulane University School of Medicine, New Orleans, Louisiana

LEANDRA GODOY, PhD
Assistant Professor of Pediatrics, Child Health Advocacy Institute, Children's National
Health System, Washington, DC

RACHEL S. GROSS, MD, MS, FAAP
Assistant Professor, Department of Pediatrics, Associate Fellowship Director for
Academic General Pediatrics, Department of Pediatrics, Children's Hospital at
Montefiore, Albert Einstein College of Medicine, Bronx, New York

BRITTANY A. GURNEY, MA
Project Manager, Trauma Informed Care Program (TIC), Laboratory Manager, Behavioral
Health Integration Program (BHIP), Department of Pediatrics, Montefiore Medical Group,
Bronx, New York

LAUREN A. HALICZER, MA
Doctoral Student, Department of Clinical Psychology and Brain Sciences, University of
Massachusetts Amherst, Amherst, Massachusetts

EMILY HARRIS, MD, MPH
Assistant Professor of Psychiatry, Clinical-Affiliate of General and Community Pediatrics,
Division of Child and Adolescent Psychiatry, Department of Psychiatry and Behavioral
Neuroscience, Cincinnati Children's Hospital Medical Center, University of Cincinnati,
Cincinnati, Ohio

NICOLE HEILBRON, PhD
Department of Psychiatry and Behavioral Sciences, Duke University School of Medicine,
Durham, North Carolina

ROBERT J. HILT, MD
Professor, Department of Psychiatry and Behavioral Sciences, University of Washington,
Seattle, Washington

KATHERINE HOBBS KNUTSON, MD, MPH
Assistant Professor, Department of Psychiatry and Behavioral Sciences, Duke University
School of Medicine, Durham, North Carolina

ELIZABETH HORSTMANN, MD
Associate Physician, Department of Psychiatry and Biobehavioral Sciences, Semel
Institute for Neuroscience & Human Behavior, David Geffen School of Medicine at UCLA,
Los Angeles, California

CHRISTOPHER HOUCK, PhD
Director of Research, The Hasbro Children's Partial Hospital Program, Associate
Professor of Psychiatry and Human Behavior, The Warren Alpert School of Brown
University, Providence, Rhode Island

PATRICIA IBEZIAKO, MD
Assistant Professor, Department of Psychiatry, Harvard Medical School, Department of
Psychiatry, Boston Children's Hospital, Boston, Massachusetts

JAMES JACCARD, PhD
Professor, Co-Director of Center for Latino Adolescent and Family Health, Silver School of
Social Work, New York University, New York, New York

PETER S. JENSEN, MD
Professor, Director of Training and Research, Child and Adolescent Psychiatry,
Psychiatric Research Institute, University of Arkansas for Medical Sciences, Little Rock,
Arkansas; President, Chief Executive Officer, The REACH Institute, New York, New York

KIMBERLY KELSAY, MD
Department of Psychiatry, Pediatric Mental Health Institute, Children's Hospital Colorado,
University of Colorado School of Medicine, Aurora, Colorado

LISA KHAN, Ed.M.
Director, Patient-Centered Mental Health in Pediatric Primary Care Program,
The REACH Institute, New York, New York

ALLISON R. LOVE, PhD
Postdoctoral Fellow, Psychiatric Research Institute, University of Arkansas for Medical
Sciences, Little Rock, Arkansas

JOSEPH LUCAS, PhD
Social Science Research Institute, Duke University, Durham, North Carolina

D. RICHARD MARTINI, MD
Chair, Department of Psychiatry and Behavioral Health, Primary Children's Hospital,
Chief, Division of Pediatric Psychiatry and Behavioral Health, Professor of Pediatrics and
Psychiatry, Department of Pediatrics, University of Utah School of Medicine, Salt Lake
City, Utah

GARY R. MASLOW, MD, MPH
Assistant Professor, Department of Psychiatry and Behavioral Sciences, Program
Training Director Child and Adolescent Psychiatry Fellowship, Co-Chief, Division of Child
and Family Mental Health and Developmental Neurosciences, Department of Psychiatry
and Behavioral Sciences, Assistant Professor of Pediatrics, Primary Care Pediatrician,
Duke University School of Medicine, Durham, North Carolina

JENNIFER A. MAUTONE, PhD
Roberts Center for Pediatric Research, Child Development and Behavioral Health Clinic,
Assistant Professor, Department of Psychiatry, Perelman School of Medicine, University
of Pennsylvania, Philadelphia, Pennsylvania

JACK NASSAU, PhD
Chief Psychologist, The Hasbro Children's Partial Hospital Program, Clinical Associate Professor of Psychiatry and Human Behavior, The Warren Alpert Medical School of Brown University, Providence, Rhode Island

WANJIKU F.M. NJOROGE, MD
Program Director, Child and Adolescent Psychiatry Fellowship, Department of Child and Adolescent Psychiatry, Children's Hospital of Philadelphia, Assistant Professor, Department of Psychiatry, Perelman School of Medicine, University of Pennsylvania, Philadelphia, Pennsylvania

McLEAN POLLOCK, PhD, MSW
Department of Psychiatry and Behavioral Sciences, Duke University School of Medicine, Durham, North Carolina

JOANNA QUIGLEY, MD
Clinical Assistant Professor of Psychiatry, Department of Psychiatry, University of Michigan, Ann Arbor, Michigan

ANDREW D. RACINE, MD, PhD
System Senior Vice President and Chief Medical Officer, Montefiore Health System, Executive Director, Montefiore Medical Group, Bronx, New York

MARCY RAVECH, MSW
Executive Director, Massachusetts Child Psychiatry Access Programs, Massachusetts Behavioral Health Partnership, Beacon Health Options, Boston, Massachusetts

MONIQUE RIBEIRO, MD
Instructor, Department of Psychiatry, Harvard Medical School, Departments of Psychiatry and Anesthesiology, Perioperative and Pain Medicine, Boston Children's Hospital, Boston, Massachusetts

MICHELLE L. RICKERBY, MD
Psychiatric Director of Med/Psych Services and The Hasbro Children's Partial Hospital Program, Clinical Professor of Psychiatry and Human Behavior, The Warren Alpert Medical School of Brown University, Providence, Rhode Island

MICHAEL L. RINKE, MD, PhD
Medical Director of Pediatric Quality, Division of Pediatric Hospital Medicine, Montefiore Medical Center, Albert Einstein College of Medicine, Bronx, New York

PAUL M. ROBINS, PhD
Department of Child and Adolescent Psychiatry and Behavioral Sciences, Children's Hospital of Philadelphia, Professor, Department of Psychiatry, Perelman School of Medicine, University of Pennsylvania, Philadelphia, Pennsylvania

KENDRA ROSA, MPH
Department of Psychiatry and Behavioral Sciences, Duke University School of Medicine, Durham, North Carolina

CHASE SAMSEL, MD
Instructor, Department of Psychiatry, Harvard Medical School, Department of Psychiatry, Pediatric Transplant Center, Boston Children's Hospital, Department of Psychosocial Oncology and Palliative Care, Dana-Farber Cancer Institute, Boston, Massachusetts

BARRY D. SARVET, MD
Chair, Department of Psychiatry, Baystate Health, Professor and Chair, Department of Psychiatry, University of Massachusetts Medical School-Baystate, Springfield, Massachusetts

ABIGAIL SCHLESINGER, MD
Associate Professor, Department of Psychiatry, Western Psychiatric Institute and Clinic, University of Pittsburgh, Pittsburgh, Pennsylvania

SANDRA SEXSON, MD, DFAACAP, DFAPA, FACPSYCH
Professor and Chief, Child, Adolescent, and Family Psychiatry, Psychiatry and Health Behavior, Professor, Pediatrics, Medical College of Georgia, Augusta University, Augusta, Georgia

KRISTEN STEFUREAC, MSW
Department of Psychiatry and Behavioral Sciences, Duke University School of Medicine, Durham, North Carolina

JOHN H. STRAUS, MD
Medical Director, Special Projects, Massachusetts Behavioral Health Partnership, Beacon Health Options, Boston, Massachusetts

AYELET TALMI, PhD
Departments of Psychiatry and Pediatrics, Pediatric Mental Health Institute, Children's Hospital Colorado, University of Colorado School of Medicine, Aurora, Colorado

BARBARA KEITH WALTER, PhD, MPH
Department of Psychiatry and Behavioral Sciences, Duke University School of Medicine, Durham, North Carolina

ARIEL A. WILLIAMSON, PhD
Behavioral Sleep Medicine Fellow, Sleep Center, Children's Hospital of Philadelphia, Center for Sleep and Circadian Neurobiology, Perelman School of Medicine, University of Pennsylvania, Philadelphia, Pennsylvania

LAWRENCE S. WISSOW, MD, MPH
James P. Connaughton Professor of Community Mental Health, Division of Child and Adolescent Psychiatry, The Johns Hopkins University School of Medicine, Baltimore, Maryland

Contents

> Telemedicine with child psychiatry specialists is a useful tool for collaborative and integrated care systems. This article reviews the workforce and care process rationale for using child psychiatric telemedicine for collaborative care, and discusses practical ways to address the technical challenges that arise when using telemedicine. Different systems of using telemedicine that are discussed include child psychiatry access programs, collaborative and integrated care use of telephone consultations, televideo consultations, and televideo care delivery. Telemedicine can also be used for collaboratively conducted but care review requested by third-party consultations with treatment providers or care teams.

> The Massachusetts Child Psychiatry Access Program is a statewide public mental health initiative designed to provide consultation, care navigation, and education to assist pediatric primary care providers in addressing mental health problems for children and families. To improve program performance, adapt to changes in the environment of pediatric primary care services, and ensure the program's long-term sustainability, program leadership in consultation with the Massachusetts Department of Mental Health embarked on a process of redesign. The redesign process is described, moving from an initial strategic assessment of program and the planning of structural and functional changes, through transition and implementation.

> Integrated mental health services within health care settings have many benefits; however, several key barriers pose challenges to fully implemented and coordinated care. Collaborative, multistakeholder efforts, such as health networks, have the potential to overcome prevalent obstacles and to accelerate the dissemination of innovative clinical strategies. In addition to engaging clinical experts, efforts should also include the perspectives of families and communities, a grounding in data and evaluation, and a focus on policy and advocacy. This article describes how one community, Washington, DC, implemented a health network to improve the integration of mental health services into pediatric primary care.

Integrated health care models attempt to cross the barrier between behavioral and medical worlds to improve access to quality care that meets the needs of the whole patient. Unfortunately, the integration of behavioral health and physical health providers in one space is not enough to actually promote integration. There are many models for promoting integration and collaboration within the primary care context. This article uses the experience of the Children's Community Pediatrics Behavioral Health Services system to highlight components of collaboration that should be considered in order to successfully integrate behavioral health within a medical home.

Training combining the disciplines of pediatrics, psychiatry, and child and adolescent psychiatry dates to World War II, but formal combined programs began more than 3 decades ago as the Triple Board Program and 10 years ago as the Postpediatric Portal Program. Triple board training was rigorously examined as a pilot program and ongoing surveys suggest that it provides successful training of physicians who can pass the required board examinations and contribute to clinical, academic, and administrative/advocacy endeavors. As evidence grows, showing the value of integrated care, physicians with combined training will offer a unique perspective for developing systems.

Integrated behavioral and mental health systems of care for children require multidisciplinary team members to have specific competencies and knowledge of the other disciplines' strengths and practice needs. Training models for multidisciplinary professionals should consider the developmental level of trainees. The authors describe a model of flexible scaffolding, increasing intensity, and depth of experience as trainees gain skills and knowledge.

This article focuses on the cross-discipline training competencies needed for preparing behavioral health providers to implement integrated primary care services. After a review of current competencies in the disciplines of child and adolescent psychiatry, psychology, and social work, cross-cutting competencies for integrated training purposes are identified. These competencies are comprehensive and broad and can be modified for use in varied settings and training programs. An existing and successful integrated care training model, currently implemented at Children's Hospital of Philadelphia, is described. This model and the training competencies are discussed in the context of recommendations for future work and training.

The heuristic model of family-based integrated care (FBIC) was developed from 1998 to 2016 in the context of the development of the Hasbro Children's Partial Hospital Program (HCPHP) along with the development of a family therapy training program for Brown University child psychiatry and triple board residents. The clinical experience of the HCPHP team in treating more than 2000 patients and families in combination with the authors' experience in training residents for diverse practice settings highlights the usefulness of the FBIC paradigm for interdisciplinary family-based treatment for a broad range of illnesses and levels of care.

An estimated 1 in 5 children in the United States meet criteria for a diagnosable mental disorder, yet fewer than 20% receive mental health services. Unmet need for psychiatric treatment may contribute to patterns of increasing use of the emergency department. This article describes an integrated pediatric evaluation center designed to prevent the need for treatment in emergency settings by increasing access to timely and appropriate care for emergent and critical mental health needs. Preliminary results showed that the center provided rapid access to assessment and treatment services for children and adolescents presenting with a wide range of psychiatric concerns.

Emergency departments (EDs) can offer life-saving suicide prevention care. This article focuses on the ED and emergency services as service delivery sites for suicide prevention. Characteristics of EDs, models of emergency care, ED screening and brief intervention models, and practice guidelines and parameters are reviewed. A care process model for youths at risk for suicide and self-harm is presented, with guidance for clinicians based on the scientific evidence. Strengthening emergency infrastructure and integrating effective suicide prevention strategies derived from scientific research are critical for advancing suicide prevention objectives.

Comorbid behavioral and physical health conditions are accompanied by troubling symptom burden, functional impairment, and treatment complexity. Pediatric subspecialty care clinics offer an opportunity for the implementation of integrated behavioral health (BH) care models that promote resiliency. This article reviews integrated BH care in oncology, palliative care, pain, neuropsychiatry, cystic fibrosis, and transplantation. Examples include integrated care mandates, standards of care, research, and quality improvement by child and adolescent psychiatrists (CAPs) and allied BH clinicians. The role of CAPs in integrated BH care in subspecialty care is explored, focusing on cost, resource use, financial support, and patient and provider satisfaction.

Evaluations of integrated care programs share many characteristics of evaluations of other complex health system interventions. However, evaluating integrated care for child and adolescent mental health poses special challenges that stem from the broad range of social, emotional, and developmental problems that need to be addressed; the need to integrate care for other family members; and the lack of evidence-based interventions already adapted for primary care settings. Integrated care programs for children's mental health need to adapt and learn on the fly, so that evaluations may best be viewed through the lens of continuous quality improvement rather than evaluations of fixed programs.

This study examined how to design, staff, and evaluate the feasibility of 2 different models of integrated behavioral health programs in pediatric primary care across primary care sites in the Bronx, NY. Results suggest that the Behavioral Health Integration Program model of pediatric integrated care is feasible and that hiring behavioral health staff with specific training in pediatric, evidence-informed behavioral health treatments may be a critical variable in increasing outcomes such as referral rates, self-reported competency, and satisfaction.

A multidisciplinary team approach to care, as well as robust care coordination services, are primary components of almost all integrated care delivery systems. Given that these services have limited reimbursement in fee-for-service payment arrangements, integrating care in a fee-for-service environment is almost impossible. Capitated payment models hold promise for supporting integrated behavioral and physical health services. There are multiple national examples of integrated care delivery systems supported by capitated payment arrangements.

Mental health integration in primary care is based on creating an environment that encourages collaboration and supports appropriate care for patients and families while offering a full range of services. Training programs for primary care practitioners should include sessions on how to build and maintain such a practice along with information on basic mental health competencies.

Pediatric primary care providers (PPCPs) are increasingly expected to know how to assess, diagnose, and treat a wide range of mental health problems in children and adolescents. For many PPCPs, this means learning and performing new practice behaviors that were not taught in their residency training. Typical continuing education approaches to engage PPCPs in new practices have not yielded the desired changes in provider behavior. This article summarizes behavior change principles identified through basic behavior science, adult education, and communication research, and discusses their application to a patient-centered pediatric primary care mental health. curriculum.

CHILD AND ADOLESCENT PSYCHIATRIC CLINICS

THE CLINICS ARE AVAILABLE ONLINE!
Access your subscription at:
www.theclinics.com

Preface

Healthy Minds–Healthy Kids: Integrating Care

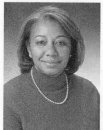 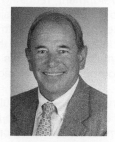 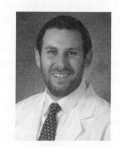

Tami D. Benton, MD   Gregory K. Fritz, MD   Gary R. Maslow, MD, MPH
Editors

Integrating mental health and primary care services has the potential to reshape and substantially improve the delivery of health care. Certainly, the health care system in the United States has a long way to go: although we were number one among 11 developed nations in terms of health care expenses, we were dead last when it came to access, equity, efficiency, quality, and indices of healthy lives. By involving primary care providers in the assessment and treatment of "garden variety" mental health problems, the workforce of mental health professionals, currently woefully inadequate to meet the demand for services, can be dramatically expanded.

Available evidence suggests that families would prefer to receive their mental health services in their familiar and accessible primary care setting. Primary care providers are typically well known and trusted by families, with no burden of stigma to deal with. They also have the advantage of knowing family members over time, in periods of sickness and health; they know the family's strengths and vulnerabilities. What primary care providers tend to *lack* that often impair their effectiveness with mental health issues are knowledge, confidence, and interest: important issues that will need to be addressed as the integrated care movement progresses.

Until recently, most of the publications regarding integrated care seem to be in the adult realm. The widely cited studies based on the Impact Model of Collaborative Care have consistently documented improved outcomes and financial savings, typically in adults with serious chronic medical illnesses and depression or other psychiatric disorders. Too often the assumption seems to be that if we figure out integrated care for adults, the approach can readily trickle down to children and adolescents.

Child Adolesc Psychiatric Clin N Am 26 (2017) xv–xvii
http://dx.doi.org/10.1016/j.chc.2017.08.001
1056-4993/17/© 2017 Published by Elsevier Inc.

childpsych.theclinics.com

The problem is that, as with most things, the requirements for an integrated care system for children and adolescents are different from adults. Children tend to be healthy, and most primary care visits are for health maintenance or acute treatment. Mental disorders are by far the costliest pediatric conditions, in contrast to diabetes and heart disease for adults. The potential to identify early signs of psychological problems, intervene early, and *prevent* serious, chronic adult dysfunction is a unique opportunity for pediatric integrated care. Children's dependency on adults, especially parents, is a central fact of development, requiring the focus to be on a *family*-centered medical home. It is also important to consider how to provide integrated care in all medical settings, since most children with physical conditions receive medical care from pediatric specialists with whom they build long-term relationships. Finally, the financial underpinnings and sources of return on investment are very different for a pediatric compared with an adult integrated care system.

This issue recognizes these critical differences and seeks to pull together the knowledge and experience of a diverse group of experts in pediatric integrated care. The authors focus on four areas: integrating mental health into community networks; training the mental health workforce; integrating care in diverse clinical settings; and preparing medical providers for integrated care by addressing financial barriers and educational needs.

These are exciting times to be working at the blurring boundary between pediatrics and psychiatry. The stigma of mental illness, while far from gone, has decreased substantially, and the demand for services continues to go up. Mental health parity remains to be fully executed, but as a legal issue it has been decided: psychiatric disorders must now be treated equally with medical illness. The turmoil of health care reform presents ample opportunities for new ideas, and integrated care is one of the most promising. We believe this issue will be materially useful to child mental health and medical professionals as we explore new territories of pediatric integrated care.

Tami D. Benton, MD
Chair, Department of Child and Adolescent Psychiatry and Behavioral Sciences
Children's Hospital of Philadelphia
Associate Professor of Psychiatry
Perelman School of Medicine at the University of Pennsylvania
3440 Market Street, Suite 410
Philadelphia, PA 19104, USA

Gregory K. Fritz, MD
Division of Child and Adolescent Psychiatry
Department of Psychiatry and Human Behavior
Warren Alpert Medical School
of Brown University
E.P. Bradley Hospital
Rhode Island Hospital/
Hasbro Children's Hospital
Bradley Hasbro Children's Research Center
Coro West, Suite 204
1 Hoppin Street
Providence, RI 02903, USA

Gary R. Maslow, MD, MPH
Duke University Child and Family Studies Center
2608 Erwin Road, Suite 300
Durham, NC 27705, USA

E-mail addresses:
bentont@email.chop.edu (T.D. Benton)
gfritz@lifespan.org (G.K. Fritz)
gary.maslow@duke.edu (G.R. Maslow)

Telemedicine for Child Collaborative or Integrated Care

Robert J. Hilt, MD

KEYWORDS

- Telemedicine • Telepsychiatry • Consult • Collaborative • Mental health
- Child psychiatry • System of care • Information security

KEY POINTS

- Telemedicine helps collaborative and integrated care systems access specialized child psychiatric resources that may not otherwise be available.
- Telemedicine is a broad field that includes televideo connections between treatment providers, televideo connections between a provider and patient, electronic communication, and telephone connections between providers.
- Technical challenges for telemedicine include addressing the security of both site and signal transmission, quality of connection speed, screen size and position, and reimbursement requirements.
- Telemedicine can be used for child psychiatry access programs, third-party request consult programs, and collaborative and integrated care systems.

INTRODUCTION

Pediatric primary care is a key site for behavioral health disorder detection, care coordination, and treatment. Most families in need of behavioral health care bring their kids to pediatric primary care practices for support, rather than reaching out themselves to the specialty mental health care system. In the United States, about three-quarters of all young people with mental health disorders get care from their primary care providers, whereas the specialty mental health care system ultimately serves less than 1 in 4 children who could benefit from specialty mental health treatment.[1,2] A continually increasing family and care system request for primary care to deliver the first steps in child mental and behavioral health care has been recognized for more than 2 decades.[3]

Disclosures: Dr R.J. Hilt has received grant support from Center for Medicare and Medicaid Services (CMS), the National Institute of Health, has been a consultant for Optum, and directs child psychiatric consultation services for Washington and Wyoming Medicaid.
University of Washington, M/S CPH, PO Box 5371, Seattle, WA 98105, USA
E-mail address: robert.hilt@seattlechildrens.org

Child Adolesc Psychiatric Clin N Am 26 (2017) 637–645
http://dx.doi.org/10.1016/j.chc.2017.05.001
1056-4993/17/© 2017 Elsevier Inc. All rights reserved.
childpsych.theclinics.com

Abbreviation	
CPAP	Child psychiatry access program

Primary care providers report that they experience significant difficulties with the referral process, for instance in 1 study only about one-third of providers believed that their patients would frequently follow through on recommendations to seek specialty mental health care.[4] Unfortunately, for a variety of family, workforce, and insurance reasons, a simple referral out of primary care and into specialty mental health care often means that no care will be delivered. Integrating collaborative mental health care programs right into primary care settings offers an opportunity to ensure a much broader population of children get access to high-quality early detection, assessment, and treatment, which can then meet the "triple aim" of improving care, improving health, and lowering costs of care.[5]

A system of integrated mental health care relies on distributing some degree of new mental health expertise and services into the workflow of primary care practices. However, bringing mental health care expertise into primary care offices presents many challenges; for instance, not every primary care practice should be expected to employ its own mental health experts, available every day under their roof. One way to more flexibly bring mental health services into primary care practices is the use of telemedicine.

Telemedicine is a broad and evolving field, and as such the term telemedicine has received more than 100 different definitions over time in peer-reviewed publications.[6] In brief, telemedicine can be thought of as the application of medical expertise or services via a remote care delivery or support pathway. An example of a longer but quite inclusive telemedicine definition by the World Health Organization is,

> The delivery of health care services, where distance is a critical factor, by all health care professionals using information and communication technologies for the exchange of valid information for diagnosis, treatment and prevention of disease and injuries, research and evaluation, and for the continuing education of health care providers, all in the interests of advancing the health of individuals and their communities.[7]

So in the realm of mental health, telemedicine could include telephone based support for practitioners, remotely reviewed patient care interactions, interactive electronic communications, and 2-way live videoconferencing for peer support or patient evaluations (**Box 1**). Telemedicine has been growing in popularity and acceptance within all areas of medicine over the years, particularly for psychiatry. This is because there are a few aspects of psychiatry that lend themselves very well to the use of telemedicine.

Box 1
Some common varieties of telemedicine services

- Treatment delivery via 2-way interactive televideo
- Patient consultation via 2-way interactive televideo
- Provider care discussions via 2-way interactive televideo
- Collaborative mental health provider support via telephone
- Primary care provider consultation via telephone
- Electronic communication for consultation/collaboration purposes

Psychiatric care providers are relatively unique in that with only rare exceptions they are not expected to physically touch their patients to provide best practice services. Verbal and visual assessments with child and parent, which can occur via telemedicine, are all that need to be used to engage with patients appropriately, obtain full diagnostic accuracy, and provide most types of treatment services. This makes using 2-way tele videoconferencing for clinical assessments and treatment delivery a reasonable mode of psychiatric treatment.

Another reason for an increasing popularity of child telepsychiatry in particular is the shortage and maldistribution of child psychiatrists. The American Academy of Child and Adolescent Psychiatry reports there are only about 8300 practicing child psychiatrists in the United States, which represents a severe national shortage.[8] Every state in the country has a significant workforce shortage, although some states (especially the predominantly rural states) are much worse off than others.[8] Beyond this general workforce shortage, child psychiatrists tend to locate their practices in the more urban areas of a state, leaving the less population dense areas and areas of low socioeconomic status with significantly reduced access.[8,9] Telemedicine makes it possible for families to access child psychiatrists in a system of care where there are not any child psychiatrists available. For the psychiatrists who live and work in urban areas, it allows them to more easily provide support or services to primary care practices and families located in underserved, rural areas.

TECHNICAL CONSIDERATIONS FOR TELEVIDEO TELEMEDICINE

The telemedicine field typically focuses on using 2-way interactive televideo technology for the provision of direct patient care services. To provide direct televideo psychiatric care services, there are certain requirements to be able to approximate the experience of an in-person encounter (**Box 2**).

One requirement is confidentiality, that both provider and patient need to be assured that their interaction is not being overheard by uninvited others. This consideration starts with the physical locations of both the provider and the patient or family, that they need to be conducting their interactions in rooms where no one unwanted is viewing them or listening to them. Initially, this was inherently addressed by both the patient and the provider using dedicated videoconference equipment that was housed in clinical care offices. But with improvements in technology, home computers, tablets, or cell phones are capable of supporting a video conference in locations which may not be very room secure. For instance, an adolescent could have a video conference interaction from their home to a treating psychiatrist, which may be overheard by siblings or parents in the next room without your awareness or knowledge.

Box 2
Televideo basic technical considerations

- Private room for the televideo system
- Signal transmission that is compliant with the Health Insurance Portability and Accountability Act
- Broadband connection (>384 Kbs upload preferred)
- Screen, camera, and microphone in comfortable positions
- Provider credentialing if using a hospital-based site
- Plan for addressing in-session technical problems

The other confidentiality issue is technological, namely, that interactions via electronic means need to be performed in a secure manner so that your session cannot be easily hacked into or viewed by others. Videoconferencing occurs through a general Internet connection, and as such there are potential issues with information security, just like everything else that happens on the Internet. Providers looking to conduct remote care patient appointments need to ensure that their telemedicine connection equipment and connection pathway are compliant with health information protection laws like the Health Insurance Portability and Accountability Act.[10,11] This assurance can happen through using secured point-to-point dedicated teleconferencing systems, which are still relatively expensive to purchase and install, or by using a program that secures the video conference signal between 2 connecting devices.[12] There are many companies offering this service now that, in essence, creates a secured electronic meeting room for tablets, smartphones, webcam computers, or dedicated conferencing equipment to connect and synchronize for a video encounter.

To conduct a patient care interaction that reasonably approximates what it is like to interact in the same room together, there should be both good audio and video quality. Internet connection speed has a major impact on audio and video quality; for instance, upload speeds of 384 Kbps or higher are preferred.[13] Slow connection speeds are more prone to image pixilation, freezing, and audio quality breakdowns, which impair the ability to interact.[12] Using high-quality microphones and video cameras that are added on to a computer may give a superior experience than cameras or microphones that come integrated in purchased devices. Ideally, providers would have the ability to control/zoom the patient-side camera (to better see facial expressions, look at pictures that a child has drawn, etc), which is generally only possible through dedicated video conference equipment. Providers need be prepared for having technical problems during a televideo session, which they would need to either troubleshoot themselves (such as rebooting the system) or ask a technology support person to provide assistance.[14]

Screen size is another consideration, because an interaction on something like a 40-inch video monitor could be more natural and engaging than an interaction occurring with a small tablet or smartphone screen. Providers also need to be aware that having to physically hold a tablet or smart phone in such a way as to maintain proper camera angles during an extended interaction could be awkward. As such, if something like a tablet is being used, putting the tablet on a stand on a table while interacting is preferable.

If one is delivering televideo telemedicine services that are either originating from a hospital or delivering services to a hospital or a hospital-based clinic, that hospital will with only rare exceptions require that all televideo providers be specifically credentialed to provide services in that facility.[15] So even if providing only rare consultations or assessments to that hospital or hospital-based clinic, the credentialing process is essentially the same as required for fully joining that hospital's staff. This can make the provision of televideo care that is either originating from or dialing in to non–hospital-based clinics, which therefore do not have that additional credentialing hurdle, a more attractive option.

Beyond these technical issues, to perform treatment services via televideo telemedicine, the treating provider will need to be able to bill for their services. Many but not all insurances will reimburse for televideo appointments conducted as equivalent to in-person appointments, which providers may need to explore. Notably, even if the provider is reimbursed, this is a "zero-sum game," which does not offer providers any fiscal or time incentive to engage in telemedicine over delivering in person care.[16] Another approach could be that for a particular health system's integrated care practice, they could implement an alternative or reformed payment structure that supports the telespecialist's time in an attractive way.[16] For instance, a health system could reimburse all of a provider's time dedicated to telepsychiatry service delivery, independent of completed visits/billing claims, or provide salary support for remote site providers to conduct brief virtual communications or case reviews with care managers or other members of the care team.

USES OF TELEVIDEO TELEMEDICINE

Televideo telemedicine has been shown to be an effective way to deliver treatment services. A significant volume of research now supports that telepsychiatry can provide comparable diagnostic accuracy, treatment alliance, treatment outcomes, and both patient and provider satisfaction as does in-person care delivery.[13,17] Further, providing behavioral health treatment in a more convenient to access location for the family via televideo can increase the success rate of primary care referrals to specialty care. Without telemedicine or collaborative care system access, only around one-half to two-thirds of children referred by primary care to an outside specialty mental health provider will attend even a single treatment appointment, and there is another significant drop-off in those who will attend multiple treatment sessions at outside mental health clinics.[18]

Performing televideo patient care within a primary care practice can also benefit the integrated care process if both scheduling and clinical documentation are performed within the health care home's own record systems. Although having a shared clinical record does not by itself guarantee that collaboration and communication will occur, it does make it easier for primary care and specialist providers to collaborate around patient care.[16]

In addition to treatment delivery, televideo telemedicine can be used in an integrated system of care to perform otherwise difficult to access consult appointments, which can specifically assist the primary care provider's diagnostic process and care planning for treatments that primary care providers would then deliver themselves.[14] There is an integrated care system advantage for using televideo to perform consults over using televideo for treatment delivery, because doing so maintains the accessibility of specialists.[16] A limited amount of specialist televideo time would otherwise become quickly filled with clients for whom the specialist provides ongoing care services. If at least some of the specialist's time is reserved for consultations, primary care will always be able to receive specialist input on challenging diagnoses or treatment planning. Providing telepsychiatry appointments changes where children can receive their diagnostic or treatment services, but it does not inherently improve how many children can be served by a limited number of child mental health specialists.

TELEVIDEO TELEMEDICINE FOR COLLABORATIVE CARE

Integrated care and collaborative care are terms that are sometimes used interchangeably, but, as the Substance Abuse and Mental Health Services Administration has defined them, we should view them as distinct. Integrated and collaborative care exist along a spectrum of integrated service delivery designs, for which collaborative care represents a lower level of overall behavioral health integration.[19] Integrated care as opposed to collaborative care involves a greater emphasis on practice-supported care coordination, care tracking, and care delivery than what is typical for collaborative care, and integrated care requires an in-office behavioral health coordinator or behavioral health provider to operate. For instance, in integrated care a practice-embedded behavioral health provider or coordinator performs tasks like maintaining a registry of behavioral health cases, monitoring patient clinical outcomes, coordinating care delivery, and helping the health care home to adjust treatment to achieve patient- and family-centered goals of care.[16,19]

Televideo telemedicine can be used in different ways in an integrated care system. Providing telemedicine behavioral health treatment within a primary care office, even if it is just of a short-term variety, is a significant boon for the young people cared for in that clinic. As noted for workforce reasons noted, this may not be possible to offer for all primary care patients in need of behavioral health services. An on-site care coordinator for the integrated care program working with the clinic's primary care providers could control access to their televideo treatment resource. Generally speaking, it is clearer for care processes to have upfront agreements about which categories of clients can use the health system's teleprovider (for instance, specifically available just for depression and anxiety care).

Televideo telemedicine can also be used to perform consult evaluations in integrated care, to help the team decide if the child would be well served by an integrated care treatment (such as for attention deficit hyperactivity disorder or uncomplicated depression), or if the child has a disorder of higher clinical severity, which would instead be best served with care centered at a specialty mental health center (such as bipolar or a psychotic disorder).[1] Televideo can also be used for collaboration among team members. For instance, a child psychiatrist could use a televideo connection when performing caseload review discussions with on-site behavioral health providers or coordinators, or could use televideo to discuss specific cases with primary care providers.

OTHER WAYS TO USE TELEMEDICINE FOR COLLABORATIVE CARE

Telemedicine service delivery systems for collaborative/integrated care do not just include televideo appointments. Telephones represent the oldest form of telemedicine technology that still has the advantages of being highly reliable, widely accessible, and capable of delivering a useful collaborative care connection between providers. Telephone consultation access programs have exploded in popularity across the country in the last decade because of their ability to easily spread a limited child psychiatry resource across a wide variety of practice settings and geography for a limited per-capita investment.[20–22]

Child psychiatry access programs (CPAPs) have as their core unit of service rapid telephone access for patient-specific or general educational consultations with a child psychiatrist. To use this type of telemedicine support, primary care providers can call a service line for assistance with any behavioral health cases that they see, ideally would immediately discuss the case over the phone with a child psychiatrist, and then before the child leaves their office that day they can implement a treatment plan that has collaborative assistance from the psychiatrist.[20,23,24] Some form of CPAP service is currently available in more than one-half of the US states.[22]

Most CPAP telephone consultations will result in a recommendation that the child engage in a new psychosocial intervention, which may require referral assistance for the family to be able to follow through with the advice.[23,24] Providing referral services to community mental health providers is, therefore, a common element for most CPAPs. How that referral service is delivered can vary, in that some programs provide referral advice just to primary care providers, whereas another program's referral service may directly work with parents to assist them in making appointments.

There are many different variations of CPAPs that add different elements on to what is typically the core telephone access component. For instance, based on funding sources, access programs may be just for the providers within a specific health care system, whereas other programs may be available to every provider statewide.[22] CPAPs may specifically enroll community providers to use the service, or may not require formal provider enrollments. Educational events could be offered for providers, and distributing written clinical practice guides may be another program offering.[23] CPAPs may or may not send providers written summaries of each telephone consult discussion. Some CPAPs offer in-person or televideo consultations, and some will offer short-term counseling treatment.[22] CPAPs generally avoid offering short-term medication management services, because experience shows that if a CPAP psychiatrist starts prescribing for a family it becomes difficult to transition the care and prescriptions back to primary care.[20,25] Prescribing a medication changes the role of a psychiatrist from consultant to ongoing care provider, which families, and sometimes primary care providers too, can have difficulty stopping.

THIRD-PARTY REQUESTED TELEMEDICINE CONSULTATIONS

Everything described so far regarding telemedicine for collaborative or integrated care assumes that these interactions are actively sought out by primary care practices. But there are other entry pathways for child psychiatric specialists to become engaged in collaborative care. A third party like a health system, health care insurer, or child care overseeing agency (eg, foster care or schools) may request child mental health specialist consultations to collaborate around patient care. When third parties seek such a consultation over a very broad geographic reach, telemedicine is often a practical delivery pathway.

Prescribers typically have a dislike for health systems or insurers requiring that a second opinion consultation happen about one of their patients. This is an understandable perspective; for instance, if a second opinion medication review is performed by a nonclinician who applies rigid checklist review criteria as a barrier to medication access and does not offer the clinician any helpful care support, then that is clearly not a collaborative care consultation. But it does not have to be that way.

Clinical specialists may instead deliver second opinion consultations with the primary goal of offering helpful diagnostic suggestions and clinical care support/advice for what are inevitably the providers' most difficult to manage patients (by virtue of meeting some kind of trigger for review). If performed in this fashion, third-party requested telephone or televideo consultations can be received by treating providers as truly collaborative and helpful. One example is mandatory second opinion medication reviews using child psychiatrists for telephone-based care discussions in 2 different Western states that have been found to both be generally well received by the provider communities and lead to very significant changes in community prescribing practices without a reliance on reviewers saying "no" to prescription authorizations.[26,27] Another example is a program of child psychiatrist televideo consultations with foster care children to local, rural social service teams, which was again a well-received service that led to significant improvements in the children's care plans (eg, foster children more successful at remaining in their home communities).[26]

SUMMARY

To best serve the needs of the whole population of young people already going to primary care practices for help, child psychiatric knowledge and expertise should be leveraged beyond one-on-one patient care delivery into pathways of delivering collaborative and integrated care. Telemedicine can be an essential strategy to help providers and families in remote locations engage in more accessible and higher quality psychiatric care services. Child psychiatrists and other child mental health specialists can deliver telemedicine consultations, tele-case reviews, remote provider trainings, brief televideo treatment, or telesupport for integrated care providers, which greatly expands the impact any single child mental health specialist can have for the population of children in need of services.

Telemedicine in all of its forms listed is likely to see steady increases in use as a tool to assist collaborative and integrated care programs for young people. Continual improvements in technology and increased acceptance of remote communication may in our future bring health care consumer demands for in-home telemedicine service delivery via tablets and even smart phones, which will present both unique treatment opportunities and many new challenges for practitioners of child psychiatry.

REFERENCES

1. Martini R, Hilt R, Marx L, et al, for the American Academy of Child and Adolescent Psychiatry. Best principles for integration of child psychiatry into the pediatric health home. 2012. Available at: http://www.aacap.org/App_Themes/AACAP/docs/clinical_practice_center/systems_of_care/best_principles_for_integration_of_child_psychiatry_into_the_pediatric_health_home_2012.pdf. Accessed March 21, 2017.

2. American Academy of Child and Adolescent Psychiatry Committee on Health Care Access and Economics Task Force on Mental Health. Improving mental health services in primary care: reducing administrative and financial barriers to access and collaboration. Pediatrics 2009;123(4):1248–51.

3. Committee on Psychosocial Aspects of Child and Family Health, American Academy of Pediatrics. The new morbidity revisited: a renewed commitment to the psychosocial aspects of pediatric care. Pediatrics 2001;108(5):1227–30.

4. Williams J, Palmes G, Klinepeter K, et al. Referral by pediatricians of children with behavioral health disorders. Clin Pediatr 2005;44(4):343–9.

5. Talmi A, Muther E, Margolis K, et al. The scope of behavioral health integration in a pediatric primary care setting. J Pediatr Psychol 2016;41(10):929–37.

6. World Health Organization. Report on the second global survey on eHealth. 2010. Available at: http://www.who.int/goe/publications/goe_telemedicine_2010.pdf. Accessed March 21, 2017.

7. World Health Organization. A health telematics policy in support of WHO's Health-For-All strategy for global health development: report of the WHO group consultation on health telematics, 11–16 December. Geneva (Switzerland): World Health Organization 1998; 1997. Available at: http://apps.who.int/iris/handle/10665/63857. Accessed March 21, 2017.

8. American Academy of Child and Adolescent Psychiatry. Child and adolescent psychiatry workforce crisis: solutions to improve early intervention and access to care. 2013. Available at: https://www.aacap.org/App_Themes/AACAP/docs/Advocacy/policy_resources/cap_workforce_crisis_201305.pdf. Accessed March 21, 2017.

9. Thomas KC, Ellis AR, Konrad TR, et al. County-level estimates of mental health professional shortage in the United States. Psychiatr Serv 2009;60(10):1323–8.

10. Rodriquez-Feliz JR, Roth MZ. The mobile technology era: potential benefits and the challenging quest to ensure patient privacy and confidentiality. Plast Reconstr Surg 2012;130(6):1395–7.
11. HealthIT.gov. Health IT legislation and regulations. Available at: https://www.healthit.gov/policy-researchers-implementers/health-it-legislation. Accessed March 21, 2017.
12. Myers K, Cain S, American Academy of Child and Adolescent Psychiatry Work Group on Quality Issues. Practice parameter for telepsychiatry with children and adolescents. J Am Acad Child Adolesc Psychiatry 2008;47(12):1468–83.
13. Hilty D, Yellowlees PM, Parrish MB, et al. Telepsychiatry: effective, evidence-based, and at a tipping point in health care delivery? Psychiatr Clin North Am 2015;38(3):559–92.
14. Gloff NE, LeNoue SR, Novins DK, et al. Telemental health for children and adolescents. Int Rev Psychiatry 2015;27(6):513–24.
15. Joint Commission on Accreditation of Healthcare Organizations. Final revisions to telemedicine standards. Jt Comm Perspect 2012;32(1):4–6.
16. Fortney JC, Pyne JM, Turner EE, et al. Telepsychiatry integration of mental health services into rural primary care settings. Int Rev Psychiatry 2015;27(6):525–39.
17. Myers KM, Palmer NB, Geyer BA. Research in child and adolescent telemental health. Child Adolesc Psychiatr Clin N Am 2011;20(1):155–71.
18. Gopalan G, Goldstein L, Klingenstein K, et al. Engaging families into child mental health treatment: updates and special considerations. J Can Acad Child Adolesc Psychiatry 2010;19(3):182–96.
19. SAMHSA-HRSA Center for Integrated Health Solutions. A standard framework for levels of integrated healthcare. 2013:1–13. Available at: http://www.integration.samhsa.gov/integrated-care-models/A_Standard_Framework_for_Levels_of_Integrated_Healthcare.pdf. Accessed March 21, 2017.
20. Sarvet B, Hilt R. Child and adolescent psychiatry in integrated care settings. In: Raney LE, editor. Integrated care: working at the interface of primary and behavioral health care. Arlington (VA): American Psychiatric Publishing; 2015. p. 63–90.
21. Gabel S. The integration of mental health into the pediatric practice: pediatricians and child and adolescent psychiatrists working together in new models of care. J Pediatr 2010;157(5):848–51.
22. National Network of Child Psychiatry Access Programs. Existing programs: member organizations by state. Available at: http://nncpap.org/existing-programs.html. Accessed March 21, 2017.
23. Hilt RJ, Romaire MA, McDonnell MG, et al. The partnership access line: evaluating a child psychiatry consult program in Washington state. JAMA Pediatr 2013;167(2):162–8.
24. Straus JH, Sarvet B. Behavioral health care for children: the Massachusetts child psychiatry access project. Health Aff 2014;33(12):2153–61.
25. Connor DF, McLaughlin TJ, Jeffers-Terry M, et al. Targeted child psychiatric services: a new model of pediatric primary clinician-child psychiatry collaborative care. Clin Pediatr 2006;45(5):423–34.
26. Hilt RJ, Barclay RP, Bush J, et al. A statewide child telepsychiatry consult system yields desired health system changes and savings. Telemed J E Health 2015;21(7):533–7.
27. Barclay RP, Penfold RB, Sullivan D, et al. Decrease in statewide antipsychotic prescribing after implementation of child and adolescent psychiatry consultation services. Health Serv Res 2017;52(2):561–78.

Massachusetts Child Psychiatry Access Project 2.0
A Case Study in Child Psychiatry Access Program Redesign

Barry D. Sarvet, MD[a],*, Marcy Ravech, MSW[b], John H. Straus, MD[b]

KEYWORDS

- Child and adolescent psychiatry • Collaborative care
- Child psychiatry access programs • Mental health integration

KEY POINTS

- The Massachusetts Child Psychiatry Access Program is a statewide public program offering dedicated resources of telephone consultation, expedited assessment, care navigation support, and training to pediatric primary care providers across Massachusetts.
- Opportunities for improvement in the performance of the program identified through a systematic strategic assessment included the need to provide outreach to pediatric practices, to redefine the care navigation support provided by the program, and to improve the consistency and efficiency of the program services.
- Outreach practice consultation is a new function of the program designed to help pediatric practices achieve mental health process improvement goals and to address specific primary care provider training needs.
- The landscape of pediatric practice in Massachusetts has changed substantially over the past 12 years since the initial design of the program: pediatric practices are increasingly organized into networks, adopting the patient-centered medical home model, and embedding behavioral health clinicians into the primary care team.
- Programs require periodic iteration in order to address environmental changes, to debug programmatic vulnerabilities, and to make improvements based on analysis of the program's performance.

Conflicts of Interest: The authors have no conflicts of interest to disclose.
a University of Massachusetts Medical School-Baystate, 759 Chestnut Street, WG703, Springfield, MA 01199, USA; b Massachusetts Child Psychiatry Access Programs, Massachusetts Behavioral Health Partnership, Beacon Health Options, 1000 Washington Street, Suite 310, Boston, MA 02118, USA
* Corresponding author.
E-mail address: barry.sarvet@baystatehealth.org

Child Adolesc Psychiatric Clin N Am 26 (2017) 647–663
http://dx.doi.org/10.1016/j.chc.2017.05.003
1056-4993/17/© 2017 Elsevier Inc. All rights reserved.

INTRODUCTION TO THE CHILD PSYCHIATRY ACCESS PROGRAMS MOVEMENT

Inadequate access to mental health care for children and families has been a vexing problem in communities across the United States.[1-3] Pediatric primary care providers, working at the front lines of the health care system, confront the unmet needs of children with mental health problems on a daily basis; however, lacking appropriate training and access to referral resources, they are frequently ill-prepared for this role.[4-6] For common health problems arising in other systems of the body, primary care providers receive basic clinical training in residency in the prevention, early detection, diagnostic assessment, initial management, and follow-up care of patients. Primary care practices are also typically connected, informally or formally, to a network of specialist colleagues and ancillary resources for the care of patients with non–mental health conditions. Primary care providers commonly have staff members within their practice assisting them in providing this care. None of these conditions are consistently present for children with mental health conditions.

In 2004, the Massachusetts Child Psychiatry Access Project (MCPAP),[7,8] the first of a series of system-level public mental health programs that have come to be called child psychiatry access programs (CPAPs), began to address this gap. CPAPs are programs designed to provide a range of scaffolding resources for a defined set of pediatric primary care practices enabling them to address mental health problems for children and families in a manner comparable with common non–mental health problems. The set of primary care practices are most often defined geographically, according to municipal boundaries based on public funding specifications, although CPAPs can be directed to practices according to health system or network affiliation. CPAP teams are organized in a hub/spoke configuration with pediatric practices. The services provided by CPAPs address both knowledge and service coordination gaps for primary care teams and may include the following:

1. Informal so-called curbside telephonic consultation to primary care providers (PCPs) by child and adolescent psychiatrists (CAPs) and/or other children's mental health specialists
2. Direct expedited clinical assessment of patients, either in person or through a tele-video resource
3. Assistance with referrals and care navigation for the implementation of a mental health care plan
4. Provision of continuing medical education programming for PCPs

Since 2004, the CPAP model has spread widely throughout the United States. At present, CPAPs are operating in 28 states, and according to data compiled by the National Network of Child Psychiatry Access Programs it is estimated that PCPs for more than one-third of children in the United States (approximately 24 million) currently have access to child psychiatry consultation resources.[9]

THE MASSACHUSETTS CHILD PSYCHIATRY ACCESS PROJECT EXPERIENCE 2004 TO 2016

Over 12 years, MCPAP has developed into a robust, statewide, geographically based CPAP offering collaborative support to all pediatric PCPs in Massachusetts. This article refers to the period from October 2004 through December 2016 as MCPAP 1.0. During this time, the program was geographically configured with 6 regions, each with a team consisting of a full-time equivalent (FTE) of a CAP (consisting of several individuals), a behavioral health clinician (social worker/licensed mental health counselor), and a care coordinator. This staffing provided a close, collaborative relationship with many of the providers in the team's region. These personalized relationships allowed consultants to customize recommendations according to variations in PCPs' level of interest, ability, and comfort in managing behavioral health problems. With this staffing, usage grew (**Fig. 1**). In fiscal year (FY) 2016, MCPAP 1.0 consulted on 7302 youth and 65% of pediatricians used the consultation line at least once, some more than monthly. Survey data showed a remarkable impact on PCP experience of behavioral health practice (**Fig. 2**). Survey respondents reported a comfort managing attention-deficit/hyperactivity disorder (ADHD), depression, and anxiety but not substance use (**Fig. 3**).

With widespread, robust use of MCPAP 1.0 by PCPs, the legislature has, since 2004, provided full support ($3.3 million in the budget of the Department of Mental Health). Stakeholders, especially family advocates, the Children's Mental Health Campaign,[10] and the Department of Mental Health (DMH), were a constant source of support. In 2014, the legislature mandated the commercial insurers to financially contribute to the state in proportion to its use by covered plan subscribers in order to ensure long-term sustainability. Also in 2014, using funds from the Centers for Medicare & Medicaid Services (CMS) State Innovation Model (SIM) grant, the program was able to spawn a related program, MCPAP for Moms, providing similar services for obstetricians/gynecologists, adult PCPs, and general psychiatrists to improve access to care for postpartum depression.[11] As of December 31, 2016, MCPAP for Moms has provided help to 2252 women and the DMH appropriation was increased in FY2016 to replace SIM grant funding.

THE NEED FOR REDESIGN

Although MCPAP 1.0 continued to have high levels of usage and satisfaction among enrolled PCPs, ongoing review of program performance and environmental changes led to some concern regarding the program's long-term sustainability.

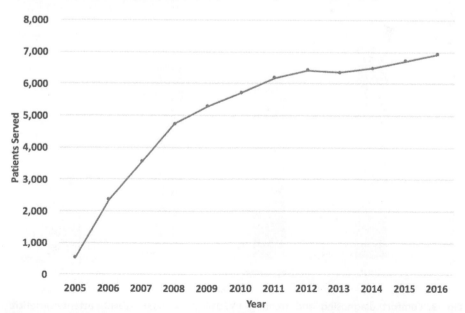

Fig. 1. Annual number of patients served in MCPAP.

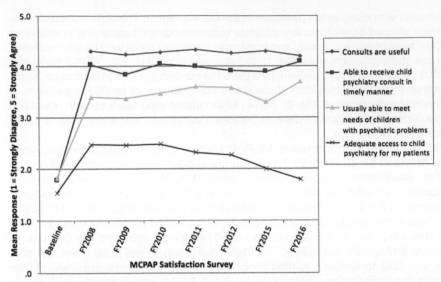

Fig. 2. Mean MCPAP satisfaction survey responses. Baseline, fiscal year (FY) 2008 through FY2016 (N = 563 in FY2016).

Program Performance Issues

Care coordination

The MCPAP 1.0 method of care coordination consisted of the MCPAP care coordinator talking with the family to determine their needs, checking availability of several community resources, and then providing referral information directly to the family.

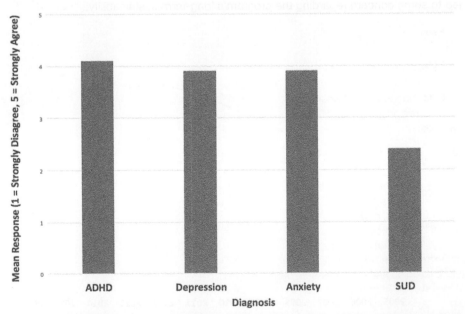

Fig. 3. Comfort diagnosing and treating FY2016 (N = 563). ADHD, attention-deficit/hyperactivity disorder; SUD, substance use disorder.

In 2015, a care coordination follow-up activity was developed to determine whether or not the referral successfully resulted in receipt of services and, if not, to provide further assistance to the parent. In the course of this work, the program was unable to reach the family about 50% of the time. Of those families reached, approximately 50% had not received the service for a variety of reasons, including, most commonly, difficulty securing a convenient appointment time or a change in a parent's perception of the need for the appointment. This finding led to the recognition that effective care coordination is not a so-called one-and-done event but a process requiring continuous engagement. Furthermore, it was acknowledged that MCPAP 1.0 contained neither adequate resources nor the continuous relationship with the family required for effective care coordination. This one-and-done care coordination service provided by MCPAP 1.0 was, at best, ineffective, and may paradoxically have given primary care practices a false sense of security, leading them to withdraw their attention from the support and referral tracking inherent in their role as a patient-centered medical home.

Multiple Massachusetts Child Psychiatry Access Projects

Performance data regarding volumes of service provided by the 6 MCPAP teams showed wide variation in the usage of MCPAP services within and across teams. Some PCPs interacted with MCPAP multiple times per day and others rarely, if ever, requested MCPAP services. The experience of the program for PCPs interacting frequently with MCPAP was qualitatively different than that for the PCPs who called rarely. Also, the program noted significant cross-team variation in PCP-adjusted volumes of services provided, suggesting variation in MCPAP performance in the engagement of PCPs. Some of the variation in usage could be explained by differences in internal or local resources available to PCPs; however, it was known that many of the practices rarely using MCPAP were lacking in these resources.

Inconsistency in response times

The MCPAP 1.0 team configuration required the CAP on each team to multitask between answering the phone line for consultations, doing face-to-face evaluations, and assisting practices with educational opportunities. At times, multitasking was leading to response times of more than 30 minutes for phone consultations and excessive waiting times for face-to-face consultations, and there was rarely enough time to provide outreach to practices for the purpose of improving engagement and providing practice-based education. Changes in team configuration toward consolidation would be required in order to efficiently allocate CAP time exclusively for these MCPAP services.

Environmental Change: Pediatric Primary Care Networks and Behavioral Health Integration

When MCPAP was originally designed and implemented, accountable care organizations (ACOs) had not yet been formed, and, with the exception of federally qualified health centers, pediatric primary care sites in MA rarely included colocated or integrated behavioral health clinicians. Over the ensuing years, there has been significant growth of primary care networks across the state. These networks have begun to leverage resources to help primary care practices to earn performance incentives and shared savings within value-based contracts. Recognizing the unfavorable impact of behavioral health problems on overall health and health care cost, networks have been developing their own strategies to address unmet behavioral health needs in their defined populations. In this context, increasingly, practices have been embedding behavioral health and care coordination staff within their practice teams. For example, the Pediatric Physicians Organization at Children's (PPOC) is a network of 96 pediatric primary care practices located throughout Massachusetts.[12] The PPOC, in collaboration with the Department of Psychiatry at Boston Children's Hospital, has developed a robust strategy for helping member practices to improve their performance in addressing behavioral health needs. The strategy included the development of a "learning community" model of training, clinical practice standards for treatment of common psychiatric disorders, and support for integrated behavioral health clinicians. Originally designed to forge collaborative relationships with independent primary care practices, it was recognized that MCPAP would need to learn how to collaborate with primary care practice networks. In the case of the PPOC, this would mean that MCPAP consultants would need to be involved in the PPOC learning community in order to ensure that their recommendations were consistent with the PPOC practice guidelines and referral practices. In addition, MCPAP consultants would need to provide consultation not exclusively to PCPs but to primary care teams, including integrated behavioral health clinicians and care coordinators.

THE REDESIGN PROCESS: ASSESSMENT, RECOMMENDATIONS, REPROCUREMENT

Massachusetts Behavioral Health Partnership (MBHP), a Beacon Health Options company, is contractually responsible to the Massachusetts Office of Medicaid and the Massachusetts DMH for the administration of MCPAP and delivery of MCPAP services by health care institutions operating the MCPAP teams. In consultation with DMH, MBHP engaged an external consultant, DMA Health Strategies, to conduct a comprehensive assessment of MCPAP and make recommendations to inform the program's long-term strategic plan.

Assessment

The assessment was designed to evaluate how well MCPAP had been meeting its purpose: to ensure that all children in the Commonwealth have access to psychiatric consultation when needed and to help pediatric PCPs manage the behavioral health needs of their patients. Four key questions were developed to be answered by structured interviews using a written protocol, analysis of program data and reports, and review of peer-reviewed publications about MCPAP (**Box 1**). The assessment was conducted over approximately 4 months.

Groups of key stakeholders were identified for the interviews, including PCPs (MCPAP users); MCPAP leadership and team staff; health system leaders representing ACOs, physician organizations, guilds, and trade associations; government

---

Box 1
Assessment questions

Strategic assessment research questions

1. How efficiently and effectively is MCPAP performing its current functions and are there alternative ways to perform these functions?

2. How are pediatric primary care practices managing patients' behavioral health care, what additional supports do they need, and from where should these be provided?

3. How are primary care practices serving youth changing, and how is this likely to affect what they need to manage behavioral health care?

4. How will changing forms of payment and organization affect what primary care practices serving youth need to manage mental health care over the next 5 years?

stakeholders; and others such as legislative and program advocates. More than 50 structured interviews were conducted. In order to provide all 47 MCPAP team staff with an opportunity to contribute to the assessment, the consultant developed a Web-based survey to obtain their input. The survey resulted in a 68% response rate. Eleven years of program data and reports were analyzed, including monthly and quarterly encounter activity, team productivity, response times for consultation, number of children served, PCP enrollment, PCP usage rates, and provider experience survey responses. The MCPAP leadership team, DMH, and the external consultant engaged in a series of meetings, including a full-day retreat to review interim and final results of the strategic assessment. Findings were divided into 2 categories: (1) review of MCPAP performance data, and (2) stakeholder perspectives on program performance and environmental changes. Key findings on MCPAP performance can be found in **Box 2**. Key findings on stakeholder perspectives are summarized in **Table 1** and **Box 3**.

Stakeholders have consistently projected that the shortage of child psychiatry will not improve in the foreseeable future. Consequently, PCPs serving youth, even those affiliated with ACOs or health systems, thought that they would continue to need psychiatric consultation. Stakeholders also consistently reported that MCPAP is well positioned to assume a leadership role in developing best practices for primary care behavioral health and supporting practices with integrating behavioral health into their practices. Some thought that MCPAP should definitely take more responsibility for providing services in areas of the state where the wait for community-based child psychiatry can reach up to 9 months.

Notably, stakeholders pointed out that the emergence of organized systems of care such as ACOs presents new challenges and opportunities for MCPAP. For example, as PCPs bring behavioral health clinicians and care coordinators into their

---

Box 2
Massachusetts Child Psychiatry Access Project performance

MCPAP performance highlights

Program has achieved near-universal enrollment of pediatric primary care practices across the state.

The number of unique PCPs using MCPAP is steadily growing but considerable variation in usage exists across regions.

The number of children served has increased over time.

Reasons for contact have remained consistent over time, although contacts for access to community resources has increased.

Most MCPAP contacts result in the PCP continuing to manage patients' behavioral health care and to serve as the prescriber when medications are involved.

A common concern among stakeholders is unreliable throughput for external referrals.

PCPs are consistently highly satisfied with MCPAP's response time and the usefulness of consultations, and think that they are able to meet the needs of children with psychiatric problems.

PCPs frequently express wish for MCPAP to improve network availability for specialty psychiatric care for patients with complex needs.

There is considerable variation across regional hubs in the number of children served despite roughly equivalent funding and covered population size.

PCPs consistently rate the quality of consultation to be high across regional hubs.

Table 1
Massachusetts Child Psychiatry Access Project stakeholder perspectives on program performance and features

Strengths	Weaknesses
Responsiveness to PCP requests High quality of consultation Responsive to families' needs Knowledge of regional resources Longevity of MCPAP team	Use of MCPAP by pediatric practices is uneven[a] Some PCPs concerned that medications are recommended too readily[b] Need for increased support for special populations: (1) autism spectrum disorders, (2) infant/early childhood mental health, (3) adolescent substance abuse Families need more help than MCPAP provides to ensure follow-up with external referrals Inconsistent operational performance of teams stemming from multitasking obligation of single on-duty CAP per team (telephone consultation, face-to-face consultation, training, orientation) Lack of data on children's race and ethnicity prevents determination of possible treatment disparities

MCPAP Features Thought Necessary	MCPAP Features Thought Not Necessary
Universal access: independent of payer, independent of provider network Timely response High-quality consultation Accessible psychiatric assessments Resource and referral Knowledge of local resources Primary care/specialist relationships	Teams sited in academic medical centers Existing configuration of regional catchment areas

[a] May or may not represent weakness because some PCPs have alternative resources.
[b] Statistics show that more than 50% of contacts with PCPs do not result in a child being on medication.

practices, they may need less help with basic diagnostic consultation and referral support from MCPAP. In contrast, integrated behavioral health providers are expected to increase the overall involvement of primary care practices in mental health delivery, and thereby generate an increased demand for psychiatric consultation regarding patients who do not respond to first-level intervention. Stakeholders agreed with program leadership that, in order to be responsive to enrolled practices across multiple networks, MCPAP will need to be familiar with a diverse spectrum of behavioral health integration models as well as a variety of network-specific protocols and resources.

Recommendations

The set of strategic recommendations for future program development that resulted from the assessment are summarized in **Box 4**. Overall, the recommendations underscored the need for MCPAP to pursue strategies for increasing consistency in operational performance and to improve engagement with both network and non-network primary care practices. The assessment recommended increased attention to PCP

Box 3

Massachusetts Child Psychiatry Access Project stakeholder perspectives on environment

The changing landscape of pediatric primary care services in Massachusetts

1. Many practices are in varying stages of colocating or integrating behavioral health clinicians into their practices; however, some are not considering this at all.

2. Individual providers, large and small groups, networks, physician organizations, and health systems recognized the importance of behavioral health integration for population health and are either considering or beginning to develop behavioral health integration strategies.

3. Spurred by Massachusetts Health Policy Commission, practices are increasingly seeking National Center for Quality Assurance (NCQA) PRIME accreditation for the adoption of the patient-centered medical home model.

4. Movement toward alternative payment models with incentives for behavioral health integration will continue, although there is concern that pediatrics have a lower priority than adult medicine, at least for commercial payers.

5. Increasing frequency of behavioral health presentations in primary care setting in context of persistent access challenges and shifting role of primary care system for chronic disease management.

6. Administrative and financial barriers to behavioral health integration faced by primary practices include lack of sustainable financing, affiliation with more than 1 care system with different models of integration, and/or no affiliation with a care system that can support the necessary infrastructure.

7. Some primary care practices serving youth remain uninterested in moving toward greater integration of behavioral health.

Box 4

Strategic assessment recommendations

Performance improvement

1. Improve engagement of PCPs with MCPAP services.

2. Increase consistency in service provision and quality across teams.

3. Further develop consultation and training for PCPs and their practice teams.

4. Develop a strong capacity for telepsychiatry videoconferencing.

5. Improve service to families.

6. Communicate with payers and key stakeholders.

Potential strategies for program enhancement

1. Expand scope of consultation beyond individual patient needs to address practice needs in relation to behavioral health integration.

2. Clarify role of MCPAP in addressing inadequacy of community-based psychiatry networks.

3. Support behavioral health staff in PCP practices.

4. Reduce the number of teams in order to improve consistency of operation and operational efficiency.

5. Offer MCPAP services to schools.

6. Develop clinical standards for behavioral health in primary care.

7. Consider extending MCPAP program model to support primary care/specialist collaboration in order to address knowledge/service gaps in other areas of health care delivery.

training and education as well as practice-level consultation to support process improvement initiatives to improve primary care mental health service delivery. Increased provision of telepsychiatry was recommended in order to improve accessibility of face-to-face consults for families. The assessment also suggested that reduction in the number of teams could offer advantages of improved efficiency of operation as well as consistency of program deliverables across the state. Recommendations to expand MCPAP consultation to schools as well as extension of the MCPAP model to address other areas of health care delivery beyond children's mental health were taken under advisement pending opportunities for expanded funding.

Although it was not possible to adopt all of the recommendations, MCPAP leadership and DMH agreed that a redesign of the program would be necessary, toward the goal of building on strengths and essential features of the program and addressing challenges and relative weaknesses of the program identified in the strategic assessment. Given that the scope of the redesign would encompass changes in team number, geographic catchment areas, staff roles and responsibilities, and program deliverables, it was necessary to conduct a transparent and competitive reprocurement process following standard guidelines for public programs.

Reprocurement

Recognizing the significance of the impending transition, MBHP and DMH collaboratively decided to release a request for information (RFI) to both (1) begin the process of informing stakeholders that MCPAP would be making changes to the program, and (2) provide an opportunity for stakeholders to react to and provide feedback regarding program changes under consideration. The RFI was distributed to the MCPAP team leadership, MCPAP PCP Advisory Committee, Beacon Health Options regional leadership, key government stakeholders, and MA Children's Mental Health Campaign (advocacy group), and was made available on the MCPAP Web site. Responses were received from the MA Health Policy Commission and the institutions currently providing MCPAP 1.0 services. After consideration of the feedback included in the responses, MBHP and DMH finalized the specifications for MCPAP 2.0 and incorporated them into a request for proposals (RFP) directed to provider organizations with the ability to operate MCPAP teams according to outlined specifications.

An RFP Review Committee was constituted with representatives of both MCPAP central administrative leadership and DMH, as well as subject matter experts from 2 other states with similar consultation programs. Despite broad publicity surrounding the RFP, only 2 proposals were received. Each of the 2 proposals contained a plan for creating a consolidated team composed of original MCPAP 1.0 institutions working collaboratively (as encouraged in the RFP). The combined geographic regions of the 2 proposed teams covered the entire state. Each of the 7 institutions that had been delivering MCPAP 1.0 were included in one of the 2 proposed teams. There were no proposals from organizations not previously involved in MCPAP. The proposed teams included 1 for the western/central region of the state (including Baystate Medical Center and UMass Memorial Hospital) and 1 for the entire eastern region of the state with subteams in the north (including Massachusetts General Hospital for Children and North Shore Medical Center and Massachusetts General Hospital) and south (including Boston Children's Hospital, McLean Hospital, and Tufts Medical Center). After a process of negotiation, a 2-team program structure was finalized. Contracts were executed between each of the institutions and MBHP in preparation for transition to MCPAP 2.0 in January, 2017.

MASSACHUSETTS CHILD PSYCHIATRY ACCESS PROJECT 2.0: KEY ELEMENTS AND CHANGES

The program redesign was intended to build on the strengths of the original MCPAP design and to better position the program for long-term growth and sustainability, rather than to radically alter the fundamental nature of the program. Consequently, many of the core services of MCPAP 1.0 were preserved in the redesign. Also, the overarching goal of the program remained the same: to improve access to mental health care for children by supporting and strengthening the role of PCPs in addressing the children's mental health needs. However, numerous substantial changes were made to the structure, staffing, and functioning of the program (**Table 2**).

Structural Change

As noted earlier, the operation of 6 MCPAP teams across the state of Massachusetts was associated with some inefficiency and inconsistency of practice. It was decided that consolidation of the program structure resulting in a smaller number of teams was desirable. This consolidation would result in a smaller number of call centers; however,

Table 2
Massachusetts Child Psychiatry Access Project 1.0 to 2.0: key changes

	MCPAP 1.0	MCPAP 2.0
Number of Call Centers	6	3
Number of Teams	6	2
Staffing Roles for Each Call Center	1.0 FTE child and adolescent psychiatrist Behavioral health clinician Care coordinator	2.0 FTE child and adolescent psychiatrist Behavioral health clinician Resource and referral specialist Program coordinator
Core Services	Telephone consultation Face-to-face consultation Care coordination	Telephone consultation Face-to-face consultation Resource and referral (2 levels) Outreach practice consultation
Telephone and Face-to-face Consultation	Customized to individual need of PCP Guided primarily by clinical judgment of consultant Offered primarily to PCP	Customized to individual need of consultee Recommendations made explicitly in reference to clinical guidelines when possible Offered to PCP and/or embedded behavioral health provider
Care Navigation	Labeled care coordination Implied role of ongoing contact with family to support successful engagement with services	Labeled resource and referral Stratified into 2 levels according to patient severity and risk: Level 1: referral resource information provided to practice Level 2: directly assist family in securing appointment For both levels, practice is responsible for care management role of referral tracking, monitoring care plan
Practice Liaison	Ad hoc, not explicit program service	Formalized role CAP time set aside to engage in practice outreach, formal needs assessment

planners did not wish to centralize operations to the extent that local relationships between teams, individual consultants, and PCPs would be jeopardized. The final structure after the reprocurement resulted in 2 teams, each covering half of the geographic area of the state. The eastern team, including 2 subteams, along with the west/central team, created 3 separate call centers to cover the entire state. Each of the 3 call centers would be twice as busy as the 6 original call centers, requiring CAPs on duty for telephone consultation to devote their attention exclusively to this function. Consolidated teams allowed the program to have 2 separate child psychiatrists on duty at a given time: 1 to staff the telephone consultation line, and 1 to conduct scheduled face-to-face consultations and outreach visits to primary care practices (practice liaison service). Larger consolidated teams required collaboration between institutions in order to cover larger regions and multiple sites to provide a convenient location for face-to-face evaluations. In addition, the development of telepsychiatry resources for face-to-face evaluations, to further address geographic barriers across the larger regions of the consolidated teams, was specified in the redesign.

Each of the teams and subteams includes a 0.1 FTE medical director role to promote effective collaboration and to ensure optimal coordination of service across sites. Team medical directors work with the central medical director to ensure consistency, efficiency, and collaboration across institutions in alignment with MCPAP standards of practice.

Change in Care Navigation Support

The original care coordination function of MCPAP was modified and renamed resource and referral (R&R). Two levels of R&R service may be provided according to the patient's clinical complexity and acuity. For the first and most basic level, the MCPAP staff member takes basic clinical, insurance, and demographic information about the patient from the primary care practice. The staff member also inquires about the type of service needed, the preferences of the family regarding location and other variables, and insurance coverage. With access to a statewide database, the R&R staff member provides the practice with a short list of appropriate resources along with referral instructions. For the second level of R&R, provided exclusively for more urgent and/or complex cases, after clinical telephone consultation, the R&R staff member works directly with the parent to help secure a specific appointment with the recommended clinical service. Both levels of R&R differ from the original MCPAP care coordination in that the primary care practice is asked to maintain ongoing engagement with the family regarding the treatment plan. Although inconsistently delivered across the teams, the original MCPAP care coordination service carried an implication that the program would follow along with the patient to ensure successful engagement in treatment, and that there was no need for the primary care practice to devote ongoing attention to the treatment planning and referral process. Because each original MCPAP team was accountable to approximately 225 practices, this was neither feasible nor desirable given that successful care coordination ordinarily requires a continuous relationship with the family, which is a fundamental aspect of the patient-centered medical home.

Outreach to Primary Care Practices

In the original MCPAP design, most of the service to the PCPs required some initiative on the part of the providers to request help from the program. By design, minimal effort was required in the form of a call to a special hotline; nonetheless, it is surmised that many of the practices rarely using the program are especially in need of improvement in their mental health care service delivery. Lack of motivation to engage in mental health issues could contribute to low MCPAP usage; however, lack of facility and comfort in mental health delivery was often thought to be an underlying factor. As a result, the MCPAP 2.0 redesign includes an outreach function for the purpose of supporting practice-based improvement processes in the area of children's mental health. Each practice is different in its readiness and motivation for change and specific needs and priorities for improvement. As a result, the outreach practice consultation service is designed to begin with a practice-based needs assessment. Examples of process improvement goals that may be addressed include improvement in mental health screening; development and use of clinical registries; implementation of measurement-based care; optimizing roles of medical assistants and nurses in order to improve team-based mental health care; strategies to use embedded mental health providers to implement models of integrated care; and improving behavioral health billing/documentation practices. In order to deliver this consultation, the CAPs on each team spend a portion of their time serving as practice liaisons for a defined set of primary care practices. Within this role, the CAPs schedule periodic meetings with each practice to provide practice-based consultation focused on the goals described earlier. Practice liaisons are responsible for being well informed in existing improvement initiatives and integration models deriving from practices' network affiliations in order to ensure that their work is aligned with these network functions. In keeping with this, network practices are grouped together in their assignments to their CAP practice liaisons.

Clinical Practice Guidelines and Peer Review

Quality and performance improvement were featured prominently in MCPAP 1.0 and included detailed analysis of encounter activity and regular surveys of PCPs in order to assess PCP engagement, program impact, program responsiveness, and team productivity. For MPCAP 2.0, in the interest of improving the quality of mental health treatment of children in the primary care setting, the clinical quality of the consultation process has been established as a major area of focus. To this end, the program redesign includes a process for the development of a set of clinical practice guidelines. Building on substantial efforts made in this field by the department of psychiatry at Boston Children's Hospital, a set of MCPAP-endorsed guidelines for primary care–based mental health practice is slated for development during the first year of MCPAP 2.0. These guidelines will cover the most common mental health problems presenting in the primary care setting. With their adoption, the guidelines will help to ensure that recommendations made to PCPs in telephone consultations, face-to-face consultations, and training sessions are aligned with agreed-on standards of evidence-based practices, and appropriately adapted for the primary care setting. The guidelines will be used in training and orientation practices for MCPAP consultants. Peer review of documentation of face-to-face consultation and recordings of telephone consultations will be performed on a regular basis to assess the degree to which consultants' clinical recommendations are concordant with these guidelines.

TRANSITION AND LAUNCH OF MASSACHUSETTS CHILD PSYCHIATRY ACCESS PROJECT 2.0

After acceptance of the team proposals and execution of contracts with institutions was complete, a comprehensive plan was developed to prepare for the transition to the new program design (**Table 3**). Concurrently, each team began working on the development of processes for collaboration between their member institutions in order to operationalize the program in its new form.

Table 3 Plan for the transition to the new program design	
MCPAP 2.0 Transition Plan	
MCPAP staff orientation, training, and team building	Retreat Individual team meetings
Infrastructure	Phone Document sharing
Documentation	Database changes Reporting changes
Service delivery	Protocol development Teams' geographic changes Practice reassignments
Communication	Orient PCP advisory committee members Prepare articles for MCPAP and American Academy of Pediatrics (AAP) newsletters Produce and hold monthly webinars for PCPs Official notification to enrolled PCP practices

A retreat was held in mid-December to bring MCPAP staff together, provide a venue to discuss program changes, and begin the process of team building. Each of the institutions involved in the consolidated teams and call centers had used different procedures for delivering MCPAP services. Joined together in the new team structure, the institutions needed to resolve these differences in order to jointly conduct operations and collaboratively staff consolidated call centers. In this regard, it was helpful that MCPAP 2.0 program specifications were more detailed than those of the previous version.

The transition to consolidated teams also required communication and information technology infrastructure changes, including upgrading from conventional phone lines to a voice-over Internet protocol phone system for improved call routing and analytics, as well as a secure document-sharing program to support cross-institution communication. In addition, the encounter database, MCPAP Live, which had been used since the beginning of the program, needed to be updated to support cross-institution collaboration.

Throughout the month before launch, program coordinators, R&R specialists, and behavioral health clinicians received group training to prepare them for new program procedures and to train them in the use of the new communication and information systems. This group continues to meet biweekly for ongoing transitional support.

MCPAP leaders oriented enrolled PCPs and practices through a variety of channels over 2 months before MCPAP 2.0. These channels included newsletters, webinars, information posted on the MCPAP Web site, and presentations at relevant meetings. Orientation content included rationale and description of key program changes, clarification of team assignments, and instructions for accessing MCPAP services. Every enrolled practice received a welcome packet including a letter with the practice's team assignment and new access phone number, an overview entitled "MCPAP 2.0: What is Changing and What You Need to Know," a list of team staff, new provider brochures, and notepads with the new team name and access number printed on them.

INITIAL IMPRESSIONS AND CHALLENGES GOING FORWARD

The transition to MCPAP 2.0 was fairly smooth. Engagement of PCPs with the program as reflected in frequency of requests for clinical consultation suggests that there has been no significant disruption in relationships between PCPs and the program. Occasional episodes of miscommunication between sites resulted in negative feedback from PCPs. Although a small number of PCPs expressed initial disappointment with changes in team assignment and discomfort related to the need to establish new relationships with unfamiliar MCPAP consultants on the consolidated teams, these issues were quickly resolved. Anecdotal feedback to date from MCPAP staff, PCP Advisory Committee members, and informal conversations with enrolled PCPs has been uniformly positive.

Groups of MCPAP central administration and regional team staff meet regularly to continue developing and clarifying policies, protocols, roles, and responsibilities, which has created a shared comradery and spirit of problem solving. A new medical leadership committee composed of central, team, and subteam medical directors meets biweekly. In addition to providing a central point of contact for support, feedback, and input on clinical issues arising from daily operations, the work plan for the medical leadership committee includes the development of MCPAP clinical practice guidelines, developing procedures for the new practice liaison role, and the further development of peer review methodology to improve the quality of clinical consultation.

There is some initial concern that the anticipated increase in efficiency associated with the MCPAP 2.0 team structure has yet to be realized. Furthermore, some of the teams have struggled to maintain compliance with the program standard of offering face-to-face evaluations within 2 weeks because of staffing transitions. As a result, the implementation of practice liaison activities has been pushed back several months in order to ensure that services for patients are being delivered in a timely manner. It is anticipated that increased efficiency in the use of child and adolescent psychiatry time by virtue of the batching of telephone consultations through consolidated call centers and elimination of multitasking will be realized with the stabilization of new MCPAP processes, thereby allowing CAP time to be allocated to the new practice liaison role. Also, the use of clearly defined triage protocols to guide the use of face-to-face consultation is expected to free up CAP time needed for practice liaison work. Data systems will be leveraged for tracking team performance in these areas in order to monitor these transitional issues and to ensure successful phase-in of the outreach practice consultation service.

SUMMARY

On first learning about the MCPAP model, students often imagine that there is a finite number of questions that PCPs might ask about their patients and wonder whether the program would eventually put itself out of business once pediatricians over time received answers to all of the questions. After 13 years in service, this does not seem to be the case. To the contrary, usage data suggest that the program is needed as much as ever. Even pediatricians who have used the program frequently for years continue to use the program regularly for clinical consultation questions. Although these MCPAP high users are observed to have developed significant growth in child psychiatry knowledge and skill over time, it has been an informal observation that their questions remain pertinent and reflect increased clinical sophistication. The remark attributed to Albert Einstein, that "the more I learn, the more I realize I do not know," seems to be applicable in this instance. Although common children's mental health problems can often be managed appropriately with basic clinical protocols, clinical presentations in child psychiatry are frequently ambiguous, and it seems that the availability of an experienced specialist for consultation is of continuing utility for PCPs across a wide range of degrees of mental health knowledge, skill, and confidence. In contrast, it is anticipated that demand for the R&R services of the program may be partially offset by ongoing growth of integrated behavioral health programs that include practice-based care coordination. Careful tracking of the use of MCPAP core services will be used to ensure that various MCPAP resources are appropriately allocated to best address the needs of enrolled pediatric primary care practices.

The wide dissemination of the MCPAP model, the strong ongoing public and private support for the program, and the sustained high level of use of the program by PCPs suggest that the program continues to strike a chord with both PCPs and policy makers. The program, configuring a structured relationship between PCPs and teams of specialists, provides a scalable and cost-effective process for collaboration that has been highly regarded across the United States.

Programs require iteration not only to address environmental changes but to debug programmatic vulnerabilities and make improvements based on analysis of the program's performance. In the case of MCPAP, needs for improvement in core services along with changes in the landscape of pediatric primary care practice provided an imperative for change. The changes made do not change the essential nature of the program. The program continues to provide a statewide infrastructure for consultative relationships designed to address gaps in knowledge and service coordination for PCPs. This next iteration of MCPAP is intended to position the program for future growth and sustainability by improving the efficiency and consistency of the program services, providing more outreach to pediatric practices, adapting the model of the program to support primary care networks and practices organized to provide a patient-centered medical home for their patients, and introducing methods to promote adoption of clinical practice standards.

ACKNOWLEDGMENT

The authors wish to thank the following individuals for their contributions to the work described in this report: Christina Fluet, MA Department of Mental Health; Heather Strother, MPH, MA Department of Mental Health; Wendy Holt, DMA Health Strategies.

REFERENCES

1. Kataoka SH, Zhang L, Wells KB. Unmet need for mental health care among U.S. children: variation by ethnicity and insurance status. Am J Psychiatry 2002; 159(9):1548–55.
2. US Department of Health and Human Services. Mental health: a report of the surgeon general. Rockville (MD): US Department of Health and Human Services; 1999.
3. Thomas CR, Holzer CE. The continuing shortage of child and adolescent psychiatrists. J Am Acad Child Adolesc Psychiatry 2006;45:1023–31.
4. McMillan JA, Land M Jr, Leslie LK. Pediatric residency education and the behavioral health crisis: a call to action. Pediatrics 2017;139(1):e20162141.
5. Horwitz SM, Storfer-Isser A, Kerker BD, et al. Barriers to the identification and management of psychosocial problems: changes from 2004 to 2013. Acad Pediatr 2015;15(6):613–20.
6. Leaf PJ, Owens PL, Leventhal JM, et al. Pediatricians' training and identification and management of psychosocial problems. Clin Pediatr 2004;43(4):355–65.
7. Sarvet B, Gold J, Bostic JQ, et al. Improving access to mental health care for children: the Massachusetts Child Psychiatry Access Project. Pediatrics 2010; 126(6):1191–200.

8. Straus JH, Sarvet B. Behavioral health care for children: the Massachusetts Child Psychiatry Access Project. Health Aff (Millwood) 2014;33:2153–61.
9. The National Network of Child Psychiatry Access Programs. Available at: http://www.nncpap.org/existing-programs.html. Accessed April 27, 2017.
10. The Children's Mental Health Campaign. Available at: https://www.childrensmentalhealthcampaign.org/about. Accessed April 27, 2017.
11. Byatt N, Biebel K, Moore Simas TA, et al. Improving perinatal depression care: the Massachusetts Child Psychiatry Access Project for moms. Gen Hosp Psychiatry 2016;40:12–7.
12. The Pediatric Physicians Organization at Children's. Available at: http://www.ppochildrens.org. Accessed April 27, 2017.

Using Effective Public Private Collaboration to Advance Integrated Care

Lee S. Beers, MD[a],*, Leandra Godoy, PhD[a],
Matthew G. Biel, MD, MSc[b]

KEYWORDS

- Mental health • Primary care integration • Health network • Collective impact

KEY POINTS

- Health network approaches that promote multidisciplinary and cross-agency collaborations can be an effective way to promote the integration of mental health services in primary care.
- Clearly defined goals, an investment of resources, a broadly representative group of stakeholders, and a culture of evaluation and improvement are critical to collaborative success.
- Involvement of parents and families in strategic planning and feedback is an essential component of effective integration.

BACKGROUND

Integrated mental health services within health care settings have many benefits, such as improving care coordination, service delivery, treatment engagement, and patient health outcomes, and reducing stigma and costs.[1–4] Nevertheless, despite the many benefits of integrated care, the increasing number of organizations endorsing this approach,[5–7] and the growing prevalence of this model, several key barriers continue to pose challenges to integrated, coordinated care between primary care and mental health care providers and agencies. Such barriers include patient privacy concerns (eg, concerns about sharing sensitive information between medical and mental health providers), payment and sustainability challenges (eg, uncertainty about how best to bill for mental health services or obtain insurance authorization, lack of reimbursement

Disclosure Statement: The authors have nothing to disclose.
[a] Child Health Advocacy Institute, Children's National Health System, 111 Michigan Avenue Northwest, Washington, DC 20010, USA; [b] Department of Child and Adolescent Psychiatry, Georgetown University School of Medicine, 2115 Wisconsin Avenue Northwest, Suite 200, Washington, DC 20007, USA
* Corresponding author.
E-mail address: lbeers@childrensnational.org

Child Adolesc Psychiatric Clin N Am 26 (2017) 665–675
http://dx.doi.org/10.1016/j.chc.2017.06.003
1056-4993/17/© 2017 Elsevier Inc. All rights reserved.

policies that support collaborative care team approaches), and logistical barriers, such as limited provider time and space needed to integrate new clinicians.[6,8] These barriers limit the extent to which integrated care practices are adopted, a common issue in implementation and dissemination of best practices. This article describes how one community, Washington, DC, identified and addressed these challenges through a collaborative, multistakeholder approach.

THEORETIC FRAMEWORK

Collaborative, multistakeholder efforts have the potential to overcome prevalent obstacles to integrated care and to accelerate the dissemination of innovative clinical strategies and require a deliberate and strategic approach. Bringing together key experts and influencers into a health network, a relatively informal coalition of organizations and agencies with common goals focusing on specific but complex health system challenges, can provide the foundation from which a strategic approach and/or more formal partnerships may emerge.[9]

However, effecting systemic change is often difficult, slow, and frustrating, and many such networks are unprepared for the challenges of this work. Complexity science is a theoretic framework that "provides the insight that systems are comprised of inter-related parts that interact in non-linear, potentially unpredictable ways," which can be conceptually applied to these networks to improve system outcomes.[10] A transparent and deliberate recognition of this system complexity, with a particular focus on improving system interdependencies, including resources available, work processes, and the relational infrastructure between individuals, is critical. Proctor and colleagues[11] describe a model for implementation research in mental health services that captures these interdependencies. The authors propose that this model can be extended to network development. The framework describes the evolution of moving an evidence-based (or evidence-informed) practice, such as integrated care, through implementation and dissemination strategies, ultimately resulting in improved outcomes. Key assumptions in this model that are required for change include knowledge and expertise at the individual level; cooperation, coordination, and shared knowledge at the team level; structure and strategy at the organizational level; and effective reimbursement, legal, and regulatory policies at the system level.[11]

Collective Impact (CI) is a commonly used framework within communities to operationalize these concepts for the purpose of systems improvement. The 5 key conditions of CI are a common agenda, shared measurement, mutually reinforcing activities, continuous communication, and infrastructure support. These key conditions can create an environment for rapid and sustainable change. CI initiatives typically move through 3 phases of implementation, including initiation, organizing for impact, and sustaining action. Building on these elements, CI initiatives are most successful when they integrate strong governance, a sustained focus on strategic planning, meaningful community involvement, and an infrastructure for evaluation and quality improvement.[12,13] Particularly for initiatives designed to have longitudinal and broad reaching impacts, the concept of CI can provide an important framework for creating an environment based on improvement and evaluation, which then leads to systemic change.

THE DC COLLABORATIVE FOR MENTAL HEALTH IN PEDIATRIC PRIMARY CARE

Washington, DC is a city characterized by significant disparities in wealth and health. The Centers for Disease Control and Prevention–sponsored 500 Cities project reports that the 32 highest-income census tracts of Washington, DC had median household earnings of $110,000, whereas the 32 lowest-income census tracts had median household earnings of $32,000.[14] Adults from DC's poorest communities were twice as likely to be obese as those from the wealthiest communities and were more than twice as likely as those in the wealthiest neighborhoods to report experiencing consistently poor mental health for more than 2 weeks, and 3 times as likely to report consistently poor physical health. Lower-income residents also struggle to obtain medical and mental health care, because health care resources are more difficult to access in the city's poorer communities.[14] According to 2015 US Census Bureau calculations, the total population of DC in 2015 was approximately 672,000, with 118,300 children under the age of 18 (17.6% of the population).[15] Forty-eight percent of the population identifies as African American, 36% as white, 10.6% as Hispanic or Latino, and 4.3% as Asian. Approximately 74,000 children in Washington, DC receive health insurance through Medicaid, accounting for approximately 63% of the city's children.[16] Fewer than 2% of children in DC are uninsured.[17]

Faced with concerns regarding the adequacy of access to mental health services for children, particularly low-income children, in Washington, DC, and catalyzed by a published report identifying gaps in children's mental health service delivery, in 2012, a health network focusing on the integration of mental health into pediatric primary care was formed.[18] Ultimately, this health network became the DC Collaborative for Mental Health in Pediatric Primary Care ("DC Collaborative"), a multi-institution coalition of stakeholders, including local government agencies, health systems, and nonprofit advocacy groups, that aims to improve the integration of mental health within primary care. Key goals are to support primary care providers (PCPs) and the families they serve, provide education and training, promote and support clinical endeavors in integrated care within the District, and engage in policy and advocacy efforts. Importantly, at the same time the DC Collaborative was formed, other citywide efforts focused on improving access to mental health care for children were emerging and expanding; city leaders had identified mental health care for children as a key policy priority, which provided important synergies and created a ripe environment for CI.

To address infrastructure support needs and system interdependencies, the DC Collaborative organizationally includes a Working Group, whose members donate their time in-kind, that is responsible for the planning, implementation, and evaluation of all activities; a Community Advisory Board (CAB), which oversees the Working Group by providing feedback that is integrated into decision making; and a Project Team that provides day-to-day, operational support. The Project Team grew from 1 to 2.5 full-time employed staff members over 3 years and is responsible for the operations of the DC Collaborative. This team is hired and housed at one of the partner agencies in order to decrease administrative complexity and foster relationships between Project Team members. The DC Collaborative is interdisciplinary with representation from psychiatry, pediatrics, psychology, policy, advocacy, and public health. Core members of the DC Collaborative Working Group include 2 academic medical centers (Children's National Health System [CNHS] and MedStar Georgetown University Hospital [MGUH]), a local child advocacy agency (the Children's Law Center), the DC Chapter of the American Academy of Pediatrics, and several local government agencies, including the DC Departments of Health, Behavioral Health, and Health Care Finance. The CAB includes more than 30 diverse organizations representing health, mental health, educational, and parent advocacy groups. Initial funding was through both a state Title V grant and a local family foundation; continued funding was obtained from diverse sources, including local and philanthropic grants and in-kind institutional support.

The DC Collaborative has championed several citywide integration efforts since its inception in 2012. First, the network has supported District-wide efforts to promote routine, annual mental health screening in primary care through several key actions:

1. Making recommendations to the DC Department of Behavioral Health regarding recommended pediatric and postpartum mental health screening tools,[19]
2. Leading a 15-month, citywide, Quality Improvement Learning Collaborative (QI-LC) to improve mental health screening practices,[20] and
3. Providing ongoing support and technical assistance to pediatric practices to promote mental health screening.

As these supports were implemented citywide, the number of developmental/behavioral health screens billed to DC Medicaid increased 5-fold from 5020 in Fiscal Year (FY) 13 (October 1, 2012–September 30, 2013) to 26,608 in FY 16 (October 1, 2015–September 30, 2016). The largest increase in screening rates (by approximately 2.5-fold) was seen between FY 14 (9,599, October 1, 2013–September 30, 2014), and FY 15 (22,762, October 1, 2014–September 30, 2015), coinciding with the implementation of the QI-LC between February 2014 and June 2015. To the authors' knowledge, no other major initiatives focused on developmental/behavioral/mental health screening were occurring during that time.

Second, the DC Collaborative developed a comprehensive child and adolescent mental health resource guide to aid PCPs in identifying community-based agencies to which they can refer children and families in need of mental health services.[19] This guide is available free on-line through a training Web site hosted by the DC Department of Health Care Finance and is regularly updated every 4 to 6 months by the project team. The guide is frequently accessed by a wide variety of users, as per online analytics.

Third, the DC Collaborative led the development, planning, and initiation of the District's child mental health access program, DC MAP (Mental Health Access in Pediatrics),[21] a member of the National Network of Child Psychiatry Access Programs (www.nncpap.org). As one of the earliest goals of the DC Collaborative, this initiative was a priority for grant writing and solicitation of in-kind support. Infrastructure planning for the DC MAP program was primarily funded by a 2-year Title V grant, which largely supported staff time. As partners in this planning process and in recognition of the potential impact such a program could have, the local public mental health agency solicited contractors to implement the program; one of the lead members of the DC Collaborative was awarded the contract in partnership with a second lead member. Activities during the first year included a 3-month startup phase (which was accelerated by the preceding 2 years of infrastructure planning), a 6-month pilot phase, and ultimately full implementation of the program in September 2015. Startup activities included reviewing and consulting with other child mental health access programs nationally, developing local protocols and procedures, determining staffing, and building appropriate infrastructure, such as a phone system, Web site, and secure Web-based database. The team continues to participate in ongoing rapid-cycle quality improvement processes in order to continually enhance services. The DC MAP team, which is staffed jointly by CNHS and MGUH mental health providers (psychiatrists, psychologists, social workers, care coordinator), provides free services to all pediatric practices in DC, including telephone consultation with child mental health experts (within 30 minutes), in-person clinical evaluations for patients with critical diagnostic uncertainty, community resource referrals, and mental health training and support. Team members meet regularly to discuss clinical cases, program outcomes, and improvement cycles.

The DC Collaborative also promotes policies and legislation that support sustainable integration of mental health services in primary care settings. As examples, members of the group were key advocates in the passage of the "Behavioral Health System of Care Act of 2014," a piece of local legislation that mandated the creation of a child mental health access program (which became DC MAP). Members have also advocated for continued support for reimbursement to PCPs for conducting standardized mental health screening. In sum, the DC Collaborative has supported several important citywide mental health integration efforts and continues to serve as a hub for innovative, cross-sector strategies aimed at improving the integration of mental health in pediatric primary care within DC.

KEY ELEMENTS OF SUCCESSFUL IMPLEMENTATION

Although the accomplishments of the DC Collaborative were facilitated by a positive local climate, they were grounded in a systems-based and collaborative approach. Given the complex challenges of effectively integrating mental health services into primary care in a sustainable way, meaningful involvement of cross-sector and multidisciplinary teams, including both governmental and nongovernmental stakeholders, is critical. Each member of the collaborative effort brings unique knowledge and leverage, allowing for multifactorial influences and barriers to be addressed. Educational content and service delivery are enhanced by valuing and including both academic expertise and "real world, on the ground" clinical experience, and by integrating the expertise of both pediatric primary care and mental health clinicians. In addition, government and nongovernment collaborators working together create important synergies, by creating opportunities to leverage different types of supports and in different ways; for example, government collaborators may have more direct influence on regulatory policy. However, nongovernment collaborators may be able to act more nimbly and responsively.

Community Engagement and Leadership

Emerging opportunities to design and implement strategies around integration of mental health care in pediatric primary care also offer a special chance to include the perspectives of the families and communities served by health care systems.[22] Many of the inadequacies of the current "status quo," in which mental health care is too often inefficient, inaccessible, and disconnected from other medical care, are acutely and personally felt by families and communities. These inadequacies are exacerbated by structural factors that make health disparities and culturally incompetent care quite evident in pediatric mental health care.[23] Given these sobering realities, there is a particular urgency to include the expertise and perspectives of families and community members in designing integrated care initiatives.

To actively include the voices of families and communities in planning new clinical strategies within private-public efforts, those same families and communities must have the opportunity to be coleaders within those partnerships. An increasingly rich literature describes the critical ingredients of effective engagement and empowerment of community partners in public health endeavors.[24] These ingredients include a range of approaches, such as building trusting relationships with communities over time and giving multiple opportunities for community members to provide insight and suggestions that are meaningfully included in decision-making processes. These approaches can be considered components of a culturally competent approach to partnership with communities and can be foundational in community engagement efforts around both identifying relevant clinical strategies and in formulating research questions through community-based participatory research.[25]

Within the work of the DC Collaborative, active partnership with the communities and families the authors were hoping to serve was a critical component of their efforts. This partnership took several forms. The process of assessing community needs, from the standpoint of addressing barriers to care experienced by community members, was an important first step that occurred through focus groups, and key informant interviews. This feedback informed the creation of a CAB with representation from family serving agencies and parent advocacy organizations, and also including parents from the local community. Input from these organizations and individuals provided crucial insight into the lived experiences of families who struggled to access mental health care, and particularly illuminated structural challenges (such as transportation) and communication breakdowns (such as perceptions that pediatric PCPs were more interested in discussing physical health concerns rather than mental health concerns with parents). Equally powerful were needs assessments conducted with community pediatrics providers who practiced in settings that were not formally aligned with the academic medical centers leading the Collaborative. These practitioners highlighted their frustrations around expectations that they meet the mental health needs of their patients without receiving adequate training, support, or access to helpful referrals. Although none of this feedback was surprising, it was instrumental in determining the priorities of the Collaborative, particularly orienting the authors to the need to create training for providers that addressed communication strategies with patients and enhanced effective use of screening tools to begin to build capacity to address mental health concerns.[22]

Furthermore, input from family advocacy organizations and other community members was not limited to identifying challenges in current approaches to care; these organizations made insightful and practical suggestions about solutions that should inform any integrated care strategies. For example, families and community members were clear and explicit in identifying primary care as their most trusted source for health information and hoped to discuss mental health interventions, including but not limited to pharmacologic interventions, with their primary providers. In addition, these partners highlighted the positive impact of organizations that provided structured family navigation and peer-to-peer support services to families who were referred for mental health services. The authors were strongly encouraged to incorporate these adjunctive support services into integrated care efforts. Their efforts to document and communicate this feedback to city leadership was a critical element of their campaign to obtain public funding for integrated care efforts, because they were able to provide evidence of the strong community voices supporting pediatric primary care as a crucial platform for addressing mental health.

Evaluation of Impact

Collaborative efforts to advance integrated care should respond to identified needs and priorities in a given community and service setting and also must demonstrate clinical effectiveness and economic efficiency in order to build a case for support and sustainability. Evaluation efforts can be included in every facet of collaborative partnerships in order to demonstrate impact. These efforts should begin with baseline assessments that draw from existing data sources, supplemented by targeted needs assessments as previously described. For example, drawing on publically available information, such as Medicaid data about service usage in both primary care and specialty mental health care, provides important perspectives on care delivery. In a specific primary care clinical setting, data inquiries about clinical activities, such as mental health screening, prescribing of psychiatric medications, and referral to specialty mental health care services, are very informative. In settings in which some steps toward integrated care have been taken, for example, the colocation of mental health providers in a primary care clinic, data about the billing, and service patterns of those providers, can demonstrate where additional unmet needs may exist.

In the work of the DC Collaborative, these types of baseline data inquiries set the stage for a process of rapid-cycle intervention and evaluation that allowed the authors' team to demonstrate impact over relatively short time periods. As previously described, rising local public interest in improving access to mental health screening and assessment in pediatric primary care was a prominent catalyst for the DC Collaborative's efforts. The baseline data obtained from existing sources and needs assessments that indicated (1) low rates of documented mental health screening in pediatric primary care and (2) strong interest on the part of PCPs in enhancing their capacities to address mental health concerns, were the impetus to implement the aforementioned QI-LC to address the challenge of increasing rates of screening. This Learning Collaborative built on existing quality improvement infrastructure to create an active partnership with PCPs interested in taking on the challenge of increasing screening in their practice settings.[26] The approach included monthly chart review and reporting to encourage a continuous and data-driven approach to improvement.

Using this approach, the authors were able to illustrate a striking increase in rates of screening for mental health concerns at well visits across a range of pediatric primary care sites in DC, from a baseline rate of 1% to an end of project screening rate of 74%.[20] This outcome importantly served dual purposes for the team: both to demonstrate that training could positively impact provider behavior and to emphasize the need to further enhance the mental health support provided to PCPs as they respond to the increased identification of mental health concerns. The authors' case for the importance of public funding for a DC child psychiatry access program (ultimately to become DC MAP) was made more compelling by these results. A similar process of rapid cycle, consistent, and data-informed review of program services and usage has been integrated into the DC MAP evaluation plan and is used to drive program changes and improvements.

In addition to using data to inform decision making around training, program development, and clinical practice, more process-oriented data can inform the successful creation and sustaining of collaborative partnerships. Specifically, teams should regularly evaluate their own effectiveness, engagement, and success at collaboration through internal assessment procedures that are structured and anonymous; the DC Collaborative uses a standardized, Web-based survey every 12 to 18 months for this purpose. These processes can be critical in highlighting tensions or conflicts within multistakeholder teams that can potentially derail progress. These collaborative efforts can have "blind spots" that can impede effective action if left unaddressed. For example, challenges around communication, cultural competence, and racial or ethnic equity around program development are crucial to understand and address in many communities and clinical settings. Collaborative efforts need to be proactive and curious about understanding these challenges in order to achieve sustained impact.

POLICY AND ADVOCACY

Just as service delivery can be enhanced by a collaborative approach to building systems, so can policy and advocacy efforts designed to increase the sustainability and effectiveness of mental health integration into primary care. The diversity of knowledge and experience of the multidisciplinary group can help identify barriers and service gaps, but can also help better identify effective solutions. The engagement of families and care providers can help to identify concerns that might not otherwise have been recognized or addressed. The importance of the family and community voice in this process cannot be underestimated; as noted, as potential or actual recipients of the intended services, they have indispensable insight into what is and is not working in the mental health system of care.

Bringing together stakeholders with expertise including but not limited to care delivery, financing, quality improvement, advocacy, and legal issues can facilitate innovative problem solving. For example, pediatric providers involved with the aforementioned QI-LC expressed a desire to have a better way to track if their patients had improved access to care and/or improved outcomes after concerns were identified through standardized mental health screening. The DC Collaborative worked together, particularly involving the clinicians on the team and the state Medicaid agency, to develop a system of identifying and tracking patients with at-risk screens using an individualized modifier to be submitted at the time of billing for the particular screen or component of the well child visit. Uptake of this modifier was slow to implement; barriers to its use and tracking are currently being investigated and addressed using the principles of continuous quality improvement, allowing a stepwise progression toward achieving the long-term goal of improving access to care for children.

Alternately, the involvement of multiple stakeholders and institutions can sometimes be a barrier to identifying or implementing effective policy solutions. Individuals or organizations may have differing priorities, disagree on potential solutions, or may be competing for funding. In addition, they may have different levels of risk they are willing to assume when advocating for a particular position, or on a particular topic, particularly if the issue is controversial or politically charged. Importantly, governmental employees are typically not able to engage in advocacy on behalf of their agency or in their official roles and may need to recuse themselves from these discussions, despite the fact that they may have valuable information to contribute. In all of these situations, a clear understanding of the long-term goals and priorities of the group can help resolve conflicts. In addition, it should be made clear at the beginning of the collaboration that there may be times when an individual organization's priorities may not be able to be addressed because of the implications for the entire group. Rarely, an external mediator may be needed, or the group may decide not to engage in a particular issue because agreement cannot be reached among the stakeholders.

RECOMMENDATIONS AND SUMMARY

Overall, the experience of the DC Collaborative for Mental Health in Pediatric Primary care demonstrates that health network approaches that promote multidisciplinary and cross-agency collaborations can be an effective way to effect complex health systems change, such as the integration of mental health services in primary care. However, although the value of this approach may be clear, implementation is often more difficult. Differing priorities, resources, and availability can sometimes doom collaboration before it even begins. An effective and individualized infrastructure designed to meet the needs and the capacities of the group is essential. Defining priorities and long-term goals from the outset can help to avoid later pitfalls. In addition, although resources are typically limited for this type of initiative, identifying essential needs and planning for how to support them allow for smoother progression. Based on this experience, and the above review of the literature, the authors propose the following elements as key to success of this type of collaboration:

- A clearly defined and articulated vision of the priorities of the network, including an understanding of what activities and issues are within the scope of the group, but also which activities are not. Ideally, the whole group should be involved in crafting this vision to ensure greater commitment and investment; overarching goals should be regularly revisited to ensure relevance and effectiveness.

- A thoughtfully planned and broadly representative group of stakeholders who have an understanding of their role in the collaboration, to include community members and families. Careful consideration should be given to who is included and how; in general, inclusivity is preferred. However, there may need to be a small group of key decision makers who communicate more frequently and carry a greater share of the workload. These members in particular should be able and willing to work collaboratively, have adequate influence to effect change within their own organization, and commit to meeting regularly and following up on tasks between meetings.
- Attention to the relationships developed both internal and external to the network, with a particular focus on trust, interdependence and positive peer influence. Stronger relationships can enhance system performance and provide important synergies.[9]
- A modest investment of staff and resources committed by all partners to ensure that the goals of the group are able to be met. There are many factors that influence the degree to which this is possible; however, a greater investment can dramatically increase the effectiveness of the collaboration. Strategically, showing impact with smaller amounts of investment can sometimes be leveraged for greater investments moving forward. External funding through mechanisms such as grants or philanthropic donations can be very helpful, but it is important to have diversification of both financial and in-kind support to ensure sustainability of the efforts and prevent dependence on a single source of funding.
- A culture of decision making based on data, evidence, and continuous quality improvement to ensure the group is adequately responding to the needs of the community and team members. Evaluation should be built into all project activities; the effectiveness and functioning of the collaborative team should be regularly evaluated as well, ideally using structured and anonymous tools.

Systemically improving access to mental health services for children is a formidable challenge with which communities understandably struggle. The uncertainty surrounding potential changes to health care reform, availability of safety-net supports for communities, and funding for program implementation and research make the importance of collaborative vision and collective effort even more acute. As the African proverb so eloquently states, "When spider webs unite, they can tie up a lion." The DC Collaborative for Pediatric Primary Care is a demonstration of how a sustained and collaborative focus can improve the integration of mental health services into primary care.

REFERENCES

1. Asarnow JR, Rozenman M, Wiblin J, et al. Integrated medical-behavioral care compared with usual primary care for child and adolescent behavioral health: a meta-analysis. JAMA Pediatr 2015;169(10):929–37.

2. Huffman JC, Niazi SK, Rundell JR, et al. Essential articles on collaborative care models for the treatment of psychiatric disorders in medical settings: a publication by the Academy of Psychosomatic Medicine Research and Evidence-Based Practice Committee. Psychosomatics 2014;55(2):109–22.

3. Kolko DJ, Campo J, Kilbourne AM, et al. Collaborative care outcomes for pediatric behavioral health problems: a cluster randomized trial. Pediatrics 2014;133(4): e981–992.

4. Committee on Psychosocial Aspects of Child and Family Health and Task Force on Mental Health. Policy statement–the future of pediatrics: mental health competencies for pediatric primary care. Pediatrics 2009;124(1):410–21.

5. Foy JM, Kelleher KJ, Laraque D, American Academy of Pediatrics Task Force on Mental Health. Enhancing pediatric mental health care: strategies for preparing a primary care practice. Pediatrics 2010;125(Suppl 3):S87–108.

6. American Academy of Child and Adolescent Psychiatry Committee on Health Care Access and Economics Task Force on Mental Health. Improving mental health services in primary care: reducing administrative and financial barriers to access and collaboration. Pediatrics 2009;123(4):1248–51.

7. World Health Organization. Integrating mental health into primary care: a global perspective. Switzerland: World Health Organization; 2008. Available at: http://www.who.int/mental_health/resources/mentalhealth_PHC_2008.pdf. Accessed July 22, 2017.

8. Ginsburg S, Foster S. Strategies to support the integration of mental health into pediatric primary care. Washington, DC: National Institute for Health Care Management Research and Educational Foundation; 2009. Available at: https://www.nihcm.org/pdf/PediatricMH-FINAL.pdf. Accessed July 22, 2017.

9. McPherson C, Ploeg J, Edwards N, et al. A catalyst for system change: a case study of child health network formation, evolution and sustainability in Canada. BMC Health Serv Res 2017;17(1):100.

10. Leykum LK, Lanham HJ, Pugh JA, et al. Manifestations and implications of uncertainty for improving healthcare systems: an analysis of observational and interventional studies grounded in complexity science. Implement Sci 2014;9:165.

11. Proctor EK, Landsverk J, Aarons G, et al. Implementation research in mental health services: an emerging science with conceptual, methodological, and training challenges. Adm Policy Ment Health 2009;36(1):24–34.

12. Hanleybrown F, Kania J, Kramer M. Channelling change: making collective impact work. Stanf Soc Innov Rev. 2012. Available at: https://ssir.org/articles/entry/collective_impact. Accessed April 13, 2017.

13. Kania J, Kramer M. Collective impact. Stanf Soc Innov Rev. 2011. Available at: https://ssir.org/articles/entry/collective_impact. Accessed April 12, 2017.

14. Centers for Disease Control and Prevention. 500 cities: local data for better health. Available at: https://chronicdata.cdc.gov/health-area/500-cities. Accessed April 12, 2017.

15. United States Census Bureau. Available at: https://www.census.gov/quickfacts/fact/table/DC,US/PST045216. Accessed April 12, 2017.

16. Medicaid and CHIP Payment and Access Commission. MACStats Washington, DC: Medicaid and CHIP Payment and Access Commission. Available at: https://www.macpac.gov/wp-content/uploads/2015/12/MACStats-Medicaid-and-CHIP-Data-Book-December-2015.pdf. Accessed April 12, 2017.

17. American Academy of Pediatrics Analysis of the Henry J. Kaiser Family Foundation. Medicaid income eligibility limits of children ages 0-18, 2000–2016. 2016.

18. Brink R. Improving the children's mental health system in the District of Columbia. Washington, DC: Children's Law Center; 2012.

19. District of Columbia's HealthCheck provider education system. Available at: https://www.dchealthcheck.net/. Accessed April 11, 2017.

20. Beers LS, Godoy L, John T, et al. Mental Health Screening Quality Improvement Learning Collaborative in Pediatric Primary Care. Pediatrics 2017, in proco.
21. DC Map – Mental health access in pediatrics. Available at: http://www.dcmap. org/. Accessed April 11, 2017.
22. Biel MG, Anthony BJ, Godoy L, et al. Collaborative training efforts with pediatric providers in addressing mental health problems in primary care. Acad Psychiatry 2017. [Epub ahead of print].
23. Jellinek MS, Henderson SW, Pumariega AJ, et al. Cultural competence in child psychiatric practice. J Am Acad Child Adolesc Psychiatry 2009;48(4):362–6.
24. Roussos ST, Fawcett SB. A review of collaborative partnerships as a strategy for improving community health. Annu Rev Public Health 2000;21:369–402.
25. Wallerstein NB, Duran B. Using community-based participatory research to address health disparities. Health Promot Pract 2006;7(3):312–23.
26. John T, Morton M, Weissman M, et al. Feasibility of a virtual learning collaborative to implement an obesity QI project in 29 pediatric practices. Int J Qual Health Care 2014;26(2):205–13.

From Theory to Action
Children's Community Pediatrics Behavioral Health System

Abigail Schlesinger, MD[a],*, Jacquelyn M. Collura, MD[b,1],
Emily Harris, MD, MPH[c], Joanna Quigley, MD[d]

KEYWORDS

- Integrated care • Primary care • Pediatric behavioral health
- Behavioral health workforce

KEY POINTS

- Successful models of integration must first consider the needs of the providers and the capacity of the system to meet these needs.
- Providers and administrative early adopters and collaborators must endorse the model of integrated care.
- Successful integrated care therapists must have both general health and mental health expertise and a willingness to be flexible when responding to the needs of the practice and patients.
- Psychiatrists in integrated health care settings need unique skills related to interprofessional communication, patient stabilization, and system-level consultation.

INTRODUCTION

In 1977, Dr George Engel advocated for the biopsychosocial approach and questioned the silos of physical and psychosomatic medicine. Unfortunately, decreased communication between primary care and mental health care providers was reinforced by the exclusion of mental health care from health plans and privacy laws.[1]

Disclosure Statement: The authors have nothing to disclose.
[a] Department of Psychiatry, Western Psychiatric Institute and Clinic, University of Pittsburgh, Pittsburgh, PA, USA; [b] NW Permanente, PC, Physicians and Surgeons, Portland, OR, USA; [c] Clinical-Affiliate of General and Community Pediatrics, Division of Child and Adolescent Psychiatry, Department of Psychiatry and Behavioral Neuroscience, Cincinnati Children's Hospital Medical Center, University of Cincinnati, College Hill Campus ML 6015, 5642 Hamilton Avenue, Cincinnati, OH 45224, USA; [d] Department of Psychiatry, University of Michigan, Rachel Upjohn Building, 4250 Plymouth Road, SPC 5766, Ann Arbor, MI 48109-2700, USA
[1] Present address: 9800 Southeast Sunnyside Road, Clackamas, OR 97015-9750.
* Corresponding author. Pine Center, 11279 Perry Highway, Suite 204, Wexford, PA 15090.
E-mail address: schlesingerab@upmc.edu

Child Adolesc Psychiatric Clin N Am 26 (2017) 677–688
http://dx.doi.org/10.1016/j.chc.2017.05.004
1056-4993/17/© 2017 Elsevier Inc. All rights reserved.

childpsych.theclinics.com

Outsourcing mental health care has resulted in a problematic disparity in health care. Integrated health care models attempt to cross the artificial boundary of behavioral and medical worlds in order to improve access to quality care that meets the need of the whole person.[2] Integrating behavioral health care with primary care and/or medical subspecialties requires certain considerations above and beyond building a traditional mental health or primary care setting. This article describes lessons learned from integrating behavioral health in a large pediatric primary care group.

It has been estimated that 13% to 20% of children living in the United States experience a mental disorder in a given year, with suicide as the second leading cause of death in the 12- to 17-year age range.[3] Fifty percent of pediatric office visits involve significant psychosocial concerns requiring intervention, and 75% of children with psychiatric disorders are being brought to a pediatric primary care provider.[4] These percentages continue to grow, with estimates of cost for youth mental health services in excess of $200 billion annually,[3] not taking into consideration the cost of disability for those without access to behavioral health resources.[5] These numbers become increasingly alarming when considering time-based growth, increasing costs per untreated individual over the lifespan, and the estimate that only 20% of children with recognized mental illness receive treatment.[6] There are significant missed opportunities given that half of all lifetime mental illnesses begin at 14 years of age and three-quarters by 24 years of age.[4] This is a time when many individuals are seen regularly through primary care: 84% of US children aged 0 to 17 years are reported as having a well-child visit in a review of 2014 data with substantial growth in accessibility of pediatric primary care since implementation of the Children's Health Insurance Program.[7] Access to child and adolescent psychiatry within this setting additionally addresses often-cited barriers of fragmented and difficult-to-access care due to location and insurance carve-outs and the stigma and distrust associated with the mental health care system.[5] By initiating services within the primary care setting and involving a trusted provider in psychoeducation and warm handoffs, treatment can be implemented earlier, which is both more effective and can avoid greater costs to the individual and family's quality of life and avoid the multiple costs of hospitalizations.[6] The role of a child psychiatrist as consultant is increasingly necessary considering the relative shortage of child and adolescent psychiatrists practicing in the United States and lack of infrastructure or trainees to meet this need in the foreseeable future.[8,9]

Several models exist to address integration of behavioral health and primary care: coordinated care, colocated care, and integrated care. *Coordinated care* relies on routine screening in the primary care setting and a referral relationship between the primary care provider and behavioral health clinician. There is a mechanism in place for routine exchange of information between treatment settings, and ultimately the primary care provider delivers interventions discussed with the specialist using brief algorithms. Additionally, the behavioral health consultant can assist with community referrals for additional supportive resources. *Colocated care* models contain medical and behavioral services in the same setting. There is a referral process in place for medical cases to be seen by behavioral specialists. A unique advantage of this model is the enhanced communication between primary care provider and mental health specialist, which allows for a greater quality of care to the individual particularly in cases whereby there are longitudinal and complex behavioral health care needs. Additionally, ongoing ease of consultation between behavioral health and primary care providers enhances the knowledge and skill sets of both groups. This model is also associated with an improved show rate for behavioral health treatment. *Integrated care* implies one collaborative treatment plan with both behavioral and medical elements. A team works together to deliver care using a prearranged protocol. The unique aspect of this model that enhances overall sustainability is the use of a team composed of a physician but also use of allied health professionals including physician assistants, nurse practitioners, nurses, case managers and behavioral health therapists. Although operating under one treatment plan, the model does not depend on all players to remain within the same location, which allows for some flexibility in distributing limited resources. A database is used to track care of patients screened into behavioral health services to provide ongoing outreach and follow-up.[10,11] The focus in this article is primarily on lessons learned from implementation of an integrated model with a multidisciplinary, collaborative team using a stepped-care approach to behavioral health service access.

CONSIDERATIONS WHEN BUILDING A SYSTEM

Integrated mental health care models exist in a variety of formats and iterations.[12] Building an effective and sustainable model for implementation of integrated mental health care may begin by reflecting on attributes of the existing infrastructure: physical space, personnel, management, and resources.[13] Inherent to this is an effort to push previously independent elements of a health care delivery system (or systems) into a cooperative and collaborative space.[12] Buy-in from each component of this system is necessary: from first point of patient contacts, such as scheduling and front desk staff, to the highest levels of health care administration and management.

Defining needs for the providers and administrators and expectations of what the model will deliver is vital and often difficult. One paradigm of mental health integration in adult primary care suggests focusing on the following 6 components: identify a specific population, use measurement, target specific treatment outcomes, include care management, psychiatric supervision, and brief psychological therapies.[14] Aligning clinical and educational needs of an integrated system with the financial stability and growth of a system can be difficult to balance. Assessment of payer relationships and advocacy for appropriate reimbursement may require creativity and advocacy from the administrative and business leadership. Careful assessment of funding streams and budgets are required. Although collaborative care efforts have demonstrated reduced spending for the treatment of adult depression,[15] there is often an initial financial investment required to build an integrated delivery system. Individual providers and administration within a health care system may not have experience or comfort in aligning such efforts and may lack the communication skills or shared language to define needs and goals and execute them. A child and adolescent psychiatrist who is open to working between systems is well placed to serve as an intermediary in these relationships helping to bridge the gaps between the behavioral health world and the physical health world. Additional training and/or close collaboration with an administrative colleague is useful to assure that the clinical and financial components of the model are appropriately aligned.

Creating an efficient system is fundamental to ensuring financial sustainability as well as provider and consumer satisfaction.[16] Selecting leadership within this integrated system should reflect the goals of the integrated enterprise, the type of care and services the system wishes to deliver, and how it is going to create financial viability. Leadership should have clinical and administrative expertise as well as an understanding of the patient population needs and provider needs and an awareness of community resources and levels of care within the system. Defining ownership can inform the process: Who owns the patients? Who owns the outcome? Who owns the cost? So too can considering the goals of care: to increase access to mental health care, improve quality of care, or lower costs of care? Is it to reduce or increase referrals to subspecialty care or community mental health care? Examining these questions may lead to a more effective assessment of capacity within the existing systems.

Different players may arrive at this process with certain biases regarding what should and should not happen in a primary care setting, how mental health care should be delivered, and what should be managed within the primary care setting.[13] Primary care providers may acknowledge the burden of mental health care needs within their patient population; they may not view mental health management as a condition within their purview of long-term care/management.[17]

Integrated delivery systems must also be dynamic, capable of adjusting to changing demands over time. This includes logistical support involving scheduling and billing. It involves consideration of privacy, confidentiality, and compliance concerns across systems.[14] It involves the support of the existing electronic medical record, particularly considerations of documentation of communication, recommendations, and services that may not involve direct contact with patients but impact delivery of care. For colocation and embedded care models, there must also be flexibility in utilization and assignment of space, administrative supports to the staff, and support in patient flow. Although a goal of integrated models may be to increase the provision of mental health care within the primary care setting, inherent in this will likely be the greater or better identification of mental health needs and potentially a greater need for services. Do case managers exist within the system or shared between primary care and mental health care needs? Will the accessible behavioral health care system work in alliance with the integrated model and be open to referrals or sharing of resources? Successful adaptation may also require ongoing training and educational outreach to providers and allied health professionals within the system.

Transparent and effective communication is essential to the success of interprofessional collaboration and work.[18] Poor communication between primary care and mental health care providers is often identified as a barrier to collaborative efforts in pediatric mental health care.[19] Factors impacting communication within an integrated system are discussed in the literature.[16] Different styles and comfort levels with types of communication must also be acknowledged within the system. The types of interpersonal strategies used within integrated care models has been codified as existing in consulting, coordinating, and collaborating roles, each requiring different approaches and types of communication between providers.[18] Establishing clear avenues for communication ensures better care for patients and better provider satisfaction. This communication can exist in many different modalities[13]: one-on-one consultation in the embedded or colocated model, primary care and behavioral health clinicians, seeing patients together, or having behavioral health consultants provide quick interventions following appointments with primary care providers. The behavioral health clinician's colocation or in-person availability for curbside communication and face-to-face time can also improve provider satisfaction within integrated models.[18,20] Effective utilization of the electronic health record can also foster improved communication. Many models also use case conference models, panel review models, telephonic consultation, and tele-psychiatry.[21] As with each component of an integrated system, allotting appropriate time and resources to effective communication requires an ongoing investment.

Respecting the office culture around mental health and better understanding the providers, staff, and population served are critical in hiring and maintaining behavioral health clinicians who will interact with the practice. An oversight committee is needed to monitor the program to ensure it is reaching its global aim as well as ensuring sustainability of the program and balancing competing priorities among the financial stakeholders. When implementing a large system change, different aspects of the project may require different personnel to be involved with piloting the plan.

Integrative programs require financial, structural, and clinical components of integration to be sustainably successful. The working committee requires leadership that can represent critical components of how the change may affect the current system, both clinical and administrative. Leaders from scheduling/registration, nursing/triage, clinicians, and business managers are needed to offer insights into key processes the new program will affect. Small issues can create large obstacles if the appropriate personnel were not involved with planning and troubleshooting.

When working with large systems that support multiple practice sites, varying levels of resistance will be present. A practice that seems to have a high desire to make mental health integration work will likely be an early adopter of the new program. This practice visualizes the long-term benefits of the program and is willing to work through the obstacles to ensure its success. Early adopters often serve as a role model for the other practices that may be more hesitant to fully commit initially. Examples of potential practices that are likely to act as early adopters may have limited psychiatry resources, a pediatrician or nurse practitioner who has obtained extra training and acts as the office's peer specialist, or the office has a positive mental health culture that promotes discussing mental health concerns (displaying posters, maintains resources for families, triage protocols, or uses mental health screens).

Practices that are early adopters of change will help drive momentum and enthusiasm for the project. Remember to not exclude people who raise objections or have strong opposition to the concept, as they can provide invaluable perspective to navigate barriers.

SELECTING THERAPISTS

Just as selecting a motivated practice is critical with early successes, the therapist selection is equally important. Given the nature of the pediatric practice, the therapists will have to function with very little supervision and be able to quickly assess patients and families, determine level of intervention needed, and provide appropriate services to families and communicate readily with the referring provider. Please see **Box 1** for attributes of a therapist to asses in the interview process.

Therapists need to have mental flexibility and an interest in working in a team to adjust to needs as well as the ability to think on their feet when a clinician approaches them with a warm handoff or curbside consult about a patient. Implementation is a state of transition for the practice and therapist. They need frequent and open communication with the leadership (within psychiatry and pediatric practices). A space where therapists can openly work through interpersonal obstacles with staff or clinicians and the information is construed as feedback that provides insight for potential system failures can frame frustrations into groundwork on which to develop positive solutions. For instance, if a pediatrician disagrees with the assessments and ignores recommendations, the therapist may feel unheard and ineffective, leading to resentment. The pediatrician may have referred the family to 2 different resources because of concerns that the embedded therapist did not have perceived availability. With treatment team meetings or discussion with leadership, the therapist could be supported to approach the pediatrician directly or reframe his or her actions to reflect his or her motivation. Program leadership may need to facilitate discussions that assist with the process for the therapists and practices to meet in the middle, focusing on the mission of

Box 1
Attributes of a therapist

Clinical skills

Training in diagnoses, safety planning, and basic therapeutic skill development

Ability to assess and recommend interventions in first session

Ability to think on feet without onsite supervision during curbside consultation or requests for warm hand-offs

Ability to access off-site supervision/support appropriately

Experience

Experience with young children and adolescents

History of work in nontraditional setting or of interacting with primary care or specialty physicians

Attitudes

Perspective of the program mission and vision

View the role of the therapist as not only a therapist but also an educator and liaison for the provider, family, and specialty care resources

the program, which is to provide quality care for patients and families. Keeping open communication within the team may reduce unnecessary transfers of care and reduce the pediatrician undermining the therapeutic process inadvertently, both of which may ultimately delay patients' recovery (**Table 1**).

Table 1
Selected responsibilities of providers

Practice	Therapist	Psychiatrist
Buy-in to mission and model	Be able to provide evaluation and initiate treatment quickly	Be comfortable providing brief treatment and referral to primary care
Identify physician lead for to lead implementation of mission and model	Be skilled in evidence-based practices for common conditions	Stay attuned to behavioral health skills of pediatricians and be willing to help them progress in their skill set
Identify administrative lead (often practice or nurse manager) to follow through on nuts and bolts of implementation	Be flexible and able to adjust style to primary care setting, including possibility of being interrupted occasionally	Be flexible and able to adjust to the style and needs of the primary care setting
Support behavioral health providers as members of the team, patient check-in and scheduling patients as well as supplies	Be able to seek supervision from pediatrician, psychiatrist, or lead therapist	Have the ability to refer youths to more specialized or intensive services when needed
Provide appropriate space, including computer and telephone access	Be willing to keep a high profile with practice	Be willing to provide education to practice and therapists
Work with behavioral health providers to clarify methods of responding to phone calls	Be willing to provide education to practice	
Provide items needed to practice: screening tools, toys, child table and chairs		

SUPPORTING SUCCESSFUL PSYCHIATRY ROLES

Psychiatrists in primary care have a largely consultative approach to care, which may include brief stabilization before returning care to the medical home or referring to external resources. The psychiatrist's role in primary care is to provide diagnostic impressions/clarifications and reinforce treatment plans that may involve initiation or management of medication options. The downsides to the psychiatrist are that continuity is not encouraged in this model and the mental and emotional demands are high (with families, pediatricians, and even therapists). To meet the needs of the system at large, one therapist may cover 1 to 2 clinic practices; the psychiatrist may be responsible for psychiatric support for several therapists. Consider the demands on the psychiatrist who may be traveling to support different practices. Do they have a designated space in the office; are they getting administrative needs handled by the practice (including messages from patients); are they isolated from staff or able to interact readily? Financial incentives, location preference, and office goodness of fit may help drive productivity for the specialist. The authors' psychiatrists have noted that other activities, such as teaching, quality improvement and outcome measures, and different clinical responsibilities outside of primary care, have helped them maintain clinical and intellectual diversity so that they can function at their highest potential.

The role of a Child and Adolescent Psychiatrist (CAP) in this setting requires a level of flexibility and comfort with a variety of consultant roles. Curbside and telephone consultation is naturally invited by the colocation model and requires an ability to focus on a specific question and deliver teaching points in a concise manner.[22] Foresight to not just focus on the clinical question but also to anticipate clinical risks and provide education in a manner that invites ongoing collaboration is also key.[22] Being comfortable with the role as a temporary care provider in an individual's overall health care experience and sometimes doing so from the sidelines is an important consideration.

FROM THEORY TO ACTION: CHILDREN'S COMMUNITY PEDIATRICS BEHAVIORAL HEALTH SYSTEM

Successful integrated care efforts must respond to the needs of the patients and providers and involve collaboration between physical health and behavioral health providers. Children's Community Pediatrics Behavioral Health System (CCPBHS) began with a request from pediatricians for better access to empirically supported interventions as well as access to child and adolescent psychiatry providers. Children's Community Pediatrics (CCP) is a large network of affiliated, but financially independent pediatric practices who use a central billing office (CBO) to provide administrative and billing support. The CBO is supported financially by the individual practices. CCP currently serves more than 250,000 pediatric lives. CCP pediatricians identified the need for child psychiatry resources within their system in the mid 2000s. They joined with the Children's Hospital of Pittsburgh (CHP), which despite being a world-renowned pediatric hospital with a robust consultation-liaison service had only a small therapy department, and Western Psychiatric Institute and Clinic (WPIC). WPIC is also seen as being largely inaccessible for typical behavioral health treatment despite being one of the largest free-standing psychiatric hospitals in the United States, with robust outpatient clinics, consistently at the top of the National Institute of Mental Health's funding list.

Stakeholders from CCP, CHP, and WPIC were brought together to form an executive committee. Past integration efforts in Western Pennsylvania were reviewed, including strengths and weaknesses. A review of the literature was completed as well as review of parent and pediatrician interviews regarding treatment of common behavioral health conditions in pediatric primary care. Expectations of the behavioral health and pediatric providers were reviewed, and breakout groups were tasked with writing a mission statement and clinical pathways for review and approval by the larger group. The initial mission statement focused on providing access to high quality empirically supported interventions within the pediatric medical home. Clinical and administrative subgroups were created to focus on areas that could become potential barriers to implementation. The clinical small group, consisting of a behavioral health therapist, pediatrician, and child psychiatrist, identified what integrated model could be accomplished with the resources that were available and suggested clinical pathways. This group would ultimately be responsible for helping to vet behavioral health providers, manage the supervision of therapists, and onboard new practices. The administrative subgroup worked to centralize billing, educate individual practices about insurance issues, and clarify the scheduling pathways for patients and onboard practices. The program initially began with one pilot practice. Lessons learned from the initial pilot were used to help successful expansion. Once CCPBHS became established, the oversight committee continued to meet on a quarterly basis in order to manage fiscal, quality, and administrative issues. The meeting of this committee has been increased to monthly in times of change or perceived stresses to the system.

CLINICAL AND FINANCIAL MODEL

The CCPBHS model of short-term treatment from an embedded therapist supported by the practice with oversight and referral pathways to a child psychiatrist has proven to be fiscally sustainable. The therapists schedule 7 patients a day, with break-even behavioral health billing at 5 patients a day. Incident to medical professionals has been piloted and increases revenue as well as integration at the clinical level. Several quality initiatives have been created and supported at the practice and system level. All therapists are encouraged to work with their physicians and support staff, such as nurse triage and practice managers, to identify needs and lead lunch and learns for individual practices. The psychiatric medical director has also worked with the executive committee to institute larger quality improvement initiatives, including a 4-part educational series on the treatment of internalizing disorders and intermittent webinars on topics of interest to all embedded and primary care clinical staff. Since 2015, the behavioral health and pediatric providers are working together on an initiative to improve substance screening and implementation of substance screening intervention and referral to treatment in youths 11 to 120 years of age. Nursing and triage staff also benefit from training on triage and general behavioral health issues.

CCPBHS relies on the primary care physician, family, and therapist as the hub of services within the medical home. They work together to identify children and adolescents in need of interventions. The pediatric practices have implemented a variety of screening programs, from developmental screens for young children to depression and substance screening for adolescents and young adults, in order to improve their ability to capture behavioral health concerns. The therapist and pediatricians work closely to help mold the system to meet their needs, although they base this on the clinical pathways that have been approved and vetted through the clinical subgroup and executive committee. For example, if there are pediatricians, nurse practitioners, or physician assistants with more interest and experience with behavioral health interventions, they are encouraged to use their skills in order to maximize the amount of treatment that can be provided in primary care. There is a focus on promoting access to evaluations and referring youths out who may need to have weekly long-term treatment. The therapists are encouraged to discuss this in twice-a-month group supervision or to use their individual supervisor to discuss unique cases. This system is not meant to supplant behavioral health services but to help support the provision of services to youths within primary care. The authors think that primary care behavioral health service is in itself a unique level of care and one whose definition is only beginning to be described in the literature.[23] The psychiatric medical director provides oversight for the therapists, helps implement new initiatives, and also does direct patient care. When CCPBHS began, there was one nurse practitioner in the system who had developed an expertise in behavioral health. Over the 10 years, there have now been 4. The psychiatrists have worked with the practices in order to help define the role of the nurse practitioner.

The CCPBHS system was quickly adopted by pilot practices and within 5 years had expanded to more than 15 sites. The executive committee identified a need for training on the use of empirically supported interventions for depression and anxiety, and a 4-part series was attended by most clinicians in the system. Chart reviews revealed an increase in the use of evidence-based interventions after the completion of the series. The health care system identified that more than $1 million a year was saved by maintaining some children within their primary care site and diverting from higher levels of care. Patients engaged in the system were less likely to use acute care visits while maintaining well-child visits. The success of this model resulted in an investment of the larger system in a rollout first to pediatric medical subspecialty care, then to adult primary care, and finally to adult subspecialty care. Although each of these initiatives has been successful in their own right, the ease of implementation and ultimate success of each individual rollout can consistently be linked back to buy-in and leadership from individual behavioral health and medical specialties.

THE ROLE OF A TRIPLE-BOARDED PHYSICIAN

Several triple-boarded providers, physicians trained as pediatricians, adult psychiatrists, and child psychiatrists, have worked in CCPBH. One role that has unique opportunities and challenges is when the physician works both as a pediatrician and child psychiatrist. This role is an attractive career option after residency for triple-board trained physicians given the ability to continue direct patient care using both behavioral health and primary care skill sets. Natural boundaries set by the tiered model of care and the collaborative team make having a dual physician role possible within this system such that the psychiatrist is not the sole point of contact for all patients accessing behavioral health within one location. A provider must be credentialed at the state level with both physical health and behavioral health payers to be reimbursed as both a pediatrician and child and adolescent psychiatrist. Not all credentialing bodies allow for this dual certification; in fact, the authors needed to work with their state agencies in order to help them understand the roles these physicians play.

AREAS OF OPPORTUNITY

It can be isolating to individual providers within a primary care setting, as physical availability of like-minded behavioral health providers to process challenging cases is not as easily accessed as in a traditional behavioral health setting. The potential for isolation among the therapists and psychiatrists must be considered in order to assure that they can provide sustainable support and evidence-based treatment to children and families. In addition, the behavioral health therapist and the CAP often take on a role of informally supporting the behavioral health needs of the practice providers. Team care meetings and supervision are important to prevent provider burnout, enhance high-level evidence-based care, and allow for sustainability. Ongoing education specific to specialty care is rewarding to all team members.

Future models of pediatric integration need to consider the integration of substance use prevention, intervention, and treatment as well as the provision of care to transitional age youths. Also, youths who go to college may have unique challenges in accessing psychiatric care. The authors are having an ongoing discussion about the role that the pediatrician and behavioral health system can, or should, play as a young adult transitions to a college in a location that does not have access to behavioral health services. At this point the authors are grappling with this issue on a case-by-case basis; but a more systematic approach, including tele-medicine services, has been considered. Primary care offices are starting to implement care coordination in order to support families between visits with the pediatric medical provider. Behavioral health also has a model for collaborative care that includes a care coordinator.[24] Pediatric practices will have to grapple with how these providers work together in the most efficient manner. It may be that one provider could provide both roles, although a workforce does not yet exist that can perform both of these tasks. Finally, future models of integration will have to rely not only on in-person evaluations and treatment in primary care but also utilization of telehealth methods.

SUMMARY

The CCPBHS initiative is an effective model with mindfulness toward sustainability. Clearly the success of a primary care–based initiative requires attention to financial, clinical, and administrative issues related to implementation and maintenance. In addition, the changing nature of the health care system world requires that the system not remain stagnant to continue to adapt and meet the needs of its physicians and their patients. The addition of an Massachusetts Child Psychiatry Access Program (MCPAP) like model in 2016 with oversight by the CCP psychiatrists has also been one way that the system has grown and adapted. The authors continue to explore the role of tele-psychiatry as well as a mixed model of integration and collaborative care as a way to maximize outcomes while efficiently using resources. Clearly one resource that cannot not be neglected is the workforce. There is a limited but growing physical health and behavioral health workforce interested and able to work collaboratively. It is vital the CAPs take a leadership role in helping to train and support these providers.

REFERENCES

1. Fritsch SL, Schlesinger A, Habeger AD, et al. Collaborative care and integration: changing roles and changing identity of the child and adolescent psychiatrist? J Am Acad Child Adolesc Psychiatry 2016;55(9):743–5.

2. Richardson LP, McCarty CA, Radovic A, et al. Research in the integration of behavioral health for adolescents and young adults in primary care settings: a systematic review. J Adolesc Health 2017;60(3):261–9.

3. Perou R, Bitsko RH, Blumberg SJ, et al, Centers for Disease Control and Prevention (CDC). Mental surveillance among children—United States, 2005-2011. MMWR Suppl 2013;62(2):1–35.

4. Martini R, Hilt R, Marx L, et al. Best principles for integration of child psychiatry into the pediatric health home. Washington, DC: American Academy of Child and Adolescent Psychiatry; 2012. Available at: https://www.aacap.org/App_Themes/AACAP/docs/clinical_practice_center/systems_of_care/best_principles_

for_integration_of_child_psychiatry_into_the_pediatric_health_home_2012.pdf. Accessed July 5, 2017.

5. Hodgkinson S, Godoy L, Beers LS, et al. Improving mental health access for low-income children and families in the primary care setting. Pediatrics 2017;139(1) [pii:e20151175].

6. American Academy of Child and Adolescent Psychiatry Committee on Health Care Access and Economics Task Force on Mental Health. Improving mental health services in primary care: reducing administrative and financial barriers to access and collaboration. Pediatrics 2009;123(4):1248–51.

7. Larson K, Cull WL, Racine AD, et al. Trends in access to health care services for US children: 2000-2014. Pediatrics 2016;138(6) [pii:e20162176].

8. Kim W, American Academy of Child and Adolescent Psychiatry Task Force on Workforce Needs. Child and adolescent psychiatry workforce: a critical shortage and national challenge. Acad Psychiatry 2003;27:277–82.

9. Workforce and graduate medical education; workforce resources: child and adolescent psychiatrist workforce maps (by state). AACAP website. Available at: https://www.aacap.org/aacap/Advocacy/Federal_and_State_Initiatives/Workforce_Maps/Home.aspx.

10. Collins C, Hewson DL, Munger R, et al. Evolving models of behavioral health integration in primary care, 11. New York: Milbank Memorial Fund; 2010. p. 504.

11. Blount A. Integrated primary care: organizing the evidence. Fam Syst Health 2003;22(21):121–34.

12. Kodner DL, Spreeuwenberg C. Integrated care: meaning, logic, applications, and implications—a discussion paper. Int J Integr Care 2002;2:e12.

13. Benzer JK, Cramer IE, Burgess JF, et al. How personal and standardized coordination impact implementation of integrated care. BMC Health Serv Res 2015;15:448.

14. Kroenke K, Unutzer J. Closing the false divide: sustainable approaches to integrating mental health services into primary care. J Gen Intern Med 2017;32(4):404–10.

15. Unutzer J, Katon WJ, Fan MY, et al. Long-term cost effects of collaborative care for late-life depression. Am J Manag Care 2008;14(2):95–100.

16. Wood E, Ohlsen S, Ricketts T. What are the barriers and facilitators to implementing collaborative care for depression? A systematic review. J Affect Disord 2017; 214:26–43.

17. Kendrick T, Sibbald B, Burns T, et al. Role of general practitioners in care of long term mentally ill patients. BMJ 1991;302(6775):508–10.

18. Cohen DJ, Davis M, Balasubramanian BA, et al. Integrating behavioral health and primary care: consulting, coordinating and collaborating among professionals. J Am Board Fam Med 2015;28(Suppl 1):S21–31.

19. Cooper M, Evans Y, Pybis J. Interagency collaboration in children and young people's mental health: a systematic review of outcomes, facilitating factors and inhibiting factors. Child Care Health Dev 2016;42(3):325–42.

20. Overbeck G, Davidsen AS, Kousgaard B. Enablers and barriers to implementing collaborative care for anxiety and depression: a systematic qualitative review. Implement Sci 2016;11(1):165.

21. Sarvet B, Gold J, Straus JH. Bridging the divide between child psychiatry and primary care: the use of telephone consultation within a population-based collaborative system. Child Adolesc Psychiatr Clin N Am 2011;20(1):41–53.

22. Sarvet B, Hilt R. Child and adolescent psychiatry in integrated settings. In: Raney LE, editor. Integrated care working at the interface of primary care and behavioral health. Washington, DC: American Psychiatric Publishing; 2015. p. 63–90.

23. Bautista MA, Nuriono M, Lim YW, et al. Instruments measuring integrated care: a systematic review of measurement properties. Millbank Q 2016;94(4):862–917.
24. Kolko DJ, Perrin E. The integration of behavioral health interventions in children's health care: services, science, and suggestions. J Clin Child Adolesc Psychol 2014;43(2):216–28.

Preparing Trainees for Integrated Care

Triple Board and the Postpediatric Portal Program

Mary Margaret Gleason, MD[a],*, Sandra Sexson, MD[b,c]

KEYWORDS

- Integrated care • Combined training • Education • Triple board • PPPP

KEY POINTS

- Training that combines the disciplines of pediatrics, psychiatry, and child and adolescent psychiatry dates back to World War II, but formal combined programs began more than 3 decades ago as the Triple Board Program and 10 years ago as the Postpediatric Portal Program (PPPP).
- Triple board training was rigorously examined as a pilot program and ongoing surveys suggest that it provides successful training of physicians who can pass the required board examinations and contribute to clinical, academic, and administrative/advocacy endeavors.
- The PPPP began as a pilot program in the Accreditation Council for Graduate Medical Education monitored by the Psychiatry Review Committee, but more recently is administered under auspices of the American Board of Psychiatry and Neurology. Recent surveys suggest that, like the triple board, the PPPP graduates have high pass rates in board examinations and practice in numerous settings, sometimes in combined practices but primarily in child and adolescent psychiatry.
- As evidence grows showing the clinical and fiscal value of integrated care, physicians with combined training will offer a unique perspective for developing systems.

INTRODUCTION: RATIONALE FOR COMBINED TRAINING

The traditional path to child and adolescent psychiatry (CAP), unlike most subspecialties focused on children, goes through general (adult) psychiatry before allowing specialization in CAP. Throughout the history of CAP training, there have been efforts

Disclosure: The authors have nothing to disclose.
[a] Psychiatry and Behavioral Sciences, Pediatrics Tulane University School of Medicine, 1430 Canal Street #8055, New Orleans, LA 70112, USA; [b] Child, Adolescent, and Family Psychiatry, Psychiatry and Health Behavior, Medical College of Georgia, Augusta University, 997 St. Sebastian Way, Augusta, GA 30912, USA; [c] Pediatrics, Medical College of Georgia, Augusta University, 997 St. Sebastian Way, Augusta, GA 30912, USA
* Corresponding author.
E-mail address: mgleason@tulane.edu

Child Adolesc Psychiatric Clin N Am 26 (2017) 689–702
http://dx.doi.org/10.1016/j.chc.2017.06.007
1056-4993/17/© 2017 Elsevier Inc. All rights reserved.

childpsych.theclinics.com

to offer alternative pathways to becoming a child and adolescent psychiatrist. For example, In the post–World War II era, with the increased awareness of the importance of children's mental health in predicting response to war and the revolution in pediatric care that came with antibiotic treatments, the federal government provided funding for pediatricians to train in child psychiatry, resulting in some of the extraordinary figures of child psychiatry.[1] The topic was addressed again in the 1980s, when leaders in CAP comprehensively reviewed the state of the field and recommended that the entry into child psychiatry training and the pathways for full training and certification be more flexible. This recommendation addressed a practical need to expand the recruitment pool for CAP but also recognized the importance of developing collaborative, interdisciplinary approaches to care and maintaining a connection to physical medicine.[2] The 2 formal pathways that have developed since this call are the triple board (pediatrics, psychiatry, and CAP) programs and the postpediatric portal programs (psychiatry and CAP after full training in pediatrics). Although the primary rationale for the development of these programs was the practical issue of the workforce shortage, physicians with combined training may offer particularly useful skills in integrated care, in which being familiar with both pediatrics and child psychiatry is seen as an asset. This article describes the background of the 2 formal combined programs in CAP, reviews both published and unpublished outcomes, and considers the role of these physicians in integrated or collaborative care.

DEVELOPMENT OF TRIPLE BOARD PROGRAMS

The Triple Board Program was developed in response to the Project Future call to action for considering more flexible pathways to training in CAP. The movement to develop these programs was led by John Schowalter MD, seen by many as the "grandfather" of the triple board programs, who led the Pediatrics-Psychiatry Joint Training Committee, which included representation from the American Board of Pediatrics (ABP), the American Board of Psychiatry and Neurology (ABPN), the Committee on Certification in Child and Adolescent Psychiatry, the American Academy of Pediatrics, the American Psychiatric Association, and the American Academy of Child Psychiatry, now the American Academy of Child and Adolescent Psychiatry (AACAP).[3] Dr Schowalter led the planning, selection, and evaluation of the programs and elicited endorsement for the project from the Society of Professors of Child Psychiatry, the American Association of Directors of Psychiatric Residency Training (AADPRT), the American Association of Chairmen of Departments of Psychiatry, and the Accreditation Council for Graduate Medical Education (ACGME) Review Committees (RCs) for Psychiatry and for Pediatrics.[3] After substantial discussion and negotiation, described by Dr Schowalter as "oratory, sweat, and blood,"[3] 6 triple board programs, selected from 32 applications, opened their doors in 1986. The original training programs at Tufts, Brown, Utah, Kentucky, Mount Sinai, and Albert Einstein each admitted 2 residents per year. The programs were intended to recruit medical students who might otherwise have focused primarily on a pediatrics pathway but who were driven by an interest in physical and mental health of children. The Triple Board Program was designed to be shorter than the 8 years that training in pediatrics and separately psychiatry and CAP would require. The program required a total of 5 years of training: 24 months in pediatrics, 18 months in general psychiatry, and 18 months in CAP, requirements that remain to the present time. Because the program was a pilot, a rigorous 10-year evaluation plan was developed, with funding from the National Institutes of Mental Health. In 1995, after only 7 years, the evaluation was discontinued early, in part because of positive findings. At that time, the programs were left under the oversight of the ABPN and the ABP, although each training component program was required to be accredited by the ACGME.[4] An editorial published by Dr Schowalter[4] at the time highlighted positive outcomes of the training programs at the resident level, faculty collaboration level, and national organization level but also recognized the biases among non–triple board–involved faculty, who regularly advised medical students not to participate in the program.[4]

OVERSIGHT OF TRIPLE BOARD PROGRAMS

After the formal approval of the programs in 1995, new programs were added, with the approval of the boards, and the programs remained under the loose oversight of the 2 boards. Of the initial 6 programs, 5 remain active. Einstein closed in the early 2000s. New programs were added, including San Antonio and Hawaii, which are no longer active, and Indiana, Cincinnati, Pittsburgh, and Tulane, all of which are actively approved. The curricular requirements were reviewed in 2000, but, otherwise, oversight by the ABPN and ABP focused primarily on the new programs during this period. In the next decade, the structures around graduate medical education expanded dramatically, with changes in training requirements by the psychiatry and pediatrics RCs and more specific and detailed common program requirements by the ACGME. In 2009, as the processes for accreditation and review of residency programs became more rigorous across the ACGME, the ABPN announced a moratorium on new combined programs, including the Triple Board Program. The rationale for this decision was described as concerns about "state licensing and insurance reimbursement" for graduates of combined programs because, at the time, the ACGME Web site described the programs as "not accredited."[5] In response, the ACGME adjusted the language to the current wording describing combined programs: "components individually accredited." Note that, to the knowledge of triple board leaders, no triple board graduate was ever not able to be licensed or receive insurance reimbursement, but, in some states without combined training programs, the program or the ABPN needed to explain the status of the program to state licensing boards to facilitate the process. Over the course of the next 5 years, the ABPN and the ABP reviewed the status of the programs and determined a course of action. In 2015, the ABPN established the Oversight Committee for Combined Training, which focuses on the combined programs that involve psychiatry. The committee includes representatives from each of the combined programs, recommended by the AADPRT leadership. Program requirements were updated by the boards and all existing programs were reviewed and approved, with a plan for ongoing oversight and review of the programs by the ABPN committee. In 2017, the moratorium on new programs was lifted and proposed new triple board programs are undergoing review.

TRIPLE BOARD PROGRAM REQUIREMENTS

The 5-year programs include 2 years of pediatrics training, 1.5 years of general psychiatry and 1.5 years of CAP training. **Table 1** presents the current requirements for triple board training. For the most part, the requirements are similar to those for the categorical residents, with fewer elective opportunities. A few differences exist. For example, until recently, triple board residents had fewer months of pediatric intensive care training than categorical residents and were not required to complete a developmental behavioral pediatrics month. Longitudinal care is a strength of the 5-year training program. Throughout the 5 years, residents have a pediatric continuity clinic for at least a half day a week. Thus, it is common for a resident to pick up a pediatric patient in the newborn nursery or neonatal intensive care unit and continue to see the

Table 1
Summary of triple board rotation requirements

	Total (mo)	Inpatient	Emergency	Intensive Care	Subspecialty Care	Outpatient Requirements
Pediatrics	24	5 minimum	3	Pediatric intensive care unit (2) Neonatal intensive care unit (2)	4 specialty selectives plus Developmental behavioral pediatrics: 1 Adolescent medicine: 1 Newborn nursery: 1 Ambulatory (including community pediatrics and advocacy): 2 Supervisory months (5; at least 3 in pediatrics)	36 half-day sessions per year in continuity clinic throughout training
General Psychiatry	18	4–9			Addiction disorder service: 1	≥6 mo FTE experience plus experience treating patients longitudinally ≥9 mo
Experiences met either in general psychiatry or CAP			Experience on a service offering 24-h emergency psychiatric care (including children)		Neurology (preferably pediatric): 1 Consultation experience to medicine and at least 1 other area (legal, schools, community systems) Clinical experience with patients with intellectual disabilities, geriatrics, substance abuse disorders Experience with common psychological testing	
CAP	18	4–6 mo inpatient, residential treatment, partial hospitalization programs, or day programs				Continuous care for at least 1 y for patients seen regularly and frequently in various (specified) modalities and each developmental level

Units are months or rotation blocks.
Abbreviation: FTE, full time equivalent.
Used with permission from American Board of Psychiatry and Neurology, Inc, Buffalo Grove, IL.

patient until kindergarten. Residents are required to see general psychiatry patients for at least 9 months of longitudinal care and have 12 months of CAP longitudinal training. In many programs, residents have child psychiatry continuity patients from their post-graduate year (PGY) 3 through the end of their fifth year, if it is clinically appropriate for the patient. The curriculum also offers residents an ability to learn development and the normal variations of development, seeing children with typical development, healthy families under stress (eg, in the intensive care unit), as well as families and patients with mental disorders. In addition, triple board training offers an important opportunity to consider development throughout the lifespan, beginning perinatally with preterm infants, through to the geriatric experiences in psychiatry and neurology.

Each program offers a slightly different approach to the curriculum, with the most significant variation being the number of transitions among specialties, or the degree of integration. Originally, schedules were the 3 separate blocks (pediatrics, general psychiatry, CAP), but no programs have maintained this structure to date.[6] Programs have moved toward more integrated schedules for several reasons, including concerns about attrition to pediatrics when residents in PGY 2 considered leaving triple board, in which they had 3 additional training years and switching to categorical pediatrics, in which they would have only 1 additional training year. In addition, moving more pediatrics training to later in the training has been thought to increase the odds of passing the pediatrics boards, compared with finishing most pediatric training in PGY 2. Residents can petition to sit for the pediatric boards in their fifth year if they have completed all but their clinic requirements.

Programs have also developed innovative integrated care approaches to their training programs. Several programs offer opportunities for child psychiatry continuity clinic early in training. For example, at Utah, residents begin a mental health continuity experience in PGY 2. At Tulane, the pediatric continuity clinic is staffed by both a categorical and triple board faculty, providing support around primary care–level mental health concerns. Increasingly, triple board residents are trained by triple board faculty in core and elective rotations as well as by categorically trained faculty.

THE TRIPLE BOARD ORGANIZATION

During the pilot program of triple board, the annual retreats were intentionally developed to provide a community for the residents and faculty in triple board. The developers recognized the importance of having a professional community of residents and faculty involved in an innovative, and to some extent countercultural, program. Anecdotally, these retreats offered an important source of support for the residents who attended and for the faculty and training directors working to develop the necessary interdepartmental collaboration for a combined program. After the end of the pilot, this function was not replaced with any specific professional home for triple boarders. In 2001, Henrietta Leonard MD was awarded an AACAP Abramson Award to convene the triple board programs for a retreat, to reexamine the program training activities, and develop an organization dedicated to triple board. This organization, which became the National Association for Pediatrics, Psychiatry, and Child and Adolescent Psychiatry Training (NAPPCAPT) became the professional home for the triple board world. Over the next 10 to 15 years, the organization developed a leadership system, held biannual meetings, and developed mentoring and academic activities, including a Web site for prospective and current residents. The organization held an annual reception for interested medical students, current residents, graduates, and faculty to meet and create a professional home within the larger organizations. NAPPCAPT offered resident scholarships to the AACAP meeting and created a graduate email listserv to connect the triple boarders nationally. In addition, NAAPCAPT offered clinical presentations about pediatric medicine at the AACAP national meeting, bringing pediatric resources to child and adolescent psychiatrists. This program has been ongoing for more than 8 years, with positive feedback. Building on the contributions of the NAPPCAPT members and residents, triple board has become more integrated into existing organizations. For example, in 2013, American Academy of Pediatrics and AACAP established mutual liaisons between their residency training committees. NAPPCAPT served as a temporary professional home and organizational structure for triple board, whereas the combined training model became more accepted within the mainstream professional organizations. In 2012, AADPRT created a formal triple board caucus and, in 2016, AACAP created the Committee on Triple Board and Post Pediatrics Portal. With inclusion into the established organizations, NAPPCAPT has served its purpose as a bridge for the triple board community and will cease its independent activities. Triple boarders in the Midwest have also developed an annual summit, which is a day-long program of triple board presentations by residents and faculty, primarily from Pittsburgh, Kentucky, Cincinnati, and Indiana.

TRIPLE BOARD OUTCOMES

Outcomes of the triple board programs have been examined using varied methodologies during the history of the program. As noted earlier, the initial pilot programs underwent extensive evaluations, including personality testing, qualitative evaluations through regular retreats, and examination of in-service tests, leading Dr Schowalter to call the early cohorts "bright, adventuresome guinea pigs."

Pilot Program

The pilot program, the most systematic evaluation of the triple board training program, evaluated the training from 1986, when the first trainees enrolled, to 1995. The evaluation consisted of site visits, annual retreats for residents and faculty, recruitment data, an assessment of clinical reasoning, and postgraduate evaluations.[7] Throughout the pilot period, each program filled and 2 programs expanded from 2 to 3 residents per year. During the pilot program, residents were ranked in comparison with the categorical residents doing the same specialty work. In pediatrics, PGYs 1 and 2, on average, were ranked 6 out of 10 residents compared with pediatrics residents, PGYs 3 and 4 were ranked about 5 out of 10 residents compared with general psychiatry residents, and in PGY 5, 3.6 out of 10 compared with CAP residents. Similar findings were seen on in-service examinations, on which triple board residents scored less than the categorical pediatrics average but more than the psychiatry and CAP average. In a case-based assessment of clinical reasoning, triple boarders scored higher than the categorical CAP residents, a finding that was thought to support a qualitative assessment that triple boarders thought differently compared with categorically trained residents at all sites and across all years.[7] Of the 49 graduates in the pilot project, 44% passed the pediatric certification examination, 95% had passed the general psychiatry certification examination, and 77% had passed the CAP certification examination.

2005 Survey

In 2005, Warren and colleagues[8] reported on an updated outcomes survey of triple board graduates, with a high response rate of 81% of the identified 140 graduates between 1995 and 2003. This survey focused primarily on career paths and certification examination outcomes. Of the respondents, about 75% reported that they worked in

CAP settings, 15% in pediatrics, and 6% in general psychiatry. Approximately 38% reported that they worked in academic settings, with outpatient clinical work being the most commonly reported settings. One-third had completed or were completing postresidency fellowship training in areas such as child psychiatry specialization, infant mental health, epidemiology, forensics, addiction medicine, and neuroimaging. Pediatric certification examination pass rates increased over time, with an average pass rate of 77% among pediatric board takers. Pass rates for general psychiatry and CAP exceeded 90%. Barriers to taking board certification examinations included that it was not important for respondents' careers, which was common among the 18% of respondents who had not taken the pediatric examination, as well as worry about passing and financial concerns. Note that, in the era of oral board examinations, triple boarding, including travel, cost graduates approximately $10,000. Fewer barriers were identified for the ABPN examinations.

2012 Survey

The most recent assessment of triple board outcomes was a follow-up survey of graduates.[9] Although at that time it was estimated that 200 residents had graduated from a Triple Board Program, emails were available only for 154 because of programs closing or graduates being lost to communication from their programs. Total response rate to the Survey Monkey survey was 58%. This survey, designed by the program directors of triple board, examined preresidency status, perception of training quality, board certification status, and postgraduation activities. About 14% of the graduates had been elected into Alpha Omega Alpha in medical school, a rate higher than the rates in pediatrics (12.0%) and psychiatry (4.9%).[10] Approximately one-third reported that they would have chosen a pediatrics pathway if they had not done triple board and two-thirds would have pursued training in psychiatry. During training, intensive care training was rated as the least influential experience, but, overall, all but 1 respondent reported that the benefits of doing triple board training outweighed the drawbacks and two-thirds reported that the training was the best decision of their professional lives. In this sample, 58% had passed pediatrics boards at least once. Equal numbers had not taken pediatrics boards (13%) and failed the examination (14%). Higher rates had taken and passed the general psychiatry certification examination at least once (71%). More than half had passed the child psychiatry certification examination (58%) at least once and no one reported that they had failed the examination. Note that the higher rate of not taking the child psychiatry certification examination may be partially explained by the fact that, in the era of oral boards, it could take 3 to 4 years to take all of the examinations, even when fully successful, so some graduates would not have had an opportunity to sit for the examination. Similarly to the 2005 publication, a quarter had done postresidency fellowships and 64% worked in academics. Nearly half (44%) had published in a peer-reviewed journal. More than 1 in 4 had worked in pediatrics and about half had practiced general psychiatry. Of note, more than half had received service awards for their work in the community. Given the lower response rate in this survey, the high rates of academic achievement may overrepresent the general triple board population, because graduates in academics may be more likely to keep in touch with their residency programs and maintain a continuous email address, compared with those in practice. Overall, this sample showed that triple board was recruiting high-achieving medical students, a substantial minority of whom would not have done child psychiatry without triple board. The group was highly satisfied with their training, had acceptable board examination pass rates, and produced substantial academic contributions postresidency.

Beyond objective findings in surveys, what distinguishes triple boarders is identity.[11–13] Triple boarders who describe their career path almost universally begin with how the training shaped their professional identities. It is common for triple boarders to describe one of the most important benefits as the cross-cultural identify that comes from spending time in the cultures of pediatrics, psychiatry, and CAP as a "native" of each culture. Evidence of this identity, which allows the triple boarders to function comfortably in both settings, can be seen in the number of triple board graduates who sit on committees in both the AACAP and the AAP. In addition, the training across the various systems of pediatrics, psychiatry, and CAP provides opportunities to consider the health care system more broadly, and triple boarders are commonly found in positions of health and mental health leadership around the country. Even when triple board graduates seem to be functioning in a categorical setting, many say that their practice is undeniably shaped by the training, resulting in what they call holistic or integrated approaches to care.[13]

Similarly, in established triple board programs, the programs also influence their institutions. Residents and faculty talk of "cross-pollination," in which the effects of having a combined program influence not only the combined residents but the categorical residents as well. Combined residents tend to be viewed as resources by their categorical peers (even before they have any training in the other specialties) and the "curbside" consultations are frequent and last throughout a career. Similarly, combined programs may serve as a mechanism to develop additional research, training, or service collaboration. For example, at Tulane, senior triple board residents run an intern support group for the pediatric residents, resulting in group process training for the triple board residents and a supportive process for the pediatric residents. Having combined-trained faculty in a clinical competency committee almost always results in conversations about how a struggling resident is adjusting to life stressors or residency, with the combined faculty being asked to provide reflections or suggestions about management. Clinical programs, such as primary care mental health consultation, may develop in the context of triple board training programs. The day-to-day challenges of scheduling, resident recruitment, and professional development are significant. For a program to survive, collaboration at the level of the departmental leadership is necessary and the result may be a strengthened child-focused coalition.

DEVELOPMENT OF THE POSTPEDIATRICS PORTAL PROGRAMS

Like the Triple Board Program, the postpediatric portal program (PPPP) grew out of another AACAP initiative to increase the workforce in CAP by offering alternative pathways for entering training in the field. In 2004, then AACAP president-elect Thomas F. Anders told Psychiatric Times that the number of child and adolescent psychiatrists needed to care for America's children was insufficient.[14] As the leader of this AACAP initiative to increase recruitment into the CAP workforce, Dr Anders suggested the need to create additional pathways for entering CAP training other than the traditional 5-year psychiatry/CAP course or the more recent triple board programs described earlier in this article. Subsequently, AACAP, led by Dr Anders, sought support from the ACGME for an educational innovations project then available at the ACGME for a program that would allow an innovative pathway into training in CAP. This pathway would facilitate persons with accredited training in pediatrics to enter an abbreviated, 3-year training program encompassing both psychiatry and CAP, in a program similarly structured to the psychiatry/CAP component of the Triple Board Program. Again, with the support of other organizations, including AADPRT, ABPN, AAP, as well as CAP consumer groups, a pilot program was introduced requiring 3 years of additional training in psychiatry and CAP for applicants who had completed ACGME-accredited pediatric training. In 2007 the ACGME, through the psychiatry RC, invited up to 10 psychiatry/CAP programs to offer the 3-year training consisting of 18 full time equivalent (FTE) months in each specialty, integrated over 3 years. This effort, as Dr Anders commented to *Psychiatric Times* in 2008, "will attract board-eligible and board-certified pediatricians who wish to switch careers."[15] Initially, 4 pilot programs were approved by the ACGME: Case Western Reserve University/University Hospitals of Cleveland, Creighton/University of Nebraska, Children's Hospital of Philadelphia, and Maine Medical Center. Case welcomed the first PPPP fellows in 2007, Creighton in 2008, and Children's Hospital of Philadelphia in 2009. Subsequently Maine, after admitting 3 fellows, stopped recruiting and ultimately withdrew its program, and, more recently, a new program was approved at the Medical College of Georgia at Augusta University (MCG).

OVERSIGHT

After the formal approval of the programs in 2007 oversight was provided by a subcommittee of the Psychiatry RC, and the PPPP program directors and trainees were invited to join triple board entities that supported these abbreviated training sequences. Then, the ACGME decided it no longer would support the educational innovative projects under which the PPPP had been accepted. However, with support from the field and the Psychiatry RC, in October 2012, the PPPP was reinstated and designated as accredited by the ACGME with the Psychiatry RC continuing the oversight functions. Then, in March 2016, the ACGME RC for Psychiatry announced to all PPPP programs that they would no longer continue oversight, effective immediately, and that no new positions should be offered, and suggested that programs should contact the ABPN regarding whether the ABPN would recognize the training of the residents in the PPPP. Leadership organizations in psychiatry advocated for continuation of these programs and ultimately the ABPN assumed oversight of the programs in existence. Subsequently, in 2017, the field has opened to application for new PPPP programs, one of which is presently being reviewed. During this advocacy process it was apparent that, although the numbers of programs as well as graduates are small, this pathway does offer an alternative pathway to entry into CAP that meets the needs and interests of some fully trained pediatricians.

POSTPEDIATRIC PORTAL PROGRAM REQUIREMENTS

The 3-year PPPP programs include an FTE 18 months of psychiatry and an FTE 18 months of CAP, integrated over 3 years. **Table 2** shows the current requirements for PPPP training, which parallel the 3 years of psychiatry and CAP training in the triple board requirements. Again, the differences between the PPPP requirements and the categorical training in psychiatry and CAP are primarily related to length of training in inpatient settings and a small difference in psychiatry outpatient settings. In contrast, PPPP residents typically have longer periods for longitudinal care in outpatient settings in both psychiatry and CAP, particularly if the program starts outpatient continuity-type clinics early in the training.

POSTPEDIATRIC PORTAL PROGRAM OUTCOMES

Outcomes for the PPPP are reported here. In an earlier survey of the first 10 PPPP fellows, 9 of the 10 fellows had completed and returned surveys.[16] None had graduated at that time. The report addressed how training had proceeded and what disorders in

Table 2
Summary of Postpediatric Portal Program requirements

	Total (mo)	Inpatient	Emergency	Subspecialty Care	Outpatient Requirements
General psychiatry	18	4–9	Experience on a service offering 24-h emergency psychiatric care (including children)	Addiction disorder service: 1 Neurology (either adult or pediatric): 1 Consultation experience to medicine and at least 1 other area (legal, schools, community systems) Clinical experience with patients with intellectual disabilities and neurodevelopmental disorders, geriatrics, substance abuse disorders Experience consulting to or providing treatment in community mental health care Experience with active multidisciplinary collaboration Exposure to the most common psychological testing	≥6 mo FTE experience plus experience treating patients longitudinally ≥9 mo
Experiences met either in general psychiatry or CAP					
CAP	18	4–6 mo Can include RTP, PHP, day TX, and/or acute inpatient units		Pediatric neurology: 1 if had during pediatric training, this requirement may be waived	12 mo With opportunity to evaluate and treat patients from different age groups and see some patients continuously for 12 mo. Experience with and development of beginning clinical skills in brief and long-term individual therapy, family therapy, group therapy, crisis intervention, supportive therapy, psychodynamic psychotherapy, CBT, and pharmacotherapy.

Applicants must have completed an ACGME-accredited pediatric residency before entering a PPPP.
Units are FTE months or rotation blocks.
Abbreviations: CBT, cognitive behavior therapy; Day Tx, day treatment; PHP, partial hospitalization program; RTP, residential treatment program.
Used with permission from American Board of Psychiatry and Neurology, Inc, Buffalo Grove, IL.

CAP each was comfortable treating, which was generally comprehensive. All responding fellows planned to practice CAP on program completion, with 3 planning to practice adult psychiatry as well and 2 others undecided about adult, but only 1 fellow planned to continue practicing pediatrics. The trainees reported diverse geographic sites for practice, including urban, suburban, and rural areas across the country. All participants were pleased with their training. Challenges identified among those who entered the programs from pediatric practice, and to some extent those who entered directly out of pediatric training, included adjusting to both the lifestyle (going from practitioner to trainee) and, as one trainee put it, "going from a muckety-muck to a minion."[16] Working with adults again was also a challenge. The overall conclusion of this early survey was that this pathway had been successful in achieving its goal of attracting pediatricians into CAP training, all of whom, at that time, were planning to practice CAP.

Recent unpublished data (Sexson S, MD, 2017) regarding the graduate outcomes from the existing PPPPs are summarized in **Table 3**. As of January, 2017, there have been 20 graduates, all having achieved ABPN psychiatry certification on the first try. Twelve passed ABPN CAP certification on the first try, 6 are planning to take the examination in 2017, and 1 in 2018. One has not reported her status. There are no reports of any failures at this time. These data support high external validation through board certification that this abbreviated pathway is successful in training competent psychiatrists and child and adolescent psychiatrists. Of interest, more than two-thirds of these initial trainees entered the training program from pediatric practice, with slightly less than a third coming directly from completion of their pediatric residencies. Recent trends seem to indicate an increase in those coming directly out of pediatric practice. Present trainees are 50% from practice and 50% directly out of training. Programs have also started to receive inquiries from potential applicants early in their pediatric training, possibly indicating that some pediatric residents are looking at the PPPP much as they might see a subspecialty fellowship in pediatrics, which would similarly require an additional 3 years of training. Graduates are overrepresented in general in academic positions, with more than half serving in some academic capacity. Moreover, 7 of the 20 graduates are working in integrated care settings, integrated with pediatrics.

Table 3
Postpediatric Portal Program combined training background through January 2017

Graduates (N)	20
Passed ABPN Psychiatry First Try (N)	20: all had passed
Passed ABPN CAP First Try (N)	12: all who have taken passed (6 planning to take in 2017)
Graduates Who Had Practiced Pediatrics Before Training	14
Graduates Who Entered Directly After Pediatrics Training	6
Presently in Training (N)	13
Present Trainees Who Practiced Pediatrics Before Training	7
Present Trainees Who Entered Directly After Pediatrics Training	6
Practice Outcomes	
Academic Practice	9
Community-based Practice	8
Private Practice	5

Discussion

A growing literature highlights some of the value of integrated mental and physical health care. Common sense and empiric data support a model that moves away from a health care model built on an artificial mind-body dichotomy and even moves away from the equally problematic mind-brain dichotomy. Quality medical care has always attended to the biology of a disorder as well as the person affected by the disorder. Research across medicine has illuminated some of the mechanisms, even on the molecular level, and shown that core physiologic systems share complex interactions with emotions, behaviors, relationships, and experiences.[17] Recent, extensive review revealed that attending to the physical and mental aspects of health through effective health care integration could save $26 billion to $48 billion dollars annually in the United States, primarily by reducing facility costs and emergency room visits in adults.[18] A parallel study focused on children is underway and is also likely to reveal substantial cost savings associated with integrated care in pediatrics.[19] Recent legislation has created systemic changes toward integration of care. The Affordable Care Act explicitly directs the Agency for Healthcare Research and Quality to support education for primary care providers about mental health and the Substance Abuse and Mental Health Administration to develop programs focused on colocation of primary care and mental health services. The more recently passed 21st Century Cures Act, passed in 2016, requires funding for statewide child psychiatry consultation to pediatric primary care providers, allows for billing by both a primary care and mental health professional on the same day in Medicaid, and supports statewide teams of child mental health delivered by telehealth.[20] As of this writing, the future of the Affordable Care Act is unclear, but active advocacy from child-focused organizations, including the AACAP, has powerfully voiced the need for any future health care legislation to protect the needs of children,[21] and the potential for cost savings in integrated care efforts may be a helpful advocacy tool going forward.

Most of these integrated approaches will be led effectively by categorically trained physicians. Combined training models, including triple board and PPPP, offer a model of training physicians with a unique perspective on systems and clinical integration, and whose medical training results in internal integration as well as the ability to function across disciplines. Several triple boarders have held leadership in major health systems, both mental health and overall health, in which they address the needs of families through systems change. Still more, as shown by the recent PPPP data, are working in or leading the development of integrated care settings. Clinically, combined trainees apply an integrated approach to patient care by virtue of the training they have. As one graduate reported in the anonymous program survey,[9] when she is practicing in a child psychiatry setting, "I can't unlearn how to be pediatrician." The high rates of combined-trained physicians in academic settings and particularly in leadership positions means that the next generation of categorically trained physicians is likely to be influenced both by educators with categorical training as well as by some who have an integrated perspective.

It has been argued that combined training programs are a substantial investment of time and effort to train a limited number of physicians. A counter to that argument is that the training programs do not exist for the trainees but for the patients with otherwise unmet needs who receive child psychiatric treatment from a combined-trained physician who might otherwise have taken a different training path. It is clear that, given the unmet needs of children with psychiatric disorders, more child and adolescent psychiatrists are needed. The numbers of child and adolescent psychiatrists in the United States are increasing, although they are still nowhere near the projected need. However, in 2017, almost 1 in 7 training positions remained open after the match.[22] This gap highlights the value of alternative pathways that might produce CAP-trained physicians who did not/would not pursue the traditional path and existing positions. Additional alternative pathways to train child psychiatrists have been discussed in the field. Among these, perhaps the most revolutionary would be a stand-alone child psychiatry training path, which has not gained significant support.[23] However, the lifting of the ABPN moratorium on new programs provides the opportunity for expansion of existing models. Efforts on the part of AACAP and ABPN to make these program more visible to medical students and pediatric residents may increase the interest in these combined training pathways, ultimately adding more child and adolescent psychiatrists to a specialty in great need of additional practitioners.

SUMMARY

In the last 3 decades, combined training has grown and matured as a training model. Triple board findings suggest positive outcomes using a varied set of measures and there are also anecdotal examples. The PPPP invites a new population of physicians to enter CAP. Early outcomes evaluations show similar success to the triple board model, with trainees having very high board pass rates and significant contributions to the field as well. Both training models result in physicians with a different, and likely complementary, perspectives to categorical training. The diversity of perspectives is likely to strengthen the field and the work that is done for children and may provide a cadre of child and adolescent psychiatrists who have special expertise in integrated care.

REFERENCES

1. Schowalter J. A history of child and adolescent psychiatry in the United States. Psychiatric Times 2003.
2. Philips I, Cohen RI. Child psychiatry: a plan for the coming decades. Washington, DC: American Academy of Child and Adolescent Psychiatry; 1983.
3. Schowalter JE. Tinker to Evers to Chance: triple board update. J Am Acad Child Adolesc Psychiatry 1993;32(2):243.
4. Schowalter JE. Tinker to Evers to Chance. J Am Acad Child Adolesc Psychiatry 1989;28:829.
5. Faulkner L, Summers RE. Update for psychiatry GME programs on combined training program accreditation/approval Feb 2012. Chicago: APBN; 2012.
6. Davison B, Lowenhaupt E. Triple board training: a curricular review of U.S. combined training programs in pediatrics, psychiatry, and child and adolescent psychiatry. 18th World Congress of the International Association for Child and Adolescent Psychiatry and Allied Professions. Istanbul, Turkey, July 22-27, 2008.
7. Schowalter JE, Friedman CP, Scheiber SC, et al. An experiment in graduate medical education. Acad Psychiatry 2002;26(4):237–44.
8. Warren MJ, Dunn DW, Rushton J. Outcome measures of triple board graduates, 1991-2003. J Am Acad Child Adolesc Psychiatry 2006;45(6):700–8.
9. Gleason MM, Dunn DW, Gray D, et al. Triple board training: goals and outcomes. 59th Annual Meeting of the American Academy of Child and Adolescent Psychiatry. San Francisco, 2012.
10. Resident blog spot. AOA and PHD by specialty. 2014. Available at: http://residentcafe.blogspot.com/2014/10/percentage-aoa-and-phd-in-match.html. Accessed March 13, 2017.
11. Fritsch SL. Memoirs of a triple board pioneer. Acad Psychiatry 2009;33(2):93.

12. Larroque CM. A personal perspective on triple board certification. Acad Psychiatry 2009;33(2):96–8.
13. Gleason MM, Fritz GK. Innovative training in pediatrics, general psychiatry, and child psychiatry: background, outcomes, and experiences. Acad Psychiatry 2009;33(2):99–104.
14. Child psychiatry faces workforce shortage. Psychiatric Times 2004.
15. Anders TF. Child and adolescent psychiatry: the next 10 years. Psychiatric Times 2008.
16. Anderson AK, Ellis R, Madaan V, et al. Post pediatric portal program: progress in child and adolescent psychiatry workforce development. Paper presented at: 57th Annual Meeting of the American Academy of Child and Adolescent Psychiatry; 2010.
17. O'Connor TG, Moynihan JA, Caserta MT. Annual research review: the neuroinflammation hypothesis for stress and psychopathology in children–developmental psychoneuroimmunology. J Child Psychol Psychiatry 2014;55(6):615–31.
18. Melek SP, Norris DT, Paulus J. Economic impact of integrated medical-behavioral health care. Denver (CO): Millman, Inc; 2014.
19. Fritz GK. Presidential address: child and adolescent psychiatry in the era of health care reform. J Am Acad Child Adolesc Psychiatry 2016;55(1):3–6.
20. 21st Century Cures Act, 2016.
21. Fritz GK. AHCA letter to Ryan and Pelosi. Washington, DC: American Academy of Child and Adolescent Psychaitry; 2017.
22. National Resident Matching Program. National Resident Matching Program, results and data: specialties matching service 2017 appointment year. Washington, DC: National Resident Matching Program; 2017.
23. Davis M. Five questions with Dr. Gregory Fritz. Providence Business News 2008.

Incorporating Trainees' Development into a Multidisciplinary Training Model for Integrated Behavioral Health Within a Pediatric Continuity Clinic

CrossMark

Kimberly Kelsay, MD[a],*, Maya Bunik, MD, MPH[b],
Melissa Buchholz, PsyD[a], Bridget Burnett, PsyD[a],
Ayelet Talmi, PhD[a,c]

KEYWORDS

- Multidisciplinary training • Integrated mental health • Integrated behavioral health
- Pediatrics • Medical home

KEY POINTS

- Integrated mental health and behavioral care for children requires multidisciplinary team members to work together to provide services.
- There are few descriptions of integrated care clinics that provide training across disciplines, including pediatrics, psychology, and psychiatry.
- Attending to developmental level of trainees is a helpful organizational framework when providing targeted education and training.
- Training within an integrated clinic allows multidisciplinary trainees the opportunity to observe and understand the other disciplines' strengths and roles while simultaneously developing their own discipline-specific competencies within this model.

[a] Department of Psychiatry, Pediatric Mental Health Institute, Children's Hospital Colorado, University of Colorado School of Medicine, 13123 East 16th Avenue, Box 130, Aurora, CO 80045, USA; [b] Department of Pediatrics, Children's Hospital Colorado, University of Colorado School of Medicine, 13123 East 16th Avenue, Aurora, CO 80045, USA; [c] Department of Pediatrics, Pediatric Mental Health Institute, Children's Hospital Colorado, University of Colorado School of Medicine, 13123 East 16th Avenue, Aurora, CO 80045, USA
* Corresponding author. 13123 East 16th Avenue, Box 130 , Aurora, CO 80045.
E-mail address: Kimberly.kelsay@childrenscolorado.org

Child Adolesc Psychiatric Clin N Am 26 (2017) 703–715
http://dx.doi.org/10.1016/j.chc.2017.06.001
1056-4993/17/© 2017 Elsevier Inc. All rights reserved.

INTRODUCTION

There is increasing recognition that pediatric primary care providers should have a role in preventing, recognizing, and addressing mental and behavioral health problems. Integrated care is designed to support providers and their patients within the primary care medical home in order to achieve these goals. Integrated care models often include multidisciplinary team members. The primary care provider may be a pediatrician, family medicine provider, advanced practice nurse (APN), or physician's assistant (PA) working with nurses, medical assistants, and office staff. Behavioral health team members may include psychologists, child and adolescent psychiatrists, social workers, other behavioral health clinicians, and case managers or care coordinators who may be family navigators, community health workers, or nurses.

This complex system of care requires different skill sets from various disciplines. Pediatrics[1] and psychology[2] both have statements regarding professional competencies in primary care settings, and child psychiatry is currently formulating these competencies. (See Wanjiku F.M. Njoroge and colleagues' article, "Competencies and Training Guidelines for Behavioral Health Providers in Pediatric Primary Care," in this issue.) Although some literature exists regarding training, most descriptions have not focused on the level or types of trainees. The literature does, however, identify training gaps and program descriptions. For example, pediatric residents training in a clinic without integrated mental health clinicians reported feeling unsupported and fearful of visits involving mental health concerns and that, at times, they ignored their patients' mental health concerns.[3] Pediatric residents training alongside psychology trainees reported feeling better prepared to collaborate with behavioral health providers (BHPs) than colleagues who did not train with psychologists in an integrated setting, yet they only reported feeling somewhat more often prepared for handling behavioral health issues on their own after graduation.[4] The authors propose that targeting training to the professional developmental level of the learner is important for successfully imparting the knowledge, skills, and attitude to attain the necessary competencies. The authors describe a multidisciplinary, graduated model within a pediatric teaching clinic and lessons learned in this work.

SETTING

The integrated primary care clinic is described in **Table 1**.

Pediatric trainees and faculty provide most of the primary care within this academic pediatric primary care clinic, although APNs also serve as primary care providers within the clinic. As in similar academic institutions, medical students, family medicine residents, PA students, and other pediatric residents who have continuity clinics in external community sites provide pediatric care during their general ambulatory core month.

Table 1
Integrated pediatric clinic

Clinic Setting	Characteristics of Clinic Population	Care Provided
Urban Pediatric residency continuity clinic Affiliated with academic hospital	90% Publicly insured Many different languages spoken Many Spanish speakers Young and school age predominantly Some adolescents	Well child Sick visits

Psychology and psychiatry trainees and faculty provide integrated behavioral health care through Project CLIMB (Consultation and Liaison in Mental health and Behavior). The behavioral health team also includes a full-time licensed professional counselor who works for a community mental health center. Medical social work, family navigation, community health workers, and care coordination services are available to families when indicated.

Integrated care services were developed and implemented to better serve the needs of the community and simultaneously address the educational and professional practice competencies of the pediatric training program. As the clinic has evolved, it has also increasingly served the needs of psychology and child and adolescent psychiatry (CAP) training. The clinic continues to evolve; as new models and processes are incorporated in the clinic, care is taken to expand the workforce capacity by training providers to become competent in delivering integrated care services within other community-based systems. In addition, scholarship related to various aspects of this model has helped secure educational and clinical funding as well as provided opportunities for trainees and faculty to engage in scholarly activities.

The integrated behavioral health services and training efforts began in 2005, with grant funding from local foundations who were interested in both access to behavioral health services for underserved, hard-to-reach populations and training of pediatric health professionals in better addressing mental health, behavior, and development. The program has evolved significantly over the course of more than a decade. Following the initial development and implementation funding, behavioral health services have been sustained with billing from screening efforts, institutional support from the Department of Pediatrics leadership who recognized benefits of training and education for pediatric health professionals, grants to support expansion and training, and Department of Psychiatry funding for trainees. This article describes the current model and lessons learned as the model has been implemented and adjusted.

INTEGRATED CARE MODEL

Patients in the clinic are scheduled for appointments with their primary care pediatric provider, a faculty member, resident, or other trainee completing their core ambulatory month. The pediatric provider identifies the need to involve integrated mental health team members through the following mechanisms:

- Routine screening (eg, developmental screening,[5] maternal depression,[6] psychosocial screening, teen depression screening[7]) (**Table 2**)
- Spontaneous identification of problems that are discussed or raised in the course of a visit

Table 2 Routine screeners	
Screener	**Visit Type/Population**
Ages and Stages Questionnaire	Well-child visits/aged 2 mo to 5 y
Edinburgh Postnatal Depression Scale	All visits/<4 mo of age
Patient Health Questionnaire-9 A	All visits/11 y and older
Psychosocial Determinants of Health (clinic developed screener)	All well-child visits/all ages

- Identification of needs before visits (eg, family calls to schedule an appointment because of a concern or life event) or
- Patient enrollment in prevention programs, such as HealthySteps, (a program targeting early childhood development and effective parenting in which well-child visits are conducted jointly with both medical trainees and psychologists with opportunities for home visitation, a warm line, and groups)

The flow of the integrated visits is flexible. Most commonly, the pediatric provider identifies a problem and then leaves the room to consult with the BHP. The BHP may then spend time with the family, discuss recommendations with the pediatrician, and wrap up with a visit together with the pediatric provider or separately. For example, a family that identifies concerns with infant sleep, feeding, or fussiness may have a preliminary conversation with the pediatric provider who then consults with the BHP and requests that the BHP go in to see the family. Alternatively, the BHP may join the pediatric provider as they assess and address development and concerns during a well-child visit or a visit that is targeted around a particular issue. A common example using this model is a family with concerns regarding their child's ability to focus in school. There are also patient visits for which the pediatric provider and BHP decide together that the BHP does not need to see patients. A common example is a patient who is connected to mental health services in the community and is currently doing well. The various visit flows described earlier accommodate the patient's needs while being targeted for the learners involved as described later.

DEVELOPMENTAL APPROACH TO LEARNERS

The integrated behavioral health services program was established within a teaching clinic to help trainees learn this model of care as they are developing their knowledge and attitudes of systems and their own identity as providers. Each discipline has specific foundational knowledge and a skill set to master as well as knowledge about their role within an integrated service model. The authors describe the developmental training model as it applies to each discipline. A common tenet across all disciplines is that training opportunities intensify as the trainees gain initial competencies in their respective fields. The assumption in this setting is that significant cross-disciplinary training is necessary to develop discipline-specific competencies for work in integrated care (**Fig. 1**).

Pediatric Residents and Others Training in Pediatrics

Pediatric trainees, beginning their outpatient work, are learning to manage and balance many goals, such as mastering the timing of outpatient care, practicing problem-focused care, combing targeted and open-ended questions, learning to make differential diagnoses, learning and applying normative developmental, implementing multiple practice guidelines, and learning to build alliances with children and families while also managing the other learning demands of pediatrics and the stress of intense training. Many are also learning about resources in a new community, institutional policies and procedures, and a new electronic health record system. The initial introduction to the behavioral health team of providers combines structured introduction, didactics, and natural opportunities for collaboration within the clinic. The goal is to meet trainees at their current capacity and gradually increase their work with the integrated BHP as their confidence and capacity increases.

The universal screening protocols are often the first opportunity for collaboration with the BHPs. For example, mothers of infants 4 months old or younger are given

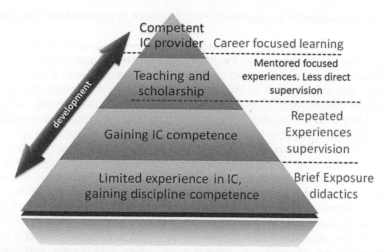

Fig. 1. Training level and educational intervention.

the Edinburgh Postnatal Depression Scale. When following the clinic protocol, residents who find an elevated score of 10 or higher on the screener come to consult with BHP. Together, the BHP and pediatric resident investigate the elevated score, asking questions about caregiver well-being and the psychosocial circumstances that may contribute to distress during the early months of parenthood. In the course of discussing the case and explaining the role of the BHP, the residents learn about other areas and topics in which they could seek behavioral health consultation from the team. Pediatric residents are supported and encouraged to get assistance from the behavioral health team for concerns around psychosocial stress, family circumstances, developmental issues (eg, feeding, sleeping, daily routines, fussiness), and mental health issues. They learn to seek help in evaluating the need for an external behavioral health referral versus providing ongoing routine support from within primary care.

As the pediatric trainees gain confidence in their role and understand the potential collaboration with the BHP, they tend to use the opportunity to work with their BHP colleagues more frequently. During the collaborative visits with behavioral health team members, including psychiatry, for problems, such as attention-deficit/hyperactivity disorder (ADHD), the BHP may lead the visit until pediatric trainees gain the necessary knowledge and skills to lead these visits on their own. Often this is a gradual process that occurs over multiple collaborative cases, whereby the BHP is available to step in at any time during the visit.

In addition to continuity clinic, residents rotate through ambulatory pediatrics for 1-month core blocks. During these blocks, there is a 1-month didactic series that includes training the residents on topics such as depression, anxiety, pregnancy-related mood and anxiety disorders, and motivational interviewing. The behavioral health team leads these didactics. During the ambulatory month, pediatric residents also receive a 3-hour presentation on general development and parenting. During this training opportunity, members of the behavioral team review general development and use specific case examples to support the residents in their conceptualization and approach to manage very common early childhood concerns that often present in the context of pediatric primary care (eg, weaning a child from a pacifier, sleep concerns, toilet training, or typical toddler tantrums). The goal of this training opportunity is to enhance the residents' competence and confidence in addressing these common concerns.

Second- and third-year pediatric residents have a weekly appointment slot in their continuity clinic schedules saved for behavioral health appointments. The training team deliberately chose the second and third year because it was thought that the knowledge and skills gained in the first year increase the comfort and potential learning from these visits in the second year. These appointments, conducted together with a child and adolescent psychiatrist, provide residents with the opportunity to assess, treat, manage, follow, and triage children and adolescents with pediatric behavioral health needs. Initially, child and adolescent psychiatrists lead these appointments, teaching the pediatric residents how to assess, identify, and manage behavioral health concerns that are commonly seen in primary care (eg, ADHD, depression, anxiety, stress reactions). Although these behavioral health issues are routinely seen and managed in primary care, residents are less familiar and often think they are not equipped to independently manage them. The experience of comanaging these cases with psychiatrists during their primary care training is intended to support pediatric residents' capacity to provide care when appropriate and triage to community-based mental health services if needed. By the end of their third year, pediatric residents demonstrate the knowledge, skills, and comfort to appropriately manage these cases.

Building on the routine primary care training, second-year residents rotate through the Breastfeeding Management Clinic with the Trifecta Model[8] whereby the psychologist meets with families who are struggling in the first month postpartum with breastfeeding, caregiver well-being, and other stressors. The clinic uses an integrated model of care with a team comprised of a pediatrician certified in lactation, a lactation nurse, and a psychologist. Behavioral health and caregiver well-being play a central role in addressing breastfeeding from a family centered perspective. The first month of life is an adjustment period for parents on many levels; when feeding is not going well, it creates a crisis situation. Even in the most supportive environments, 80% of mothers report breastfeeding difficulties.[9] The authors' Trifecta team is a model multidisciplinary threesome whereby medicine, mechanics of lactation support, as well as behavioral health consultation work well together. It is critical early in training for clinicians to see that when care is integrated it is best for both patients and for team members. Third-year residents have career-focused education elective time and can elect to spend some of this time with psychiatry and psychology as they work in integrated care. Based on pediatric residents' interests and gaps in training (eg, not having rotated in the authors' clinic), they are able to select topic areas on which to focus and shadow cases related to those topics. Providers who are planning on a career in primary care most often choose this additional training to deepen their knowledge.

Other trainees, such as family medicine residents, medical and PA students, join the pediatric residents during a core month of pediatrics as part of their training. All trainees work alongside one another in an assigned pod for the month and participate in the ambulatory didactic series. As their experience occurs within a fully integrated clinic, they are also exposed to the BHPs during the course of their work and may interact with the BHPs while administering universal screening protocols, enrolling HealthySteps families, or during behavioral consults (**Box 1**).

Psychologists

Psychology trainees at all levels (extern, intern, and postdoctoral) are trained to be members of an integrated behavioral health team. Depending on the trainees' prior experience working in pediatric health settings, trainees experience a graduated

---

Box 1
Pediatric experiences

Continuity clinic
- BHP collaboration
  Screeners
  HealthySteps
  Spontaneous problems
- 1× per week combined appointments with psychiatry

1- month ambulatory pediatrics
- Didactics
  Development
  Motivational interviewing
  Depression and anxiety
  Pregnancy-related mood disorder

Breastfeeding management clinic

Career-focused educational elective

---

program. First, they orient to working in primary care with multidisciplinary health professionals as their care-team partners. Next, they learn how to apply their behavioral health skills and tools to a fast-paced medical setting where they often see families for less time and with less frequency than is typical for outpatient behavioral health practice. Under the supervision of primary care psychologists, psychology trainees develop tools and practices that enable them to successfully support families and primary care providers in addressing a wide array of mental health, behavioral, and developmental issues. Finally, more advanced psychology trainees are able to cultivate individualized training plans that allow them to focus on populations of interest (eg, early childhood, children with special health care needs) and develop scholarship projects that complement their clinical interests.

Psychology externs are advanced doctoral students, typically in their fourth or fifth year of doctoral programs in psychology. In order to work in the primary care setting, they must have completed a year of general pediatric psychology outpatient care at the hospital. The externship experience is usually their first in primary care working on multidisciplinary teams that include pediatric health professionals. Psychology externs are oriented to the primary care model through shadowing experiences and weekly supervision. They shadow both primary care providers and BHPs in order to learn the integrated model of care. Their caseloads are generally lower than other behavioral health trainees; they work closely with the supervising psychologists in managing cases, making recommendations, and providing consultation to primary care providers. Externs are expected to deliver 2 didactic trainings for pediatric health trainees over the course of their 12-month externship.

Psychology interns, who have completed their doctoral studies in psychology, spend a year doing intensive clinical training. Interns in the primary care track spend 50% of their time providing behavioral health services in primary care, working in the general pediatric clinic and in the adolescent parents' clinic. These trainees come to the internship with a wide range of pediatric psychology experience. Many have previously worked either in primary care settings or in other pediatric health settings where they gained experience collaborating with medical professionals and interdisciplinary teams. If they are new to primary care, they are oriented similarly to the externs, with opportunities to shadow primary care and BHPs. They also receive weekly individual supervision from 2 primary care psychologists, one generalist and one focused on adolescent parents. Interns participate in education and training of pediatric health trainees by delivering between 4 and 6 didactics during their internship. Interns also engage in scholarship, typically selecting an aspect of integrated behavioral health services that is of particular interest to them, developing a project, and presenting their findings at local and national meetings.

Postdoctoral fellows have completed their doctoral degree, including a full year of clinical internship. Fellows in the authors' setting are selected for a general integrated behavioral health or an early childhood fellowship with a focus on treating the needs of very young children (aged birth through 5 years of age) in primary care settings. Primary care offers a unique opportunity for psychology trainees to interact with and treat very young children because it is the most common setting in which infants and toddlers present. Fellows rotate through clinic for 1 year and are typically in clinic between 2 and 6 half days each week. During their time in clinic, these fellows collaborate closely with the medical providers (both residents and other medical trainees and attending physicians) to meet the behavioral health needs of children. In addition to providing direct clinical care as members of the integrated team, primary care fellows engage in scholarship (30% time), such as generating scholarly research projects and posters, and developing and delivering trainings in the clinic and community related to integrated behavioral health care and education (one half-day of didactics per week). Irving B. Harris fellows, postdoctoral BHPs engaged in a yearlong Infant Mental Health and Child Development fellowship assigned to the pediatric primary care setting, also spend one full day per week in didactic training where they gain in-depth knowledge about infant and early childhood mental health. Fellows receive weekly individual supervision from primary care psychologists and are mentored by these psychologists in scholarly activities.

In addition to providing early childhood behavioral health integration services, early childhood fellows also carry a caseload of families enrolled in the HealthySteps program. HealthySteps is an evidence-based early childhood integrated behavioral health model that is embedded in pediatric primary care settings.[10] The Harris fellows work with the medical providers to identify families who would benefit from enrollment in the program and then meet with these families and the primary care provider at every well-child visit until the child is 3 years old. The goal of the model is to provide enhanced, comprehensive well-child care to children aged birth to 3 years and their families by promoting close relationships between health care professionals and parents in addressing the physical, emotional, and intellectual growth and development of young children. HealthySteps also includes home visitation services for enrolled families. One to 2 home visits are offered to each family each year. At clinic and home visits, the fellows are trained to support children and families by providing parents with information and tools to enhance their child's health and development.

Postdoctoral fellows who are being trained in the primary care clinic are expected to engage in teaching and scholarship activities, including facilitating didactic trainings and presentations to medical providers, presenting original scholarship products such as posters and conference presentations locally and nationally, and coauthoring articles with faculty. Most research conducted by trainees is related to program evaluation and quality improvement efforts. Fellows also have the opportunity to cosupervise summer research interns, public health students, and medical students in their research activities.

The early child fellows receive extensive training on the HealthySteps model. In turn, the trainees and faculty that implement the HealthySteps program use the HealthySteps strategies to enhance the medical trainees' training. Most commonly, well-child visits are conducted jointly with the medical trainees so that they can be present for the discussions around enhancing early childhood development and infant mental health. Another strategy involves bringing medical trainees on home visits with families, which provides an opportunity to observe the child and family in their natural environment (**Table 3**).

Child and Adolescent Psychiatrists

CAP trainees have had at least 3 years of general psychiatry training when they enter CAP training. During their first year of CAP training, they move from a patient-centered, individualistic approach commonly used in work with adults to a more family centered, systems-based approach for work with infants, young children, and adolescents. In order to address the mental health needs of youths, CAP trainees must master normative and atypical development, comprehensive assessment, formulation and differential diagnosis, tenets of therapeutic interventions, and psychopharmacology. Although they have mastered building a therapeutic alliance with adult patients, treating youths requires building and maintaining an alliance with youth and their caregivers. During the first year of CAP training, education regarding integrated care begins with integrated systems of care model didactics.

As CAP trainees begin the second year, they have built their knowledge and skills for working with children and families and are developmentally prepared for more intensive training regarding integrated care. CAP trainees who are interested in a career in integrated care spend a half day per week for 6 months to a year in the clinic described earlier. Competencies for this rotation include rapid triage and assessment of patients within a pediatric setting, effective use of a problem-based approach combined with return visits, collaboration and communication with other providers, encouragement of the patient-primary care relationship and skills to teach, and assess and provide feedback to pediatric trainees.

The rotation begins with shadowing other disciplines. CAP trainees shadow pediatric well-patient visits and visits whereby psychologists are collaborating with pediatric providers. They also shadow psychiatry faculty as they work with pediatric residents who are assessing and intervening regarding patient problems, such as ADHD. These later visits eventually reverse; the psychiatry faculty shadow the CAP trainees as they

Table 3
Psychology-integrated behavioral health experiences

Psychology Training Level	Integrated Behavioral Care Experiences
Psychology externs	Shadow multidisciplines Low case loads More direct supervision Weekly supervision Deliver 2 didactics to core trainees
Psychology interns	50% Clinic time More cases, less direct supervision Weekly supervision Scholarship
Psychology postdoctoral fellows	50% Direct patient care 30% Scholarship time Weekly supervision/mentorship Either primary care or EC focus EC focus: HealthySteps plus EC didactics

Abbreviation: EC, early childhood.

accompany, teach, assess, and give feedback to pediatric residents during patient visits. As the CAP trainee demonstrates competency, the CAP faculty do not shadow these visits but precept with the pediatric and psychiatry trainee.

Data
Learners
Pediatric trainees
- Two-thirds of pediatric trainees rotate through integrated continuity clinic.
- More than 180 pediatric trainees have had primary care in the integrated care clinic over 11 years.
- Thirty-five trainees have spent additional time with psychiatry/psychology.

The medical trainees who participate in home visits with HealthSteps are encouraged to reflect on the experience, including how it potentially altered the way they conceptualize and ultimately treat their patients. One trainee said the following immediately after a home visit with her patient and the HealthySteps provider: "I learned that I am not just here to provide information, but to also learn from the family about everything that is happening in their lives that will impact my patient's health."

Psychology trainees
- 6 externs
- 20 interns
- 30 fellows

Child and adolescent trainees
- Eighteen child and adolescent fellows have received didactics regarding integrated care models.
- Seven have completed the integrated experience in training.

As part of an upcoming graduate medical education self-study process, a survey of trainees found that the trainees unanimously support changing the second-year experience from an elective to a standard rotation. As of next year, all 6 CAP trainees in the second year will complete this training.

Other trainees who have participated in research and evaluation efforts with the behavioral health team
- Undergraduate research interns
- Medical students
- Public health students

Trainees that have gone on to work in integrated care settings Of the psychology trainees who worked in the authors' integrated primary care setting, more than 20% found jobs in integrated behavioral health services in a pediatric setting. Moreover, several of them were recruited to leadership positions in academic medical centers and community agencies to develop and implement integrated behavioral health programs in primary care settings.

Twenty-five percent of CAP trainees who have completed this elective have chosen jobs whereby integrated care is a significant focus of their work.

Scholarship Trainees have access to large retrospective dataset collected from an electronic medical record system using clinical informatics. Many of the projects involve quantitative and qualitative data analysis whereby trainees are mentored to apply mixed-methods approaches to understanding the types of services provided, family circumstances, and health outcomes (**Table 4**).

Table 4 Scholarship projects	
Scholarship Type	**Scholarship Topics**
>100 Presentations	Pregnancy-related mood disorders and child and family well-being
15 Publications	Screening implementation
	Children with asthma
	Children with weight management problems
	Children born prematurely
	Children with developmental needs
	Behavioral health and social determinants
	Integrated behavioral health and cultural factors
	Development of risk and protective factor coding system from EMR

Abbreviation: EMR, electronic medical record.

Patient-related outcomes Screening rates in the clinic are typically greater than 80% once screening efforts are piloted and initiated. Developmental screening is conducted at all well-child visits between birth and 5 years of age. Ongoing quality improvement efforts have enabled us to monitor screening and referral outcomes and provide guidance and training in order to ensure that children who need services are able to access community-based programs[11] Similarly, the protocol for pregnancy-related depression screening ensures that women who score 10 or greater have access to behavioral health consultation as soon as concerns are identified. Previous studies have shown that nearly 90% of mothers were screened between the newborn and 4-month well-child visit and of those whose scores were elevated, 71% had contact with a BHP around the time of their visit providing early intervention and potentially averting costs associated with untreated depression.

There are currently 427 families enrolled in the HealthySteps program. The program is staffed by 1.0 full time equivalent (FTE) of postdoctoral fellow time and 1.0 FTE licensed psychologist time. On average, the HealthySteps providers enroll 18 new families each month and conduct an average of 82 collaborative HealthySteps visits per month.

New developments in integrated systems Residents and other trainees also benefit from different initiatives and implementation efforts. Population health approaches drive pediatric primary care practices to manage patients' needs using a new empirical lens. Pediatricians are uniquely suited to engage in screening and identifying psychosocial risk factors that may affect health and wellness. However, primary care providers may not feel comfortable addressing psychosocial issues that emerge in the context of screening. In implementing psychosocial screening processes in the authors' training clinic, they relied heavily on the integrated behavioral health team to develop, pilot, secure grant funding for additional resources, implement, and evaluate psychosocial screening efforts. In order to ensure that all pediatric and behavioral health professionals and trainees had the necessary comfort and requisite skills to engage in psychosocial screening processes, the authors developed a half-day training for all staff, faculty, and trainees. The authors also conducted lunch and launch sessions to facilitate implementation and share changes from the pilot phase. By participating in these efforts, the trainees have gained skills and experience in modifying systems of care.

SUMMARY

There are many pressures driving the move toward integrated behavioral health within primary care. These pressures include workforce shortages of BHPs and difficulties with access to behavioral care, the growing science supporting the conceptualizing of health as a developmental process that begins early in life, and the move toward prevention and population-based care. Integrated behavioral health care within a teaching pediatric continuity clinic has helped to serve the needs of the community, including achieving excellent quality of care metrics, such as a high percentage of standardized screening. In addition, the clinic has been instrumental in preparing providers of multiple disciplines to competently work within integrated systems of care.

The professional development of learners likely impacts the acquisition of knowledge, yet is often not taken into account as teaching/training models of integrated care are developed. For example, learners early in their professional training are tasked with acquiring basic competencies of their discipline while also adjusting to the stressors of intense training. Exposure to the complex structure of integrated behavioral health care at this level of training could be overwhelming without scaffolding and support. However, early exposure may add the benefit of learning the strengths and challenges other disciplines face within integrated systems of care and help to establish an integrated frame of reference, before habits of practicing in silos of care have become ingrained. The authors offer a model of increasing depth of experiences and opportunities for learning as other competencies are mastered and recommend the scaffolding and structure change as providers gain knowledge and skills.

Future work in this area will benefit when each discipline provides consensus guidelines for competencies with respect to integrated care. Pediatrics has defined mental health competencies for pediatricians[1] but has not defined specific competencies related to how to practice within an integrated setting. Psychology has proposed guidelines,[2] but these are not specific to integrated settings for children and youth and, thus, are limited with respect to prevention and health promotion especially for children from birth to 5 years of age. CAP is in the process of developing guidelines and consensus. (See Wanjiku F.M. Njoroge and colleagues's article, "Competencies and Training Guidelines for Behavioral Health Providers in Pediatric Primary Care," in this issue.) Having consensus guidelines will help each discipline function within an integrated setting to enhance patient outcomes and help the work of practice or system transformation for practices/systems that are moving toward integrated care models. Consensus guidelines will also help training directors define and share best practices for educating trainees to meet competencies in providing integrated care.

Studies of both the economic and health benefits of integrated care and the educational outcomes of training within these systems will also help move this field forward. As population health management becomes a priority for the field, having integrated services to address the full continuum of prevention, health promotion and well-being, consultation, and intervention will be in even greater demand. Understanding the immediate costs and long-term health and economic benefits will be essential for building an argument to support sustainable integrated services in pediatric settings. Likewise, having information and data regarding competencies and success of graduating providers will help build support for training programs. Clinician educators need both sources of data to obtain and sustain funding for training within integrated care models.

REFERENCES

1. Committee on Psychosocial Aspects of Child and Family Health and Task Force on Mental Health. Policy statement–The future of pediatrics: mental health competencies for pediatric primary care. Pediatrics 2009;124(1):410–21.
2. McDaniel SH, Grus CL, Cubic BA, et al. Competencies for psychology practice in primary care. Am Psychol 2014;69(4):409–29.
3. Hampton E, Richardson JE, Bostwick S, et al. The current and ideal state of mental health training: pediatric resident perspectives. Teach Learn Med 2015; 27(2):147–54.
4. Garfunkel LC, Pisani AR, leRoux P, et al. Educating residents in behavioral health care and collaboration: comparison of conventional and integrated training models. Acad Med 2011;86(2):174–9.
5. Klamer A, Lando A, Pinborg A, et al. Ages and stages questionnaire used to measure cognitive deficit in children born extremely preterm. Acta Paediatr 2005; 94(9):1327–9.
6. Cox JL, Holden JM, Sagovsky R. Detection of postnatal depression. Development of the 10-item Edinburgh postnatal depression scale. Br J Psychiatry 1987;150:782–6.
7. Johnson JG, Harris ES, Spitzer RL, et al. The patient health questionnaire for adolescents: validation of an instrument for the assessment of mental disorders among adolescent primary care patients. J Adolesc Health 2002;30(3):196–204.
8. Bunik M, Dunn DM, Watkins L, et al. Trifecta approach to breastfeeding: clinical care in the integrated mental health model. J Hum Lact 2014;30(2):143–7.
9. Demirci JR, Bogen DL. An ecological momentary assessment of primiparous women's breastfeeding behavior and problems from birth to 8 weeks. J Hum Lact 2017;33(2):285–95.
10. Minkovitz CS, Hughart N, Strobino D, et al. A practice-based intervention to enhance quality of care in the first 3 years of life: the Healthy Steps for Young Children Program. JAMA 2003;290(23):3081–91.
11. Talmi A, Bunik M, Asherin R, et al. Improving developmental screening documentation and referral completion. Pediatrics 2014;134(4):e1181–8.

Competencies and Training Guidelines for Behavioral Health Providers in Pediatric Primary Care

Wanjiku F.M. Njoroge, MD[a,b,*], Ariel A. Williamson, PhD[c],
Jennifer A. Mautone, PhD[a,b], Paul M. Robins, PhD[a,b],
Tami D. Benton, MD[a,b]

KEYWORDS

- Training • Integrated practice • Primary care • Interdisciplinary training
- Competencies

KEY POINTS

- Collaborative care models in which behavioral health providers collaborate closely with primary care physicians are increasingly used to improve access to high-quality services.
- In order for behavioral health providers to function effectively in collaborative care models, they require specialized training and professional competencies.
- Cross-discipline training and professional competencies for training behavioral health providers are recommended to support the effective provision of integrated primary care services.
- Proposed training competencies include interprofessional communication, professionalism, integrated care systems practice, practice-based learning and education, preventive screening and assessment, and cultural competence.
- Child and adolescent psychiatry, psychology, and social work trainees involved in integrated primary care services should receive interdisciplinary training experiences that target these competency areas.

Disclosure Statement: The authors have nothing to disclose.
[a] Department of Child and Adolescent Psychiatry and Behavioral Sciences, Children's Hospital of Philadelphia, 3440 Market Street, Suite 410, Philadelphia, PA 19104, USA; [b] Department of Psychiatry, Perelman School of Medicine, University of Pennsylvania, 3401 Civic Center Boulevard, Philadelphia, PA 19104, USA; [c] Sleep Center, Department of Pulmonary Medicine, Children's Hospital of Philadelphia, 3401 Civic Center Boulevard, Philadelphia, PA 19104, USA
* Corresponding author. Department of Child and Adolescent Psychiatry and Behavioral Sciences, Children's Hospital of Philadelphia, 3440 Market Street, Suite 410, Philadelphia, PA 19104.
E-mail address: njorogew@email.chop.edu

Child Adolesc Psychiatric Clin N Am 26 (2017) 717–731
http://dx.doi.org/10.1016/j.chc.2017.06.002
childpsych.theclinics.com

INTRODUCTION

The past couple of decades in pediatric medicine have highlighted the challenges in providing high-quality, timely, and effective behavioral health care to all of the children that need these services.[1,2] This growing acknowledgment of the services gap for children and adolescents led to the development of multiple collaborative care models across the nation. With the development of these integrated care models, workforce training issues became more relevant as the evidence showed the ability and efficacy of providing services for children and adolescents and their families in these novel programs. With the implementation of the Affordable Care Act (ACA),[3] the American Academy of Child and Adolescent Psychiatry (AACAP), and the American Academy of Pediatrics (AAP) drafted policy statements, encouraging collaboration across disciplines and settings to provide behavioral health services to children and adolescents in primary care settings.[4–6] In recognition of the efficacy of these integrated models, and the lack of core principles in how to treat these patients, multiple professional organizations, including the American Psychiatric Association (APA), American Academy of Family Practice, AAP, and the American College of Physicians, convened in 2014 to begin to address integrated care models and training needs.[7] From these cross-discipline workgroups, multiple ideas and strategies were created to address the unique training needs of assessment, treatment, and collaboration in primary care settings.

The articles in this issue have highlighted the increasing need for effective integrated behavioral health care models to appropriately address the behavioral health needs of children and adolescents in the United States. This article focuses on the cross-discipline training competencies needed to appropriately develop and prepare the workforce that will implement these interprofessional models. The article first describes the current competencies in specific behavioral health disciplines, including child and adolescent psychiatry, child psychology, and social work. Then, training competencies for integrated behavioral health providers that cut across these disciplines are proposed. Because there are multiple ways that programs have incorporated integrated care training, this article focuses on a comprehensive set of training competencies and guidelines that can be modified for use in varied settings. A description of an existing and successful integrated care training model, Healthy Minds, Healthy Kids (HMHK), highlights how these competencies can be included in cross-discipline training. Recommendations for future work and training in integrated primary care are offered.

CURRENT INTEGRATED CARE COMPETENCIES ACROSS BEHAVIORAL HEALTH DISCIPLINES
Psychiatry

Identifying the need for comprehensive training guidelines for American medical schools, the Accreditation Council for Graduate Medical Education (ACGME)[8] developed 6 core competencies for medical education:

1. Medical knowledge
2. Patient care
3. Interpersonal and communication skills
4. Practice-based learning and improvement
5. Professionalism
6. Systems-based practice.

These competencies were further refined by individual specialty boards. The American Board of Psychiatry and Neurology (ABPN) identified milestones specific to psychiatric training attached to each of the 6 core competencies.[9]

The implementation of the ACA[3] dictated the need to improve and consolidate specific means of interprofessional practice in integrated care settings. Secondary to the substantive work of the ACGME Milestone project, and further refinement by the ABPN, the framework existed for further distillation of the milestones for specific use in developing competencies in integrated care training.[10] Ratzliff and colleagues[10] systematically outlined each of the 6 milestones, addressing the particular skills, knowledge, and awareness specific to integrated health work. Additionally, they highlighted the competencies that lend themselves to integrated work, specifically

1. Interpersonal and communication skills
2. Practice-based learning and improvement
3. Systems-based practice.

Jeffrey and Martini[11] developed a brief primer on the skills the child and adolescent psychiatrist needs to work in primary care settings. Their recommendations include specifics on how to build an integrated health team, what roles each of the disciplines play in these interdisciplinary teams, and other constituent parts that lead to successful primary care integration and collaboration.[11] They also enumerate certain skills needed by the child psychiatrist participating in these integrated care settings, including knowledge of evidence-based screening tools used specifically to target outcomes of brief interventions and the ability to consult to the primary care team, make quick decisions in the face of limited information, and act as the lead for the team. Garfunkel and colleagues[12] also noted the 3 important skills needed to participate in integrated pediatric care settings included participating in preclinic conference, availability of the trainee for discussion and consultation around cases, and exposure to the pediatric care setting and the practice culture.

In 2014, the American Psychiatric Association Council on Medical Education and Lifelong Learning drafted a report addressing the psychiatric training needs for future integrated health care practices.[7] In this seminal report, Summers and colleagues[7] described specific training models for integrated care, as well as began to outline necessary ingredients for teaching institutions. Using the Milestone Project framework, they highlighted specific milestones that could be used for evaluative feedback on integrated care rotations (**Table 1**).

Psychology

Overarching competencies within pediatric psychology were initially developed in 2003[13] and began to more clearly delineate specific skills related to professional practice within the field. Twelve topic areas were initially included:

1. Lifespan developmental psychology
2. Lifespan developmental psychopathology
3. Child, adolescent, and family assessment
4. Intervention strategies
5. Research methods and systems evaluations
6. Professional, ethical, and legal issues
7. Diversity
8. Role of multiple disciplines in service delivery systems
9. Prevention, family support, and health promotion
10. Social issues affecting children, adolescents, and families
11. Consultation and liaison roles
12. Disease process and medical management.

Table 1
Integrated Care Evaluative Examples using Child and Adolescent Psychiatry Milestones

Patient Care (PC)	Medical Knowledge (MK)	System-Based Practice (SBP)	Practice-Based Learning and Improvement (PBLI)	Professionalism (PROF)	Interpersonal and Communication Skills (ICS)
PC1: psychiatric evaluation PC2: psychiatric formulation and differential diagnosis PC3: treatment planning and management PC4: psychotherapy	MK4: psychotherapy, knowledge regarding (1) individual psychotherapies, including IPT, cognitive-behavioral, and supportive therapies; (2) family and group therapies; (3) dyadic therapies (eg, parent-child interaction therapy [PCIT])	SBP2: resource management SBP3: community-based care SBP4: consultation to and integration with nonpsychiatric medical providers and nonmedical systems	PBLI2: teaching	PROF2: accountability to self, patients, colleagues, and the profession	ICS1: relationship development and conflict management with patients and families, colleagues, members of the health care team, and other systems ICS2: information sharing and record keeping

Modified from Summers RF, Rapaport MH, Hunt JB, et al. Training psychiatrists for integrated behavioral health care. A report by the American Psychiatric Association Council on Medical Education and Lifelong Learning. 2014. Available at: https://www.med.upenn.edu/psychres/assets/user-content/documents/CMELL_ICReport_2232015 %285%29.pdf. Accessed May 23, 2017; with permission.

Together, these topic areas broadly described the roles and skills of pediatric psychologists across multiple settings.

Professional psychology has more formally been working to delineate competencies for psychology practice in primary care since 2012 with the initiation of an APA Presidential Initiative.[6] The multiple groups involved with this interorganizational work group built on the Benchmark Model,[14] which established a model for competencies for psychologists as health service providers. The psychology primary care competencies featured a biopsychosocial model, stressed the teamwork of mental health and medical providers, and provided 6 general competency clusters: professionalism, relationships, education, systems, science, and application.[15]

Pediatric psychology competencies were thereafter revised in 2014,[16] once again using the widely cited Benchmark Model.[14] These included 6 competency domains: (1) science, (2) professionalism, (3) interpersonal, (4) application, (5) education, and (6) systems, as well as cross-cutting knowledge competencies in pediatric psychology. Specific behavioral anchors within each competency domain across 3 developmental periods (readiness for clinical training experiences, readiness for internship, and readiness for entry to practice) were included, thereby allowing useful guideposts for curriculum development, clinical supervision, and professional practice development.

The general competencies within pediatric psychology[16] were subsequently applied to psychology practice in integrated pediatric primary care through the development of specific behavioral anchors.[17] These competencies focused on team-based care and improved patient experience of care (eg, quality and satisfaction), improved population health outcomes, and reduced costs (ie, the Triple Aim).[18] Again, central to the development of relevant behavioral anchors were professionalism, interpersonal skills and communication, and systems-based practice domains.

Social Work

Similar to the fields of psychiatry and psychology, within social work there have been recent efforts to increase integrated primary care training opportunities and to identify specific competencies necessary for social workers practicing in a primary care setting.[19–21] Such efforts have occurred at both the national and the local level. In 2012, the Council on Social Work Education (CSWE)[22] collaborated with the Substance Abuse and Mental Health Services Administration (SAMHSA) to launch the *Social Work and Integrated Behavioral Healthcare Project*, which aimed to increase integrated primary care graduate coursework, field placements, and related competency development in social work training programs. In the first phase of this project, social work faculty members developed master's level curriculum materials for 2 primary care-specific courses: (1) Clinical Practice and (2) Policy and Services.[22] The second and third project phases focused on developing a learning network for faculty and students involved in coursework implementation, and on increasing integrated primary care field placements for social work trainees.

Within the CSWE Clinical Practice coursework,[22] there are learning modules in the areas of multidisciplinary practice, common primary care-based assessment and intervention approaches, and cultural competence, among other topic areas. As described by Stanhope and colleagues,[21] many of the content areas covered by the CSWE courses are closely aligned with the SAMHSA–Health Resources and Services Administration (HRSA) Center for Integrated Health Solutions report on core competencies for integrated behavioral health and primary care,[23] which includes 9 broad domains that are summarized in **Box 1**.

Another primary care-related social work competency development initiative that aligns with the SAMHSA-HRSA framework is the Integrated and Culturally Relevant

---

Box 1
Broad Substance Abuse and Mental Health Services Administration and Health Resources and Services Administration core competency domains for integrated primary care behavioral health practice and field-specific skills

Core competency

1. Interpersonal communication

2. Collaboration and teamwork

3. Screening and assessment

4. Care planning and care coordination

5. Intervention

6. Cultural competence and adaptation

7. Systems-oriented practice

8. Practice-based learning and quality improvement

9. Informatics

Modified from Hoge MA, Morris JA, Laraia M, et al. Core competencies for integrated behavioral health and primary care. Washington, DC: SAMHSA-HRSA Center for Integrated Health Solutions; 2014; with permission.

Care (ICRC) field education and training model, which was developed and implemented locally by the Ohio State University College of Social Work.[19] Using community-based participatory action research methods, the program developers identified 8 key integrated primary care learning domains, each with specific social work practice competencies (**Box 2**). As noted by the ICRC program developers, these learning domains clearly map onto those described in the SAMHSA-HRSA competencies report.[23] This model is also linked to the CSWE coursework, with substantial overlap in general content areas (eg, assessment and intervention approaches, diversity or cultural competence). Importantly, in describing their model and future

---

Box 2
Social work integrated care competency domains identified in the Integrated and Culturally Relevant Care model

Learning domain

Integrated care

Technology in a health care environment

Assessment and diagnosis

Care coordination and intervention planning

Diversity

Documentation

Health care basics

Evidence-informed behavioral health interventions

From Davis TS, Guada J, Reno R, et al. Integrated and culturally relevant care: a model to prepare social workers for primary care behavioral health practice. Soc Work Health Care 2015;54(10):909–38; with permission.

---

directions for integrated primary care competency training, Davis and colleagues[19] emphasized the need to build the capacity for disseminating this primary care competency-related information and for sustaining current training initiatives for primary care-focused social workers. These efforts are especially salient given that recent research on social workers practicing integrated primary care indicates that most of these clinicians report having to learn relevant competencies on the job, without formalized training or support.[20]

INTEGRATED GUIDELINES FOR TRAINING ACROSS DISCIPLINES

Despite the development of discipline-specific, and even common, overlapping competencies across disciplines, effective pediatric health care practice demands the development of interprofessional collaborative competencies. The development and implementation of interprofessional collaborative competencies[24] was stressed early in the process of developing integrated models. Interprofessionalism, defined as a team-based collaborative, coordinated effort to improve general health, was an outgrowth of the Institute of Medicine's focus on team-based care.[25] The unique contributions that different health care professionals contribute to the primary care team were appreciated, including the development of collaborative relationships to provide healthy interprofessional teams, mutual respect, and shared values. The Interprofessional Education Collaborative Expert Panel[24] was charged with building on each profession's expected disciplinary competencies by defining competencies for effective interprofessional collaborative practice. Sponsors of this panel included the American Association of Colleges of Nursing, American Association of Colleges of Osteopathic Medicine, American Association of Colleges of Pharmacy, American Dental Education Association, Association of American Medical Colleges, and the Association of Schools of Public Health.

The values and ethics for interprofessional practice (eg, mutual respect, trust) included defining roles and responsibilities, highlighting effective interprofessional communication, and stressing use of teams and teamwork.[26] The need to move beyond profession-specific educational efforts to develop interactive learning opportunities to enhance collaboration and learning across multiple pediatric health care disciplines and professionals was strongly emphasized. Desired principles included care that is patient-centered, population or community oriented, relationship-focused, process-oriented, linked to learning activities, integrated across the learning continuum, systems-oriented, applicable across professions, outcome-driven, and described using a common language. Five cross-cutting competencies included patient-centered care, quality improvement, use of empirically based protocols, use of relevant informatics, and use of interdisciplinary teams.

Likewise, and as described above in the context of social work competencies, the SAMSHA-HRSA Center for Integrated Health Solutions recognized the lack of an overarching set of competencies guiding the work happening in integrated care settings. The Center was charged by SAMSHA-HRSA to "identify and disseminate core competencies on integrated practice relevant to behavioral health and primary care providers"[23] (see **Box 1**). Using the SAMSHA-HRSA framework, as well as the competencies identified in the 3 fields highlighted in this article, a set of broad core training competencies for all behavioral health trainees in integrated care settings was developed. These competencies are unique to overlapping aspects of training needed for interdisciplinary collaboration and are meant to be applicable to trainees in the fields of child and adolescent psychiatry, child psychology, and social work (**Fig. 1**). Building on the existing, carefully constructed frameworks, the knowledge,

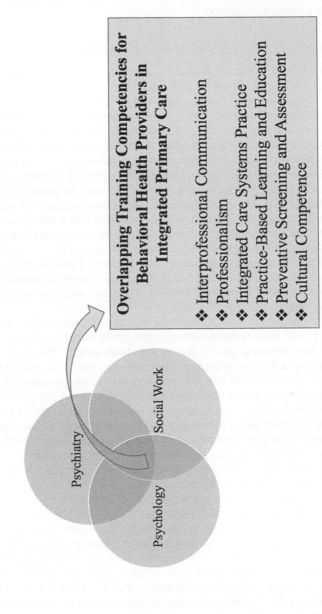

Fig. 1. Overlapping competencies for behavioral health providers in integrated primary care.

skills, and attitudes needed for interprofessional training consists of 6 competencies:

1. Interprofessional communication
2. Professionalism
3. Integrated care systems practice
4. Practice-based learning and education
5. Preventive screening and assessment
6. Cultural competence.

INTERPROFESSIONAL COLLABORATIVE PRACTICE COMPETENCIES CLUSTERS
Interprofessional Communication

The goal of interprofessional communication in integrated primary care settings is to encourage shared decision making among patients, families, and providers to promote effective team-based care. To that end, providers must demonstrate highly effective oral and written communication skills.[17,27,28] It is critical that integrated primary care providers attend to the viewpoints of multiple stakeholders (ie, patients, families, primary care physicians, other medical providers, and office staff) to be maximally effective in the primary care setting. Due to the nature of the role and setting, integrated primary care providers are better able to have frequent contact with primary care physicians; these contacts can be initiated by either provider.[29] Behavioral health trainees more familiar with outpatient settings might require targeted supervision related to the development of collaborative interprofessional relationships built on trust and mutual respect.[30] Additionally, trainees must learn to create treatment plans that extend beyond individual patients or families to include the perspectives of the primary care physician and other relevant providers (eg, members of the school team). When communicating about these plans in writing, trainees must learn how to use language that is clear and accessible to primary care physicians and that also takes into consideration confidentiality issues.[28,30]

Professionalism

This competency consists of establishing a shared professional culture and ethical or legal guidelines for practice. This is important in the integrated care setting because multiple providers are providing care and treatment of the same family, at times concurrently. It is critical that integrated primary care providers are prepared to discuss confidentiality issues because providers of different professions might approach these issues differently.[31] In integrated care settings, many of the notes and communication with providers and parents are not confidential and can be viewed by all of the providers caring for the patient in that setting. Trainees should ensure that they discuss with patients and parents the inherent differences between integrated practices and outpatient mental health, so that patients and families understand that communication is not fully confidential because primary care physicians have access to the documentation. Further discussion with trainees may include the burden placed on the providers to respect parent and patient wishes while still supporting effective team-based care.

Integrated Care Systems Practice

A comprehensive understanding of the integrated primary care context and knowledge of the different professional roles in this environment are necessary for effective practice. By definition, integrated primary care providers work in a context of multiple interrelated systems, including family, medical, school, community, and social systems. To better understand this context, trainees should obtain education in population-based health care and prevention. In addition, because there are many different professionals working within a pediatric integrated care practice, trainees should develop an understanding of the roles and values of all disciplines and members of the care team. They should also develop skills in methods to integrate contributions from and communication with team members in patient care and treatment planning. Integrated primary care practice is characterized by mutual respect and trust, as well as appreciation of the diversity reflected by each team member. Thus, shared decision-making is critical for effective patient-centered practice across behavioral health disciplines.[26] In a training context, this could be implemented through interprofessional case conferences related to mental health concerns and group discussion of specific case examples. In addition to developing shared decision-making skills, training activities related to promoting practice based on integrated care systems should include the use of informatics within integrated care practice to facilitate shared decision-making and interprofessional communication.

Practice-Based Learning and Education

This training competency reflects training needs and competency development in the interrelated areas of clinical supervision, practice-based education, and the implementation of primary care–based interventions. Teaching, training, and supervision are core educational activities across providers in integrated care settings. Interprofessional collaborative education and learning specifically requires meaningful curricular integration of interprofessional competencies related to practice at various levels in the training cycles of future practitioners. Notably, there have been recent efforts to develop training curricula unique to provider type.[32,33] However, the importance of including trainees across behavioral health disciplines in joint educational activities, specifically emphasizing biological, cognitive, affective, sociocultural, and lifespan developmental influences on children's health and illness, cannot be overstated. Additional attitudes and knowledge related to this training competency include a thorough understanding of preventive interventions and of the evolving evidence base for commonly used behavioral health interventions. An understanding of risk and resilience in community mental health is also important to inform case conceptualization and the selection of appropriate interventions for the primary care context. Finally, education in quality improvement methods is necessary to prepare trainees for evaluating intervention efforts in primary care and for making ongoing programmatic adjustments in response to the changing evidence base for clinical practice.

Preventive Screening and Assessment

This competency consists of knowledge about preventive screening and assessment tools, which is critical for both the early identification and treatment of emerging behavioral health conditions and for ongoing assessment of patient outcomes. Understanding these tools is particularly relevant for supporting collaboration with primary care physicians. Indeed, the AAP recommends that pediatricians routinely screen all children and adolescents for emotional and behavioral health concerns.[27,34] Training within this competency should broadly encompass the skills needed for appropriate measurement selection, implementation, interpretation, and communication of results.[17,23] Related to tool selection, training should focus on the psychometric properties of brief, evidence-based, and publicly available screening, as well as more targeted measures for common pediatric mental health problems, health risk behaviors, and safety (eg, the Patient Health Questionnaire depression rating scale).[23,35,36] Integrated primary care training should emphasize skills in selecting measures that are culturally and developmentally sensitive, can be integrated into the electronic medical record, and can be feasibly implemented during a fast-paced primary care visit. Furthermore, training should focus on how to use results within the context of other patient, family, and sociocultural factors to inform treatment planning, as well as methods to effectively communicate results to patients and families, and to members of the health care team.

Cultural Competence

Recognizing the importance of diversity in integrated primary care settings is another key training competency requiring a specific skill set. Pediatric outpatient settings serve patients and families of diverse racial or ethnic, linguistic, and socioeconomic backgrounds. Trainees need a clear understanding of ways to work collaboratively within diverse communities, including understanding key differences in communication styles, knowledge of behavioral health concerns, and understanding barriers to treatment that may be unique to particular families. Trainees should learn to understand how differences in childrearing practices and cultural beliefs and values may affect the way the children or families answer screening questions, report their concerns, and digest feedback from the clinical care team. Trainees must also be counseled that the services provided in the primary care sites may led to referral to a behavioral health center secondary to acuity or complexity, and the relationship and interaction with the integrated primary care team is important in fostering trust and understanding for future encounters. Other factors trainees working in primary care settings need to be familiar with include psychosocial determinants of health and the impact on the children and families' presentation.

CHILDREN'S HOSPITAL OF PHILADELPHIA HEALTHY MINDS, HEALTHY KIDS INTEGRATED BEHAVIORAL HEALTH CARE ROTATION

HMHK is the integrated behavioral health in primary care service at Children's Hospital of Philadelphia (CHOP). The team includes psychiatrists, psychologists, and licensed clinical social workers. In addition to the provision of high-quality, evidence-informed care, the team focuses on interprofessional training to support workforce development. Interprofessional training through the HMHK program currently occurs in a large, urban primary care practice in an area of Philadelphia that has been designated as a medically underserved area. The practice serves approximately 15,000 patients, of which 41.4% of are black or African American, 25.3% are white, 10.7% are Asian, and 22.5% are multiracial or of another racial group. Also, 16% of patients are Hispanic and 68.7% of patients are publicly insured. The practice comprises 22 primary care physicians and 3 pediatric nurse practitioners (representing 14.8 full-time equivalents), and 35 to 40 pediatrics residents rotate through the clinic each training year.

The HMHK rotation includes didactic and experiential learning opportunities for child and adolescent psychiatry fellows and psychology clinical child interns. The goal is to develop a training rotation for social work fellows in the near future. Trainees in psychiatry spend 6 hours each week for 6 months in the rotation and psychology trainees are placed in primary care for 16 hours per week for 1 year. Each trainee is assigned an attending supervisor within the same discipline and trainees are encouraged to discuss their cases with attending providers across disciplines.

Before their involvement in the integrated primary care rotation, trainees receive extensive supervised clinical training in assessment and diagnosis. The goal of the integrated primary care rotation is for trainees to refine their clinical practice so they will be maximally effective in the primary care setting. At the start of the rotation, trainees receive orientation focused on

1. Documentation in the electronic medical record (interprofessional communication)
2. Strategies for effective collaboration with primary care providers (professionalism, interprofessional communication)
3. Evidence-informed intervention strategies to address common presenting concerns in primary care (practiced-based learning and education)
4. Cultural competence
5. Primary care basics.

For example, trainees observe well-child visits for children of all ages (infants, toddlers, school-age, adolescent) to understand the roles and functions of pediatric primary care providers. Additionally, throughout the rotation, trainees participate in weekly interprofessional group supervision or didactic seminars co-led by a psychiatrist and a psychologist. During the seminars, trainees and supervisors focus on a specific presenting concern (eg, disruptive behavior, anxiety, sleep problems) and discuss evidence-informed strategies to address the concern. Trainees lead a case-based discussion and obtain feedback from one another and the attending providers. The discussions include a focus on relevant cultural considerations and, if ethical issues arise, these issues are discussed to highlight the unique ethical challenges that arise in pediatric integrated primary care practice.

Trainees are involved in direct patient care in a variety of ways. HMHK providers receive most referrals through a warm-handoff approach. Trainees meet the family and child the same day as a primary care office visit and they conduct a brief consultation. This warm handoff informs care coordination and intervention planning. Additionally, each trainee maintains a caseload of patients, including opportunities for new patient intakes and follow-up evidence-informed care; psychiatry fellows are also involved in medication management. All HMHK providers use a model of brief intervention (ie, 8 sessions or fewer) to provide follow-up care consistent with guidelines for integrated primary care practice.[17,23]

The HMHK is a model in which behavioral health trainees in integrated primary care can engage in interdisciplinary training and practice. Future directions for this program include the integration of social work trainees and the expansion of HMHK into additional practices, in both urban and suburban settings, which will increase the diversity of training opportunities for trainees of all disciplines.

SUMMARY AND FUTURE DIRECTIONS

It is increasingly clear that the implementation of the medical home in primary care will continue to drive integration of mental health and medical services. These changes in clinical practice will require education programs that include integrated training environments. With increasing growth of these newly integrated clinical practices, they will become the norm for clinicians from all disciplines, necessitating trainees to develop relevant knowledge and skills before entering clinical rotations. Ideally, teaching the interdisciplinary care framework would begin in the preclinical years, allowing for a more nuanced understanding before beginning the clinical rotations. Interdisciplinary collaboration and shared accountability for the care of patients in the integrated care setting will require supervised practice and evaluation of these new skills for graduate and postgraduate trainees. Thus, assessment of these competencies will require ongoing changes to the milestones in each discipline to ensure relevance.

Interdisciplinary care will be of paramount importance in providing timely and appropriate behavioral health treatment to children, adolescents, and their families. The framework presented in this article is applicable for all trainees as they rotate through pediatric primary care sites, particularly as more training programs develop core curriculums to address learning in integrated care environments. Discipline-specific differences in integrated care remain (eg, the child and adolescent psychiatrists' need to understand common illness presentation in pediatric practices, the child psychologists' knowledge of current evidence-based assessment, the social workers' knowledge of community resources) and the competencies outlined in this article do not negate the need for discipline-specific competencies. Instead, the authors suggest that these cross-discipline competencies can enhance discipline-specific skills while teaching all of the trainees a common language. Cowley and colleagues[37] reinforce the importance of trainees learning from both didactic and experiential opportunities, highlighting that the latter are key in developing content skills. The broad goal of the recommendations made in this article is to ensure that all behavioral health trainees are equipped with the skills needed to effectively treat children and their families in integrated care settings.

REFERENCES

1. U. S. Department of Health and Human Services. Mental health: a report of the surgeon general. Rockville (MD): U.S. Department of Health and Human Services, Substance Abuse and Mental Health Services Administration, Center for Mental Health Services, National Institutes of Health, National Institute of Mental Health; 1999.
2. Wang PS, Berglund P, Olfson M, et al. Failure and delay in initial treatment contact after first onset of mental disorders in the National Comorbidity Survey Replication. Arch Gen Psychiatry 2005;62(6):603–13.
3. 111 th Congress: Patient Protection and Affordable Care Act, H.R. 3590. Washington, DC, January 6, 2009 – December 22, 2010.
4. American Academy of Child and Adolescent Psychiatry. Collaboration with Pediatric Medical Professionals. 2008. Available at: https://www.aacap.org/aacap/Policy_Statements/2008/Collaboration_with_Pediatric_Medical_Professionals.aspx. Accessed March 23, 2017.
5. American Academy of Pediatrics. The future of pediatrics: mental health competencies for pediatric primary care. Pediatrics 2009;124(1):410–21.
6. Summers R, Rapaport M, Hunt J, et al. Training psychiatrists for integrated behavioral health care. Report by the American Psychiatric Association Council on Medical Education and Lifelong Learning; 2014.
7. Summers R, Rapaport M, Hunt J, et al. Training Psychiatrists for Integrated Behavioral Health Care. A Report by the American Psychiatric Association Council on Medical Edication and Lifelong Learning. 2014. Available at: https://www.med.upenn.edu/psychres/assets/user-content/documents/CMELL_ICReport_2232015 %285%29.pdf. Accessed March 23, 2017.
8. Accreditation Council for Graduate Medical Education. ACGME Common Program Requirements. 2013. Available at: http://www.acgme.org/What-We-Do/Accreditation/Common-Program-Requirements. Accessed March 23, 2017.
9. Accreditation Council for Graduate Medical Education and American Board of Psychiatry and Neurology. The Psychiatry Milestone Project. 2015. Available at: http://www.acgme.org/Portals/0/PDFs/Milestones/PsychiatryMilestones.pdf. Accessed March 23, 2017.

10. Ratzliff AH, Unützer J, Pascualy M. Training psychiatrists for integrated care. Integrated care: working at the interface of primary care and behavioral health. Washington, DC: American Psychiatric Publishing; 2015. p. 113–38.

11. Jeffrey J, Martini D. Skills for the child and adolescent psychiatrist within the pediatric primary care setting. JAACAP Connect 2016;3(3):9–14.

12. Garfunkel L, Pisani A, leRoux P, et al. Educational residents in behavioral health care and collaboration: comparison of conventional and integrated training models. Acad Med 2011;86(2):174–9.

13. Spirito A, Brown RT, D'angelo E, et al. Society of Pediatric Psychology Task Force report: recommendations for the training of pediatric psychologists. J Pediatr Psychol 2003;28(2):85–98.

14. Hatcher RL, Fouad NA, Grus CL, et al. Competency benchmarks: practical steps toward a culture of competence. Train Educ Prof Psychol 2013;7(2):84.

15. McDaniel SH, Grus CL, Cubic BA, et al. Competencies for psychology practice in primary care. Am Psychol 2014;69(4):409.

16. Palermo TM, Janicke DM, McQuaid EL, et al. Recommendations for training in pediatric psychology: defining core competencies across training levels. J Pediatr Psychol 2014;39(9):965–84.

17. Hoffses K, Ramirez L, Berdan L, et al. Building competency: professional skills for pediatric psychologists in integrated care settings. J Pediatr Psychol 2016; 41(10):1144–60.

18. McDaniel SH, deGruy FV III. An introduction to primary care and psychology. Am Psychol 2014;69(4):325.

19. Davis TS, Guada J, Reno R, et al. Integrated and culturally relevant care: a model to prepare social workers for primary care behavioral health practice. Soc work Health Care 2015;54(10):909–38.

20. Horevitz E, Manoleas P. Professional competencies and training needs of professional social workers in integrated behavioral health in primary care. Soc work Health Care 2013;52(8):752–87.

21. Stanhope V, Videka L, Thorning H, et al. Moving toward integrated health: an opportunity for social work. Soc work Health Care 2015;54(5):383–407.

22. Council on Social Work Education. Social work and integrated behavioral healthcare project. 2013. Available at: http://www.cswe.org/Centers-Initiatives/Initiatives/Social-Work-and-Integrated-Behavioral-Healthcare-P.aspx. Accessed March 23, 2017.

23. Hoge M, Morris J, Laraia M, et al. Core competencies for integrated behavioral health and primary care. Washington, DC: SAMHSA-HRSA Center for Integrated Health Solutions; 2014.

24. Barr H. Competent to collaborate: towards a competency-based model for interprofessional education. J Interprof Care 1998;12(2):181–7.

25. Institute of Medicine. Cross the quality chasm: a new health system for the 21st century. Washington, DC: National Academy of Sciences; 2001.

26. Interprofessional Education Collaborative Expert Panel. Core competencies for interprofessional collaborative practice: report of an expert panel. Washington, DC: Interprofessional Education Collaborative; 2011.

27. Foy JM, Kelleher KJ, Laraque D, American Academy of Pediatrics Task Force on Mental Health. Enhancing pediatric mental health care: strategies for preparing a primary care practice. Pediatrics 2010;125(Suppl 3):S87–108.

28. Knowles P. Collaborative communication between psychologists and primary care providers. J Clin Psychol Med Settings 2009;16(1):72–6.

29. Ward-Zimmerman B, Cannata E. Partnering with pediatric primary care: lessons learned through collaborative colocation. Prof Psychol Res Pract 2012;43(6):596.
30. van Dongen JJJ, Lenzen SA, van Bokhoven MA, et al. Interprofessional collaboration regarding patients' care plans in primary care: a focus group study into influential factors. BMC Fam Pract 2016;17(1):58.
31. Williamson AA, Raglin Bignall J, Swift LE, et al. Ethical and legal issues in integrated care settings: case examples from pediatric primary care. Clin Pract Pediatr Psychol 2017;5(2):196–208.
32. Fazio SB, Demasi M, Farren E, et al. Blueprint for an undergraduate primary care curriculum. Acad Med 2016;91(12):1628–37.
33. Huang H, Barkil-Oteo A. Teaching collaborative care in primary care settings for psychiatry residents. Psychosomatics 2015;56(6):658–61.
34. Weitzman C, Wegner L. Promoting optimal development: screening for behavioral and emotional problems. Pediatrics 2015;135(2):384–95.
35. American Academy of Pediatrics. Addressing mental health concerns in primary care: a clinician's toolkit. Elk Grove Village (IL): American Academy of Pediatrics; 2010.
36. Lavigne JV, Meyers KM, Feldman M. Systematic review: classification accuracy of behavioral screening measures for use in integrated primary care settings. J Pediatr Psychol 2016;41(10):1091–109.
37. Cowley D, Dunaway K, Forstein M, et al. Teaching psychiatry residents to work at the interface of mental health and primary care. Acad Psychiatry 2014;38(4):398–404.

Family-Based Integrated Care (FBIC) in a Partial Hospital Program for Complex Pediatric Illness

CrossMark

Fostering Shifts in Family Illness Beliefs and Relationships

Michelle L. Rickerby, MD*, Diane DerMarderosian, MD, Jack Nassau, PhD, Christopher Houck, PhD

KEYWORDS

- Family-based treatment • Integrated care • Patient-centered care
- Patient and family-centered care • Family therapy • Eating disorders
- Chronic illness nonadherence • Somatoform illness

KEY POINTS

- The heuristic model of family-based integrated care (FBIC) grounds case formulation in the context of family beliefs and relationships with a goal of productive joining with families and optimal integration of treatment across illnesses and levels of care.
- The application of the FBIC model is effective in the management of several broadly experienced challenges that occur in the management of complex pediatric illness. Some of these challenges include medical nonadherence, which leads to high morbidity and excessive health care cost, families who struggle with accepting the need for psychological intervention to optimize health outcomes, and the risk of mixed messages across disciplines of health care leading to ineffective care.
- Integrated care is effective in optimizing pediatric health outcomes.
- The HCPHP (day-treatment) model allows for intensive intervention in complex pediatric illness.
- FBIC applied in a partial hospital setting can lead to healthy shifts in family illness beliefs and relationships that support better health outcomes.

The Hasbro Children's Partial Hospital Program, The Alpert School of Medicine of Brown University, 593 Eddy Street, Providence, RI 02906, USA
* Corresponding author.
E-mail address: Michelle_Rickerby@Brown.edu

Child Adolesc Psychiatric Clin N Am 26 (2017) 733–759
http://dx.doi.org/10.1016/j.chc.2017.06.006
1056-4993/17/© 2017 Elsevier Inc. All rights reserved.

childpsych.theclinics.com

OVERVIEW
Basic Construct of Family-Based Integrated Care

The heuristic model of family-based integrated care (FBIC) was developed over an 18-year period (1998–2016) in the context of the development of the Hasbro Children's Partial Hospital Program[1] (HCPHP) along with the development of a family therapy training program for Brown University child psychiatry and triple board residents.[2] A description of the heuristic model of FBIC will provide a framework that supports the formulation of treatment needs and coordination of interdisciplinary care across illnesses and levels of care. The FBIC model allows for a meaningful, practical case formulation that is independent of specific illness, presenting symptoms, and context of care. It is also a construct that can be used in all care settings and across disciplines to help organize treatment decisions and interactions in a manner supportive of patient and family empowerment over illness.

The FBIC paradigm encourages providers to join with families around their presenting beliefs about illness and symptoms with an understanding that these beliefs may or may not be divergent from objective medical criteria and provider opinion, and may vary across patient and family members. In addition, the model supports providers in orienting themselves around the relationships between patient and family members, related to specific illness management as well as to overall functioning. With providers grounded in an understanding of patient and family beliefs and relationships in the context and needs of the illness, treatment goal setting becomes connected to the unique needs of each patient. Broadly, the goals include supporting patients and families in having accurate and mobilizing beliefs about their illness and symptoms, and supporting relationships that allow for empathy and effective support around illness needs. The process of aligning providers with these goals across disciplines and levels of care provides a stabilizing construct amidst the crises of pediatric illness while supporting healthy child developmental and family patterns.

The Primacy of Working in the Context of the Family

There is growing evidence supporting the critical impact of the family on children's mental health.[3–10] This impact is noted in research involving epigenetics, the effects of toxic stress and parental mental illness, as well as in reviews of interventions involving family-based treatment. Evidence-based psychological interventions often focus on the details of the illness or symptoms without considering context. However, these interventions are more impactful when an understanding of family systems concepts is incorporated.

In the heuristic model of FBIC, illness cannot be conceptualized outside of the context of family beliefs and relationships. In the HCPHP, family participation in treatment is central and provides a broader lens on the challenges at hand, which allows for optimization of treatment of all illnesses.

Interdisciplinary Care

The importance of comprehensive, interprofessional care for adults, adolescents, and children has been widely recognized as the ideal way to deliver care. Integrating medical and behavioral health practices leads to lower health care costs, decreased readmission rates, and improved outcomes including greater functioning and quality of life. The literature also supports the concept that mental health and medical conditions are risk factors for each other; the presence of one can complicate the treatment and outcomes of the other. This connection is supported by emerging scientific data that identify shared physiologic pathways connecting mind and body.[11]

Advantages of Day Treatment

Treating pediatric patients in a day hospital setting has a number of advantages over inpatient and outpatient treatment. This is related to the ability to combine an opportunity for intensive intervention and monitoring with the real-life challenge of illness management at home. Day-treatment models can mitigate the need for inpatient treatment in high-risk patients not responsive to standard outpatient intervention while minimizing repeat hospitalization for others.

Advantages include the following:

- Day treatment provides children at heightened medical risk with daily monitoring outside of an inpatient setting that allows for both cost savings and the comforts of home. Examples might include patients with eating disorders who require periodic nasogastric tube feedings or patients with diabetes with severely poor glycemic control who need frequent monitoring while insulin adjustments occur.
- It also allows daily psychiatric monitoring for children with heightened risk for self-endangering behavior or who are severely impaired in functional ability. This provides a secure base while supporting the process of breaking these self-destructive patterns without the regressive risk that inpatient care can engender.
- The ability of parents and extended family to participate in care in the program and at home with daily support is much expanded in day treatment versus inpatient settings. This provides a safety net that both contains caregiver anxiety and maximizes empowerment over time.
- The presence of real-life challenges in the home environment can help identify skills needed for each patient and family. These may not be as apparent during medical or psychiatric inpatient treatment. Challenges are considered "grist for the mill" in addressing all of the puzzle pieces that lead to outpatient success. Opportunities to practice skills in the home environment also increase families' self-efficacy for maintaining their goals.

The Family-Based Integrated Care Model

The FBIC heuristic model provides a framework for case conceptualization to organize interdisciplinary treatment by effectively taking into account the unique context of each patient and family. It can be applied across illnesses and patient populations and is useful for all disciplines of health care at all phases of treatment.

The Family-Based Integrated Care Graph

The FBIC graph was developed as a teaching tool that highlights the multidimensional aspects of assessing and treating a patient in the context of a family system.[2] It allows the therapist to become oriented to "where they are" in the process of joining with the patient and family with an eye toward the big picture arc of treatment. It allows for a concrete "vision" of "where we are" as well as a nonjudgmental path forward that is applicable to all families and illnesses. While providing a visual image, it also respects the complexity and fluidity involved in family dynamics. Of note is that the full range of psychological evidence–based treatment can be "mapped on" to the graph, highlighting where each intervention focuses on patient and family cognitive, behavioral, affective, and relational movement. This meta-view's consideration can magnify the impact of discrete interventions either through awareness of whether a patient and family are in a starting place that allows them to accept the intervention or by pointing toward barriers that need to be addressed to allow them to. The FBIC graph includes a cognitive dimension (eg, the presence of ongoing beliefs either shared or idiosyncratic to one family member) as well as an affective/spatial dimension (eg, relationships between family members that generate emotional states and impact the ability to problem solve). Use of this construct to orient joining and treatment efforts is not just for the "evaluation" but rather an effective construct to use throughout treatment (**Fig. 1**).

Beliefs Axis

Patient and family beliefs are powerful forces shaping behavior and emotional experience overall as well as impacting any illness challenge. Beliefs can be distorted and constraining or accurate and mobilizing. Conflict and immobilization can result when beliefs vary across family members. Beliefs are shaped by a complex set of variables, including individual experience and perception; interactions with peers, family, and social networks; and larger cultural contexts, including religion, ethnicity, and culture. Beliefs are subject to shaping and modification and consequently are a target for many evidence-based psychotherapies (cognitive behavior therapy [CBT], dialectical behavior therapy [DBT], acceptance and commitment therapy [ACT]).

From the perspective of FBIC, establishing a clear understanding of patient and family beliefs about the illness entity and associated symptoms is a key component of joining. Common orienting questions during an initial evaluation of FBIC at HCPHP might include:

- "After everything you have experienced in recent months and all of the input you have received from treatment providers what do you believe about what is causing your _____ (insert symptom)?"
- "After everything you have experienced in recent months and all of your input from treatment providers what do you believe about what is causing your daughter/son's _____ (insert symptom)?"
- "What is your understanding from input you have had from your treatment team about what is going to help you get your/your child's illness/symptoms under control?"
- "With all of your efforts with treatment so far are you encouraged, discouraged, or both?"

Key principles to consider when joining around patient and family beliefs include the following:

- It is possible to be empathic around beliefs that may be clearly distorted while also introducing a larger frame to consider.

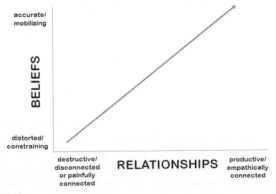

Fig. 1. The FBIC graph.

- For a parent who remains highly anxious about an as-yet undiagnosed rare medical issue that is driving a clinical presentation consistent with conversion disorder: "I hear that you remain very concerned that there is more to figure out medically. The monitoring we will do together daily will help guide our efforts. As we go forward, what is your biggest concern about how this experience has emotionally impacted your child?"
  - For a patient with refractory pain who is unwilling to speak in emotional terms: "Is this experience with your headaches the most painful, stressful thing you have ever been through?" ... "I'm glad you are here so we can figure things out. Separate from your headaches, what is the second most painful/stressful thing you are dealing with or have been through?"
- The therapy process of family members sharing existing beliefs often elucidates areas of conflict/discrepancy that are productive for treatment, explain areas of immobility, and set the stage for expanding perspective for all.
  - For parents who are clearly at odds about forces driving symptoms: "Do you mostly agree or disagree day to day on what is going to most help your son/daughter move forward in spite of his/her _____?"
  - For a family with parents more in tune with psychological factors driving physical symptoms than their child is: "Is your son/daughter surprised to hear you say how much you believe his/her anxiety is causing his/her abdominal pain to be worse?"
- Patients and families describing their illness beliefs often point toward areas in which they have received mixed messages across providers, which can serve to hamper mobilization to break symptom cycles.
  - For families in which this might be the case:
    "Does your outpatient team mostly agree with each other or do they have different opinions about what is happening for your child?" or "Do you mostly agree or disagree with how the team understands your child's illness?"

Relationships Axis

Relationships are complex evolving connections with the same range of shaping forces as illness beliefs. Within the constellation of any given family system, there is a complex web of relationships that powerfully impact each member of the family. Significantly, powerful individual variables including temperament, personality, life experience, and the presence of mental and/or physical illness impact how that individual connects with others. From the FBIC perspective, it is important to develop an understanding of the space between people that is impacted by individual, family, and larger network forces, as well as by the force of the illness entity. Interpersonal functioning within relationships is a common area of focus for a range of evidence-based treatments (interpersonal therapy [IPT]; multisystemic therapy [MST]). Expanding the support that can be derived from relationships can impact the ability to cope with illness in powerful ways.

Relationship valences can be markedly positive, significantly negative, and mixed. An overly simplified construct identifies the spatial aspect of the relationship (closeness vs distance in connection and communication) as well as the affective aspect (range from high attunement and empathy to detachment and neglect). Common questions that orient the clinician to family relationships might include the following:

- "Stress like this can pull families together, push them apart, or both. What would your daughter/son/husband/wife/father/mother say is happening with your family? What would you say?"

- "There are so many painful aspects to what you are living with from your illness. Are there some things your mother/father would rather not know, or would she/he rather you tell her what is going on even if it's really painful to hear?"

Key principles to consider while joining with patients and families around the status of their relationships include the following:

- The presence of illness and the effort required for illness management places a tremendous burden on family relationships in terms of logistics and emotional energy.
- The manner in which an illness complicates a family's routine is unique to that family.
- The time and energy spent on managing illnesses may take focus away from other significant events that need attention and discussion ("things get pushed under the rug").
- It is common for parents and children to "protect" each other by avoiding talking about the most painful details of the illness.

A simple way to assess where a family is, includes a review of "Routines, Rugs, and Risky Conversations":

- "Routines": "What is the greatest challenge for you in your daily routine related to your managing your/your child's illness?"
- "Rugs": "If we weren't spending so much time talking about diabetes/depression/the eating disorder what else would be most important for your family to spend some time talking about?"
- "Risky Conversations": "What is the scariest part of living with _____ (insert illness) that may be most difficult for your child/parent to talk about?"

It is also important to become oriented to the status and health of family relationships that existed before the illness challenge:

- We may meet children and families who had a developmentally normal and healthy pattern of relationships that have been profoundly disrupted by the immense pressure of an illness.
- We may meet children and families for whom the illness challenge pales in comparison with other life challenges. Perhaps families have lifelong severe impairment in relationship patterns that long predated the illness.
- Perhaps we meet a family who has had lifelong painful relationship patterns that are now further compromised by the pressure of the illness.

Any of these realities can be conceptualized and intervened with using the FBIC construct with interventions tuned to the family reality. Regardless of the specific illness entity, any pain/distress is eased by the presence of empathic interpersonal connections.

Interdisciplinary Value of the Family-Based Integrated Care Model

The importance of orienting oneself to the context of family beliefs and relationships is not exclusive for mental health professionals. All heath care providers can benefit from an awareness of these contextual factors. It is possible to become familiar with common belief and relationship patterns as they impact illness management and to develop a toolkit of responses without formal mental health training. This heuristic model seeks to update the "biopsychosocial model"[12] of patient formulation. Familiarity with this model allows for productive responses to common challenges for providers in treating complex pediatric illness, including helplessness in the face of severely distorted family illness beliefs and/or severely impaired relationships, frustration in treating families who struggle to incorporate a psychological understanding of their child's challenge, and the risks inherent in becoming entangled in symptom-driven decision making.

The FBIC model can help combat an expectable sense of helplessness for providers, patients, and family members in the face of powerful and life-threatening illness challenges and/or painful family relationship patterns. The meta-view of "acknowledging where the family is," even if it is a very painful, troubled place is a relief, as it naturally implies a path forward. Although the power of any particular illness entity can be overwhelming, providers can shift to feeling empowered by understanding that regardless of illness severity, they can intervene in the family system in a manner that offers relief while the patient and family lives with the illness. Forging a hopeful connection with a health care provider/provider team can often be the first step in breaking a longstanding sense of isolation derived from an illness being out of control. For parents and other family members, the message that "your understanding of your child's illness and your connection to your child are the most powerful forces in their recovery" is a message that allows for a shift from helplessness to empowerment. This helplessness is often magnified by the collateral damage of accommodation patterns already noted. Combatting this sense of helplessness is often particularly critical for therapists in training who often take on a sense of blame around the impact of illnesses on patients and families.[12]

The FBIC model can allow a productive avenue to manage patients and families who struggle to incorporate a psychological line of sight into understanding illness challenges. By assessing the status of family beliefs and relationships as a natural and expected aspect of joining with patients and families in a nonjudgmental way, rather than one that is symptom specific, a framework for the patient and family as people is created. This provides a springboard to normalize the psychological responses to illness that are not specific to a mental health diagnosis but rather inherent to life. Using the FBIC framework in discussing both medical and psychiatric illness in the same framework reinforces the construct that we are always treating the whole person in all cases. Practice with this model of case formulation and treatment discussions for non–mental health professionals allows psychological layers to become naturally embedded in illness conversations without the implication that this is a realm separate from the professional's specialized focus.

A focus on symptoms/illness outside the multidimensional context represented by the graph can grant the illness more power over the patient's and family's life rather than less. Because the FBIC model is not symptom or illness specific, it helps mitigate the dangers inherent in symptom-focused decision making. These pitfalls include making treatment decisions that do not use the right balance of medical and psychological focus, including nonproductive decisions about shifts in levels of care. More specifically, the incorporation of a psychological framework naturally leads to professionals conveying the message to families that these dimensions are valuable. With the consequent improved joining that follows, it is expectable that patients and families will be more accepting of interventions in these areas. This acceptance may allow for avoidance of unnecessary and potentially harmful interventions, such as the addition of a medication aimed at a medical etiology of symptom exacerbation that is actually believed to be more related to psychological factors. Decisions about levels of care also need to be context driven to be most productive. A common example relates to decision making around suicidality and level of care. There are situations in which context dictates that, even with intense suicidality, remaining at home with family support is the most therapeutic option. Conversely, there are other situations in which suicidality is less intense, but family relationships are less nurturing, which may necessitate an inpatient level of care. Similarly, in the realm of physical illness, the family's ability to conceptualize necessary care and mobilize around patient needs should be a critical variable in decision making around the most productive and empowering level of care at any given phase of illness.

Message Magnification Across Providers

The use of the FBIC model across disciplines allows for a productive magnification of messages given to patients and families. The graph orients providers, patients, and families to where the family system is in the treatment and recovery arc, in turn leading to conversations across disciplines around similar themes.

A patient with deeply entrenched cognitive distortions driven by their eating disorder may hear the following from different providers, both of which emphasize externalization of the eating disorder:

- A milieu therapist who encourages them to engage in a skill-building exercise focused on mindfulness might note: "When the eating disorder thoughts get really strong and painful, this is something you can try?"
- A pediatrician may say while doing a physical examination: "Even though the eating disorder is telling you not to eat, we are going to support you fighting back, because nutrition is the medicine that your body needs."

Meanwhile, the parents of the patient may hear the following, which also emphasizes externalization, as well as the importance of parents' relationships with their daughter:

- A pediatric nurse who notes after hearing of a difficult night when the patient was screaming at her parents while refusing dinner might say: "You did a really good job holding the line. Even though she didn't eat everything, the eating disorder didn't win."
- A psychologist doing family therapy with these parents may say: "As powerful as her eating disorder was last night, your relationship with her was stronger and gave the message to the illness that it is not in charge."

When anchored in the FBIC model, medical and psychological messages are integrated instead of divided. The repetition of themes is nonjudgmental, focused on the details of practical needs at hand, and directed at patient and family empowerment even during a period of the illness running rampant.

Case Example 1: Family-Based Integrated Care Case Conceptualization

Brittany is a 14-year-old girl with a restrictive-type eating disorder referred to HCPHP after a 10-day inpatient admission for medical stabilization and refeeding. When Brittany presented to the eating disorder team for an outpatient intake appointment, she was found to be critically bradycardic and symptomatically orthostatic by heart rate and blood pressure, necessitating an inpatient level of care. Brittany reported an 18-month history of restrictive eating, including calorie counting, fat and carbohydrate avoidance, and not eating at all on days that she could not exercise. In addition, she reported compulsive overexercise and water-loading. She denied vomiting, use of laxatives/diuretics/diet pills/herbal weight loss supplements/nonprescribed medications for the purpose of weight loss. Brittany reported 18 months prior she decided to "get healthy and lose a few pounds." Initially she cut out "junk food" and increased her exercise to 3 to 4 times per week. She started using a FITBIT and a weight loss app on her phone. These changes resulted in modest weight loss, and Brittany began to "feel better about herself." Approximately 6 months before admission, her parents began to have concerns that she had become extremely rigid in her eating, compulsive and excessive with exercise, and withdrawn from activities that she previously enjoyed. They also noted that Brittany appeared "too thin" and continued to feel the need to lose weight. At that time, her parents brought Brittany to her primary medical doctor who weighed her and felt reassured by a body mass index of 18.5. Over the next 6 months, Brittany became more consumed by a drive to eat "healthfully," exercise, and lose weight. Her parents remained concerned, and although she would not eat what they prepared, they allowed her to make her own food and eat what she wanted because "at least she was eating."

In this case example, Brittany's distorted cognitions about food, body, and health interfered with her ability to make healthy decisions for herself. These cognitions along with her undernourished state contributed to a depressed mood including withdrawal from peers and preferred activities. Her parents' feeling of helplessness and willingness to inadvertently collude with the eating disorder further reinforced the control it had over Brittany and the family. Despite Brittany developing some insight around the negative impact that her eating disorder had on her and her relationships, her illness remained too powerful to allow a change in her distorted cognitions and behaviors.

Family-Based Integrated Care Case Example 2: Case Conceptualization

Joann is a 14-year-old girl who lives with her parents and 17-year-old sister. She has a 20-year-old sister who attends a prestigious university. She does not have a significant medical history, has friends and plays sports, and is a good student, although she recognizes that academics do not come as easily to her as to her sister. She is currently in the eighth grade and her parents have always encouraged her to do her best, hoping that that would take some pressure off. Joann has interpreted this to mean she should work as hard as possible to achieve. She feared not being able to succeed as her sister did. Unexpectedly, as school was to resume following winter vacation, Joann developed intense abdominal pain and was not able to attend. Her parents were not initially concerned, but when the pain persisted and continued to interfere with school attendance, they began to seek medical advice, first from Joann's pediatrician and then from a gastrointestinal specialist. Each of these physicians recommended symptom-focused treatment (eg, MiraLAX for mild constipation). Joann continued to experience pain, miss school, and disengage from social activities. Joann's primary care doctor recommended counseling, but as Joann had always functioned well and did not want to reveal emotional distress to her parents, this recommendation was not followed. Instead, believing in their daughter's overall competence, they assumed that there must be an underlying medical cause for her pain. They assured Joann they would get to the bottom of her pain and sought several additional opinions from specialists who trialed her on different pain medications. Joann was seen in the emergency department and admitted to the hospital where she underwent several medical tests, all with negative results. Meanwhile, she was home from school, her sleep was disrupted due to lack of a schedule, and she more and more socially isolated.

In this case example, Joann's parents' belief that her pain was exclusively driven by an as-yet undiagnosed medical illness led to repeated visits to a variety of medical subspecialists, emergency room (ER) visits, a medical admission, and a variety of medical interventions. At the same time, very little attention had been paid to the psychosocial factors that are likely contributing to Joann's pain experience as well as to the psychological impact of her pain experience. Although all family members are worried about Joann, and are confused and frustrated about not being able to find a medical answer, the family's medical focus has made it difficult to talk about important emotional issues. Thus, although the family members share a common belief, this belief is distorted in that it does not include psychological factors. The lack of attention to this dimension has led to distance in family relationships that further escalate Joann's sense of isolation and helplessness.

Family-Based Integrated Care Case Example 3: Case Conceptualization

Caleb is a 15-year-old boy who was diagnosed with type 1 diabetes at age 13. He lives with his mother and father and 2 siblings, ages 11 and 8. He has a long history of excelling socially, academically, and athletically, qualities that his parents have fostered by encouraging his self-reliance. After being diagnosed, Caleb quickly learned to monitor his blood glucose and diet in ways that led to successful HbA1c levels. His parents, who were initially privately devastated that their son would have to manage a chronic illness each day for the rest of his life, began to feel hopeful that this would not interfere as much as they had feared. Because he effectively monitored his illness, they allowed him to manage much of his regimen independently. However, after several months of successful management, Caleb began to find it more difficult to balance his diet, exercise, and insulin, resulting in fluctuating blood glucose levels. This resulted in Caleb feeling frustrated, hopeless, and depressed. His parents, used to their son solving problems effectively on his own, continued to assume he would "figure it out." At the same time, Caleb began to believe that his illness cannot be "figured out" and gave up close monitoring and regular insulin injections, which ultimately led to long periods of very high HbA1c values, as well as an ER visit for an episode of potentially life-threatening diabetic ketoacidosis.

In this case example, Caleb's belief that his diabetes cannot be controlled has a strong impact on his mood and illness management adherence. His depressed mood likely clouds his judgment about his illness and his efficacy for managing it. Similarly, his parents' distorted beliefs that their son can handle this independently, combined with thoughts that they would not know how to help, further exacerbate the influence diabetes has on Caleb and the family. Family beliefs are constraining Caleb's ability to manage his illness. Meanwhile, Caleb's parents are empathic and concerned, but have been unable to convey support in ways in which Caleb can connect, as he has always been self-reliant. A shift toward increased monitoring in their parent-child relationship has felt like failure to all of them, leading to frustration and distance.

** Please note that case examples are derived from amalgams of a large sample of patients treated over time rather than being derived from any 1 patient or family.

THE PARTIAL HOSPITAL PROGRAM MODEL
Program Mission

The HCPHP is a collaboration of the Department of Pediatrics and the Department of Child Psychiatry of Hasbro Children's Hospital, a Lifespan affiliate. The HCPHP has been in operation since June 1998. The mission of HCPHP is to empower children, 6 to 18 years of age, and their families, to face complex pediatric illness challenges, including eating disorders, chronic pediatric illness complicated by nonadherence and/or psychiatric comorbidity, complex pain disorders, and somatoform illness such as conversion disorder. Regardless of illness, the mission is for the team to understand the illness experience and challenges unique to each child and family. In this context, the goal is to support the development of accurate and mobilizing illness beliefs as well as to support relationships between family members and with providers that are empathic and productive. Sometimes patients and families enter the program with well-delineated diagnoses, whereas in other cases there is clinical uncertainty. When FBIC is applied, the core mission can proceed in either case.

Program Development

The initial unit opened in 1998, in 2 rooms on the medical inpatient floors of Hasbro Children's Hospital with a maximum census of 6 patients ages 12 to 18. The program moved to a renovated space (approximately 5410 square feet) in 2000, along with expanded staffing that allowed for growth into 2 therapeutic milieus (one for 6–12-year-olds and one for 12–18-year-olds). The census target gradually increased from 10 patients in 2000 to 16 patients in 2014. A major expansion of physical space (3900 square feet) and staffing in 2015 increased capacity to 24 patients and allowed for the creation of 3 milieus that are age and developmentally based. All growth was driven by overwhelming need for services within the region and beyond. All renovations and expansions were hospital funded based on fiscal health of the program aside from a philanthropic fund that supported physical space renovation in 2000.

Program Beliefs

The following are HCPHP beliefs that anchor FBIC treatment for complex pediatric illness and provide a framework that encourages family belief shifts that are productive for treatment:

- Any treatment plan or decision that gives the illness less power/control over the child and family's life leads to a sense of empowerment and improved illness management.
  - Accommodation to illness symptoms that leads to avoidance and functional impairment is a feature common to pediatric and psychiatric illnesses, which leads to collateral damage for the child and family.
  - Family understanding of this reality and awareness of their ability to shift this pattern is essential to the effectiveness of many evidence-based treatments.[13]
  - The process of "externalizing the illness"[14] provides a belief shift that takes pressure off of family relationships by allowing blame to shift to empathic mobilization of support.
- Emotional expression is empowering but can be very difficult for a range of reasons.
  - Validation of child and parent emotional experience is essential to effective joining around treatment efforts.
  - It is possible to validate emotional experience without reinforcing distorted beliefs driven by illness cognitions.
- Mind and body are inextricably connected. Treating "the whole child" is essential.
  - Physical pain/distress is connected to emotional pain/distress and vice versa.
  - It is possible to address psychological distress while also attending to physical pain/distress.
- Focusing on functioning is empowering.
  - It is possible to encourage the patient's functioning while at the same time being empathic about how distressing this might be for the patient.
  - Supporting functioning does not mean that pain/distress is not "real."

- The presence of pain/distress, even more pain/distress than was there before intervention, can be an important part of moving toward physical/emotional healing and overall empowerment.
  - It is normal that when there has been longstanding pain/distress that there is fear about "pushing" on the part of patients and parents ("the fear factor").
  - Although sometimes an increase in pain/distress means that treatment is not working, other times it can mean that it is.
  - It is usual that in the process of supporting change that new "crises" are created in the family.
- Regardless of the specific illness entity, any pain/distress is eased by the presence of empathic interpersonal connections with family and health care providers.
  - Families can learn to communicate about painful things in productive versus destructive ways.

Population Served

Patients admitted to the HCPHP are between 6 and 18 years of age and have combinations of medical diagnoses as well as psychiatric diagnoses. Additional admission criteria include the following:

- Patients must be medically and/or psychiatrically stable enough to not require 24-hour hospitalization.
- If recently discharged from an inpatient medical or psychiatric unit, patients must be at high risk of rehospitalization.
- If currently treated on an outpatient basis, patients have evidence of lack of response to medical and psychiatric treatment to date and/or must be at risk of needing an inpatient level of medical or psychiatric care.
- Patients must have evidence of marked impairment of functioning (eg, inability to attend school or attend to activities of daily living).
- Patients must be able to communicate in English, even if it is not their primary language (the program can accommodate patients if their family members do not speak English).

Criteria that may preclude admission to HCPHP include the following:

- Recent history of severe aggression.
- Developmental delay of a severity that precludes engagement in the therapeutic milieu.
- Inability of the family to transport patient to and from the program and/or inability to participate in family-based aspects of care (minimum of 2 family therapy sessions per week within program hours, as well as daily communication).
- Of note is that on rare occasions HCPHP has served patients living in state custody who are in group or foster homes (in which case, group home staff or foster parents participate in program treatment).

Common *Diagnostic and Statistical Manual of Mental Disorders, 5th Edition*, diagnoses treated at the HCPHP include the following: anorexia nervosa, bulimia nervosa, avoidant/restrictive food intake disorder, pain disorder with medical and psychological factors, somatic symptom disorder, conversion disorder, major depressive disorder, obsessive compulsive disorder, generalized anxiety disorder, social phobia, and panic disorder. Less frequent psychiatric diagnoses include major depressive disorder with psychotic features, and catatonia. Common pediatric illnesses presenting to HCPHP include type I diabetes mellitus, asthma, inflammatory bowel disorders, irritable bowel syndrome, encopresis, eczema, celiac disease, pediatric cancer, seizure disorder, refractory headache, failure to thrive, and malnutrition. Less common pediatric diagnoses have included epidermolysis bullosa, lupus, Duchenne's' muscular dystrophy, sickle cell disease, and congenital syndromes, such as VACTERL association and congenital heart disease.

The HCPHP preadmission process involves an extensive review of presenting challenges and history with family members and existing providers to ensure that admission is appropriate in terms of clinical criteria as well as timing in the trajectory of treatment. An experienced full-time licensed independent clinical social worker (LICSW) is the intake coordinator with support from a full-time social work assistant (bachelor of arts degree) to coordinate patient flow and triage. The following are notable points based on experience:

- Regardless of how motivated providers may be for a patient to be admitted to the program, unless a parent/guardian makes a direct call to express interest in the program, the referral is not placed on the wait list.
- Substantial effort is used to reduce barriers to participation in the program, including mobilization of extended family or community supports to assist with transportation and support for parents to be granted leniency from employers to participate in schedule of treatment.
- Admission is voluntary, although it is not uncommon for patients to be reluctant or resistant to attend the program, in which case, program staff mobilize support for families to effectively respond to meet their child's needs.
- Rarely, patients and families are mandated by child protective services via family court to participate in the program in spite of parental resistance.

Staffing

The range of disciplines within HCPHP include pediatricians, child psychiatrists, psychologists, social workers, pediatric nurses, a psychiatric nurse practitioner, a certified nursing assistant, milieu therapists, certified teachers, unit secretaries, registered dieticians, and a diet technician. Patients also commonly require pediatric rehabilitation consultation and intervention during their stay. The program closely consults with pediatric rehabilitation staff including physical therapists, occupational therapists, and speech therapists. As billing for these services falls under outpatient services rather than the bundled rate for the program, these professionals fall under the budgets of the pediatric rehabilitation department of the hospital. Patients also have access to pediatric subspecialty consultation from hospital-based providers (also via separate billing from the program day rate), such as neuropsychology or neurology. Program staffing has proportionally increased with rising census goals over the years (**Table 1**).

Structure of the Day

The program is highly structured with the following goals:

- Having a daily schedule 7:45 AM –3:15 PM that mimics a school day (**Table 2**);
- Providing educational supports/remediation;
- Providing support for nutritional needs of patients; and
- Providing a range of psychotherapeutic supports on individual, family, and group bases.

Of note is that other services that are worked into the fabric of the daily structure include nursing and pediatric assessment or education sessions as needed, individual

Table 1
Hasbro Children's Partial Hospital Program staffing ratios

Staff	Total FTE for Average Census Goal- 22.4
Pediatric codirector	1.0
Psychiatric codirector	0.9
Clinical manager (RN)	1.0
Milieu manager (BA)	1.0
Intake coordinator (LICSW)	1.0
Chief psychologist	1.0
Staff pediatrician	1.5
Staff psychiatrist	0.9
Psychiatric nurse practitioner	1.0
Social worker (LICSW)	0.4
Social work assistant (BA)	1.0
Psychology	2.8
Milieu therapist (BA)	6.5
Pediatric nurse	4.0
Certified nursing assistant	0.9
Registered dietician	1.5
Diet technician	1.0
Program teachers	1.5
Unit secretaries	1.9
Per diem staff includes teachers, nurses, and milieu therapists	

Abbreviations: BA, bachelor of arts; FTE, full-time equivalent; LICSW, licensed independent clinical social worker; RN, registered nurse.

therapy 3 times per week, family therapy at minimum of twice per week, pediatric rehabilitation consultations and treatment as needed, and nutrition education sessions as needed. For parents, there are also 2 multifamily support groups per week that they

Table 2
Hasbro Children's Partial Hospital Program schedule

Time	Activity
7:15–7:45	Staff report (nursing, milieu therapist, certified nursing assistant)
7:45–8:15	Nursing check-in with family
8:30–9:00	Breakfast
9:00–9:30	Community meeting
9:30–10:15	Skills building curriculum (group format, milieu therapist led)
10:15–10:30	Morning snack (for select patients)
10:30–12:00	School for patients/treatment team rounds for the team
12:15–12:45	Lunch
1:00–2:00	Group therapy (clinician led)/1 day per week therapeutic art activity
2:00–2:30	Milieu activity
2:30–2:45	Afternoon snack
2:45–3:15	Nursing check-out with family

may attend. One is an open support group focused on parents' emotional processing of their treatment experience, and the other is parent training on skills that their children are taught in the program. The HCPHP Skill-Building Curriculum is a group curriculum focused on practice with coping skills informed by DBT, CBT, and relaxation training evidence-based treatments.

Admissions

Program admissions are all scheduled and occur 8:30 to 11:30 AM in a team format. When the patient and family arrive at 8:30, they are greeted by a member of the intake team (LICSW or SW Assistant) who meets with them to review the program structure and community rules and have parents sign releases for HCPHP staff to communicate with community health care providers and schools. From 9:15 to 9:30, the program teacher meets with the patient and family to obtain basic understanding of educational status of the entering student and to review the HCPHP school structure. Starting at 9:30, the primary team for the patient (nurse, pediatrician, primary therapist, and psychiatrist) meets the family and spends 60 to 90 minutes in a team admission discussion. The patient is generally present for approximately 75% of the discussion with additional collateral time for parent discussion. The primary therapist serves as the anchor for the admission discussion, which covers presenting illness challenges, medical/psychiatric and family history, psychosocial history and risk assessment, and initial treatment plan. Of note is that the primary team often has access to a significant amount of preadmission history information provided by family and previous/current providers.

Although the complexity of the patients presenting for treatment to HCPHP is high, the goal of the team admission process is not to review all areas in detail, but rather to join with the patient and family around their understanding of presenting challenges and how they are working together and with providers to address these challenges. On completion of the team portion of the admission process, the parents often have some additional conversation with the primary therapist and also spend time completing a clinical admission packet that takes approximately 30 minutes. The admission data collected include the following:

Parent data:

- Pediatric Quality of Life (PedsQL) Core and PedsQL Family Impact[15,16]
- Illness Beliefs Questionnaire (IBQ) (Appendix 1)
- Family Relationship Index (FRI)[17–20]
- Health Care Utilization (see Appendix 1)
- Screen for Child Anxiety-Related Disorders (SCARED)[21]
- Children's Depression Inventory (CDI)[22]

Patient data:

- PedsQL Core
- IBQ
- Family Relationship Index (FRI)
- Screen for Child Anxiety-Related Disorders (SCARED)
- Children's Depression Inventory (CDI)
- Eating Disorder Evaluation (EDE),[23] when applicable

On leaving the team admission discussion, the patient has a medical examination by the pediatrician and then spends time with a milieu therapist with the goal of getting comfortable before joining the milieu group. During school time of their first day, patients complete a clinical admission packet similar to that completed by parents (depending on the child's age), to obtain their perspectives as well. The patient is also assessed individually by the psychologist and psychiatrist on the admission day.

Length of Stay

The median length of stay at HCPHP over its years of operation has ranged from 18 to 20 days. Of course within this, is a range with a subpopulation of the highest-need patients being outliers in the distribution. For the subset of patients who may have a history of several lengthy inpatient admissions and multiple diagnoses, the length of stay may be as much as 3 to 4 months. These outlier patients often come from out of the region, having failed multiple intensive levels of care. Common within this subset are patients with comorbid somatoform and eating disorders, a history of complex trauma, and/or a history of alleged or confirmed medical abuse.[24]

Decisions about timing of discharge occur in collaboration with families and outpatient providers. The standard goals before discharge include the following:

- Clarity about diagnoses and optimal treatment plan
- Establishment of patient safety/stability in medical/psychiatric terms and families
- A sense of confidence that patients can continue progress in the outpatient realm

Although the hope of the team is that both patients and families have significantly moved "forward on the FBIC graph" in terms of having established an accurate and mobilizing perspective regarding their illness and having shifted to a productive relationship pattern around managing their illness, this is not always the case. It is possible that patients have shifted a lot and parents little or vice versa or neither. The reasons that lack of movement by patient and/or family does not always indicate a need for a more prolonged stay include the following:

- It is not unusual given the treatment trajectories required to shift cognitive distortions of eating disorders, depression, anxiety, and somatoform disorders that patients may still be "stuck" in maladaptive beliefs on discharge. However, if their families are understanding of this and mobilized, then moving back into the routines of life with outpatient support serves to "take power away from the illness."
- If parents remain very distorted in their own thinking about their child's illness challenges and/or continue to exhibit destructive patterns of relating to their child even with the intensive support of HCPHP, then the intervention in HCPHP may include parent referral to mental health treatment, mobilization of extended family/community support network around the child's care needs, and/or child protective intervention in collaboration with state child protective services. The key to movement in such cases is not dependent on a lengthier stay for the child at HCPHP, but a stay long enough to clarify the barriers to health with referrals appropriate to meet child and family needs on discharge.

Although uncommon, patients are sometimes discharged within a much shorter timeframe than average. Associated scenarios include the following:

- The family may become aware that they cannot logistically manage the time commitment required by the program due to competing family needs, or they demonstrate with behavior an inability to do so. In these cases, we collaborate with families about maximizing outpatient supports as well as problem-solving about what may mitigate barriers to allow their child to come back when able to participate. We find it more productive to therapeutically discharge a patient than to continue an admission while accommodating to their avoidance patterns.

- Sometimes team efforts to "create a crisis" by shifting entrenched maladaptive patient and family patterns leads to an escalation of symptoms (either medical or psychiatric or both) that the family is unable to safely manage at home. In this case, plans are made for inpatient medical or psychiatric admission to our facility with the goal of program return once stable. This is framed not as failure but as indicative of the need for more support during the most challenging phases of transformation.
- Sometimes parent beliefs are so distorted that they cannot be contained within the structure and beliefs of the program. This may be because they believe "more medical intervention is needed" or "not so much psychiatric intervention is needed." If we are unable to finesse joining within our program containment structure we prepare outpatient teams for the reality of the situation with the goal of allowing for return to intensive treatment when the parent may be more amenable. Of course in extreme cases child protective efforts may need to be mobilized.

Check-In/Check-Out

Program nurses organize check-in and check-out discussions with families. This process serves as the daily bridge between the program and families as we join to support the needs of the patients. Each milieu area has a check-in/check-out room for these conversations. In the morning, nurses meet with patients and families together to review overnight/weekend goals, hear about challenges, and reinforce the treatment process. Themes of these conversations include reminders about externalizing the illness and the importance of family teamwork, as well as support around symptom escalations being expectable while doing the hard work of breaking nonproductive patterns. Although parents often (especially early in the course of treatment) are very symptom focused, nurses always make a point to check on parents' understanding of symptom patterns (eg "What did you make of him having a worse headache last night?"). This provides an important window into where parents are in their illness belief shifts as well as providing an opportunity to reinforce program illness beliefs. Check-ins also provide an opportunity for families to pass on written records (eg, meal plan and diabetic records, program point sheet) and to pass on questions they may have for other members of the team.

Afternoon check-out is generally the nurse and parent and provides an opportunity to review the patient's functioning over the course of the day. Although symptom patterns may be reported (along with details of medical treatment), it is always anchored in the context of how the patient has functioned. This can range from a patient who is highly distressed physically and/or emotionally who struggled to accept staff help to use coping strategies, to a patient who has had great success breaking previously self-destructive and avoidant patterns to function at a higher and more independent level. The language and frame is not one of success or failure based on symptoms, but rather on acceptance of help and active coping with challenges.

Physical Space

The current program space for providing care to 24 patients (annual census goal 22.4) is 9310 square feet (**Table 3**).

Other key elements of the space plan include the following:

- Location of program space on the hospital campus for ease of access to emergency department, hospital security, hospital laboratories and imaging, pediatric rehabilitation services, and pediatric subspecialists.

Table 3
Hasbro Children's Partial Hospital Program space breakdown

Spaces	Number	Function
Lobby	1	Seating for 24 families for check-in and check-out
Front office	1	Secretarial reception window and work area and work space for nutrition team
Milieu area	3	Patient dayrooms
Check-in/out rooms	3	Check-in/out with families, family education meetings and overflow area for patients needing 1:1 interventions
Nursing station	1	Nursing work area and houses medication dispensing machine
Patient bathrooms	5	3 contiguous with milieu; 2 separate (one of which has handicapped access tub and shower)
Examination/treatment rooms	3	Pediatric/nursing examination areas and space for procedures
Family dining room	1	Therapeutic meals, group therapy and family/network meetings
Milieu therapy office	1	Work space and storage for MT team
Teacher's office	1	Shared work space for teachers
Large meeting room	1	Group therapy, network meetings, physical therapy, and admissions
"Quiet room"	1	Physical therapy, milieu overflow for 1:1 intervention and restraint area
Kitchen	2	Storage and food preparation
Team rounds room	1	Rounds, network meetings, and multifamily group
Staff lounge	1	Storage and lunch area
Clinician offices	11	Individual and family therapy

- The entire program area is badge access except for the main entry near reception that remains open during the program day but that has lock-down capability for elopement prevention.
- Multiple milieu overflow areas for when patients need to take space from the group (for treatment tasks or behavioral time-out plans).
- Access to an outdoor courtyard contiguous with the program that allows for outdoor therapeutic activities when weather permits, as well as individualized patient activity/exercise plans.
- The presence of 2 additional bathrooms noncontiguous to milieus given the frequency of toileting plans in the population served (eg, usually 3–6 patients across program who may have some version of nursing-supervised toileting schedule).
- The ability of many rooms to serve multiple functions. Most often, all communal spaces are in constant use throughout the program day (aside from 10:30–12:00 when patients participate in school, and team clinical rounds are happening).

The Milieu

Each of the 3 patient milieus serves as the anchor space for their day where they participate in milieu activities, meals and snacks, and school. Each milieu area is supervised by 2 milieu therapists per group, as well as intermittent presence of nursing staff. Key aspects of the power of the milieu include the following:

- Clear community rules are reviewed with entering patients and reinforced.
- Any newly hired program staff, newly rotating trainees, or volunteers receive an orientation before participating in any activities within the milieu.
- Although there needs to be fluidity throughout the program day for patients to leave for various treatment tasks and therapies, an effort is made for the milieu to feel like an undisrupted space. Team coordination occurs to try to avoid disrupting community meetings once started. Also, for patients on supervised meal plans, an effort is made to avoid removing them during meals and snacks unless the therapist is supervising the meal/snack for therapeutic purposes.
- An important aspect of the program experience embodied by the milieu is the process of patients (many of whom have been hospitalized or have been out of school for extended periods) practicing reintegration into a peer group.
- Having 3 milieus allows for keeping patients grouped by age/developmental ranges that maximize the impact of peer support and allow for appropriately targeted therapeutic activities. Of import is that the older teen milieu (14–18 years old) is usually the largest group (up to 10), whereas the youngest group (6–10 years old) is the smallest (usually 6). That being said, depending on the age range on the program wait list, the "youngest" milieu sometimes includes the tween age bracket. An effort is made to group the youngest patients together (so most commonly the youngest group varies between a 6–9-year-old set and a 9–12-year-old set).

Nutrition

The ability to accommodate 2 meals and 2 snacks per day allows for much-needed calorie support for patients who are the most nutritionally compromised. Although the goal is for patients to succeed with meal plans in the home environment, having the program as an anchor to gradually transition the highest-calorie meal plans to home gradually with use of evenings and weekends as test ground is welcome to families who are acclimating to the details of these intense plans. In addition to the obvious role the nutrition team and structure of HCPHP provide for severely nutritionally compromised patients, there are a range of nutrition needs that the broader population treated by the program presents.

In addition to support for standard-spectrum eating disorders, nutrition issues addressed include the following:

- Support for patients and families managing both type 1 and type 2 diabetes.
- Support for overweight patients with medical comorbidities.
- Support for nutritional repletion of patients with pediatric chronic illness (eg, cystic fibrosis, cancer).
- Management of refractory "picky eaters" with growth delays.
- Management of celiac disease and food allergies.
- Coordination regarding patients who are gastric tube dependent (often patients are referred to move off of tube dependency).

School

The role of school programming at HCPHP is to support patients' preparation for reintegration into their regular school setting. Although we are not a "school placement," teachers are certified by state parameters. The teachers work a half-time morning schedule to allow for preparation and home-school collaboration time, as well as receiving report on patient status from clinical staff before school time of 10:30 to 12:00. There is a large range of educational functioning in the patients treated in the program from highly functional students who have missed school due to health issues to low-functioning students in need of very specialized supports. In addition to the supports provided by program teachers, primary therapists are very involved in communicating with home-school personnel to collaborate about how educational and health needs can best be addressed on reentry. Common educational goals during HCPHP stay include the following:

- Keeping students on track with current work provided by home school.
- Providing remediation support for students who are far behind in school.
- Clarifying at what educational level students are functioning.
- Clarifying issues impeding educational function.
- Advocating and formulating reentry and overall educational accommodations needed for return to home school, which may be in the form of a newly formed or modified 504 plan or individualized education plan.
- Identifying needs for additional evaluation to support educational planning (psychoeducational testing, neuropsychological testing, speech and language/physical therapy/occupational therapy evaluations).

The Point System

Every patient in the program has a "point card" on which to track their participation in all aspects of the day and on which they write down their daily goals during community meeting. Point cards are developmentally modified; for tweens and teens, staff give points on a 0 to 4 graded point system, and for younger patients, a "stamp system" (0, 1, or 2 stamps for effort) is used. There are point cards for home as well, to allow for a common language and set of expectations across settings. Patients "cash in" their points in a multilevel "point store" stocked with a variety of rewards twice daily, in the morning for home earnings and in the afternoon for program earnings. Key elements of this token economy system include the following:

- It provides a concrete representation for the hard work patients are doing on their plans.
- It provides connectivity between program and home for goal setting and tracking. It is a reminder that messages and structuring/coaching from adults matters.
- Family struggles with maintaining/using the point card are reflective of larger family systems issues with communication, messaging, and maintaining limits that need attention.
- A patient's trajectory of engagement with the system over the course of his or her stay is a barometer for their "owning" aspects of their treatment and health.
- Although patients all begin with standard point cards, there is plenty of leeway to individualize them with specific goals determined by discussion among patients, families, and the treatment team.
- It is important that in collaboration with patients and families expectations/goals are expanded over the course of the stay.

The Process of Collaborative Care

The presence of a colocated interdisciplinary team is necessary but not sufficient for collaborative care. Both within the team at HCPHP and via the team's collaboration with outpatient providers and schools, there are clear means of collaboration.

Within the HCPHP team structure, a key component of care coordination occurs within the structure of multidisciplinary team rounds. Of note regarding the rounds' structure and functioning is the following:

- Team rounds occur daily. On Mondays and Fridays, all 24 patients across 3 milieus are discussed (90 minutes). On other days, a single milieu is reviewed (60 minutes). In this way, each milieu group is discussed by the whole team 3 days per week.
- All team members attend rounds on their milieu. Nurses and milieu therapists from each milieu rotate in and out on "all milieu" rounds days, whereas clinical staff (pediatrics, psychology, psychiatry) are present throughout as each member's patients are spread across milieus. Registered dieticians provide written sign outs for "all milieu days" and attend in entirety on single milieu days. Teachers attend rounds once weekly on single milieu days.
- Each discipline contributes each day in rounds. There is a specific order to stay streamlined: pediatric nurses report on check-in information and their clinical observations, nutrition input, pediatric update, milieu report, psychiatric update, and primary therapist report. Each discipline reports on their perspective to support the coordinated team effort to empower the patient and family moving forward with illness management.
- Many treatment decisions are able to be made in rounds with multidisciplinary input, although it is also common that rounds may signal an area that further discussion across disciplines is needed before a decision.
- When new admissions happen, the team rounds discussion focuses on presenting challenges, brief review of history/family context, and note on "where we are" with family beliefs and relationships. The initial treatment plan also is discussed.

In addition to team rounds, other avenues for team collaboration include the following:

- "Break Outs" are meetings of the pediatrician, psychiatrist, primary therapist, and registered dietician, as well as representatives from nursing and milieu therapy to have a more detailed discussion of a behavior plan or area of challenge for a given patient. This is also the modality used to process differences of opinion across the treatment team, as well as for complex case management planning. These meetings occur on Tuesday through Thursday after single milieu rounds between 11:30 and 12:00.
- HCPHP Leadership meeting is weekly with focus on coordinating program operations and clinical programming. In attendance are psychiatric and pediatric co-directors, clinical manager (Registered Nurse), intake coordinator (LICSW), milieu supervisor, and chief psychologist.
- A clinician weekly meeting occurs with a purpose of support around challenging cases and coordination of care across disciplines, and includes pediatrics, psychiatry, psychology, psychiatric nurse practitioner, and social work.
- Nursing, milieu therapy, and teachers have subgroup meetings coordinated by collaboration between the clinical manager and milieu supervisor.
- Monthly, all staff meetings rotate among didactic topics, case conferences, and program development collaboration.
- Semiannually all staff retreats occur for a half day and are focused on team building and program development tasks.

With regard to HCPHP team collaboration with outpatient providers and schools, the following are notable:

- Pediatricians coordinate communication with the primary care provider as well as medical subspecialists involved.

- Psychiatrists or psychiatric nurse practitioner coordinates with outpatient psychotropic medication prescriber.
- Primary therapists coordinate with outpatient therapists and schools, as well as parent providers when applicable.
- Communication occurs early in the stay, as well as in preparation for discharge.
- It is not unusual to have a team network meeting (in person and/or by phone), including a range of outpatient providers and school personnel.
- For the most complicated, high-risk patients it is common to have a follow-up network meeting approximately a month after discharge.

Patient Experience

Patients have a wide variety of therapeutic experiences across all program disciplines and the program day. The range of experiences include milieu activities including community meeting, skill-building sessions, therapeutic art experiences, and recreational activities; small amounts of unstructured time in the milieu, which allow for socialization practice under supervision; snack and meal supervision (at times individualized); nursing check-in discussions, assessment, and illness-specific education sessions; nutritional education sessions; one-on-one time with milieu therapists with guided practice for coping strategies; individual therapy with patient-specific focus (CBT, DBT, motivational interviewing, relaxation training, preparation for family therapy); family therapy sessions (may involve one or both parents, siblings, extended family); group therapy with peers; pediatric rehabilitation sessions; and education support from teachers.

Family Experience

It is not uncommon for parents (and other family members) to spend up to several hours per week with a range of program staff. Experiences include check-in and check-out discussion with nursing; nursing education sessions; nutrition education sessions; family therapy sessions, including collateral parent time and conjoint meetings with patients (with extended family network meetings or divorce counseling as indicated); school planning meetings with support from program staff; and multifamily parent groups.

Fiscal Considerations

The HCPHP program has included state and private payers from the outset with bundled rates negotiated with each payer. The proportion of patients covered by state insurance has been approximately 30% to 40% over the life of the program.

Key aspects that allowed for success with the program's initial business plan included the following:

- Establishment of a bundled day rate inclusive of most program billing (not including rehabilitation services, laboratory and other diagnostic tests, subspecialty consultation, and some pediatric billing, dependent on payer).
- Establishment of the need for program services by highlighting excessive costs of high-risk patients with repeated medical admissions (eg, patients with eating disorders requiring supervised refeeding; diabetic patients with frequent trips to the pediatric intensive care unit for diabetic ketoacidosis) who could be more optimally treated in a day hospital setting at lower cost.
- Negotiating for payment across medical and psychiatric side of payers (of note is that for 18 years, one major payer paid for program services out of the medical benefit and other payers covered costs under the psychiatric benefit).

Key aspects that have allowed for ongoing success include the following:

- The ongoing gap in integrated services for this population across the country has led to extremely high demand.
- An expanding mix of payers generated by increasing use of the program by out-of-state and out-of-region patients over time.
- Maintaining the concept of a bundled day rate.
- Effective advocacy in utilization review around these patients "not meeting typical psychiatric day-treatment criteria."

Case Example 1: Family-Based Integrated Care Treatment Course

Treatment in the FBIC model reinforced the notion of food as medicine, and encouraged family and patient to externalize the eating disorder, in turn making it more comfortable to actively fight the eating disorder in an effort to care for and support their teenager. Needing to make decisions about treatment contrary to "Brittany's wishes" was stressed. The team partnered with parents to prioritize feeding their child adequately for her needs, just as they would ensure she got the exact needed dose of chemotherapy or insulin if she had cancer or diabetes. Activity restriction was also recommended from a medical, nutritional, and psychological perspective. Being clear about expectations of treatment was essential, including communicating that it would not be expected that Brittany's perspective or motivation for recovery would change over the course of the admission. The impact of the stress of the eating disorder on family was explored, and identifying the need for parents to remain intimately involved in all nutrition-related plans while looking at other areas of a patients' life in which she could assert some independence and autonomy. Parents engaged in coached family meals, as well as nutrition education, psychoeducation sessions, and multifamily groups. Despite ongoing disagreement about the specifics of the plan, by discharge Brittany had reached her goal weight range, resulting in significant medical improvements (resolution of bradycardia and improvement in orthostasis). Of note, she identified several positive symptomatic shifts as well, including resolution of dizziness with standing; improved energy level, concentration, and attention; and healthier skin and hair. Parents noted that they were "starting to get (their) daughter back." However, significant shifts in distorted cognitions and unhealthy thinking do not occur in this phase of treatment. Psychoeducation for families about the importance of ongoing intensive, integrated treatment, as well as the persistence of a high level of supervision and support was a critical piece of the work.

Case Example 2: Family-Based Integrated Care Treatment Course

Treatment in the FBIC model in the context of the intradisciplinary day-treatment setting focused on having Joann attend the program daily, even on days when her pain was most severe. Daily contact with the nursing team, as well as frequent contact with the pediatrician who was in close contact with Joann's outpatient team, helped increase the family's trust that Joann could attend the program daily although she had been out of school for several months. The entire treatment team acknowledged that Joann's pain was real and supported the family in helping Joann increase her functioning while medical care was provided. This included participation in milieu activities and also reengaging in previously enjoyed social and recreational activities outside of the program. Attention to pain was decreased and a focus on pain coping skills was increased. Individual and family therapy focused on setting functional goals, supporting Joann in expressing her experience of anxiety and role in the family to her parents, and validating emotional stress associated with parenting a child with chronic pain. Joann began treatment with a selective serotonin reuptake inhibitor, and toward the end of treatment completed several days of school transition before leaving HCPHP. Together, these interventions positively influenced the family's beliefs about her pain (eg, that Joann could improve her functioning despite pain symptoms) and increased emotional closeness in their relationships as they better understood Joann's anxiety. Joann and her family were referred to outpatient individual and family therapy to support her and the family's progress.

Case Example 3: Family-Based Integrated Care Treatment Course

Treatment in the FBIC model encouraged family members to share unspoken beliefs and empathized with the events that had led to those beliefs (some very healthy, such as the reality of his high level of functioning as a younger child). The impact of the stress of diabetes on family relationships was a focus, as was identifying what Caleb and his parents wanted their relationship to look like at this point in their lives. Caleb's parents were able to share their uncertainty about how to help, given his resistance to their efforts and Caleb was able to share his anxiety and the changing sense of self that he experienced from being "beaten by diabetes." His parents conveyed that they did not see Caleb's struggles as indicating that diabetes had won and therefore controlled his future. Hearing their optimism that he could be healthier, Caleb became more open to support from his parents, and they negotiated acceptable involvement in his regimen. Six months after discharge from a 4-week stay on the day-treatment unit, Caleb's HbA1c showed significant improvement, and his depressive symptoms had largely resolved.

SUMMARY

The FBIC model provides a productive conceptual framework for treating complex pediatric illness. The HCPHP provides an example of operationalizing this model in the treatment of high-intensity illness challenges for patients who have failed less intensive treatment or who have required extensive inpatient medical and psychiatric care without being able to transition their health gains to the home environment.

Important implications of this model and its use in the HCPHP include the following:

- Any painful challenge/symptom/illness is improved with an empowered set of beliefs about illness and an empathic, mobilized set of relationships, which is most effectively accomplished via a family-based treatment model with integrated messages across providers.
- By intensive work with patients and families, illness beliefs and relationship patterns within families can be modified, and targeting these areas can improve treatment outcomes.
- If we are oriented to "where we are" with family relationships and illness beliefs, we will have the ability to most productively join with the patient and family and support their journey toward empowerment over the illness.
- Consistent messages from health care providers and across health care providers matter, are powerful forces influencing successful treatment, and can be effectively be guided by the FBIC model.
- Excellent provider collaboration is a strong force in supporting patient/family efficacy in illness management and securing quality of life.

Current research on treatment outcomes at the HCPHP is focused on assessment of shifts in patient and family quality of life, family illness beliefs, and health care utilization patterns from program admission to discharge, as well as 3-month, 6-month, and 1-year follow-up. Results of this research will inform continued optimization of the FBIC model as used in a day-treatment setting. Additional research on the application of this model across levels of care is essential as well, with the goal of matching the intensity of treatment intervention to a range in patient and family needs that is illness independent.

REFERENCES

1. Roesler TA, Rickerby ML, Nassau JH, et al. Treating a high risk population: a collaboration of child psychiatry and pediatrics. Med Health R I 2002;85(9): 265–8.
2. Rickerby ML, Roesler TA. Child Psychiatrists in Family Based Integrated Care. Child Adolesc Psychiatric Clin N Am 2015;24(3):501–15.
3. Patterson J, Vakili S. Relationships, environment, and the brain: how emerging research is changing what we know about the impact of families on human development. Fam Process 2014;53(1):22–32.
4. Kaslow NJ, Broth MR, Smith CO, et al. Family based interventions for child and adolescent disorders. J Marital Fam Ther 2012;38(91):82–100.
5. Retzlaff R, Von Sydow K, Behar S, et al. The efficacy of systemic therapy for internalizing and other disorders of childhood and adolescence: a systematic review of 38 randomized controlled trials. Fam Process 2014;32(4):619–52.
6. Scott S. Parenting quality and children's mental health: biological mechanisms and psychological interventions. Curr Opin Psychiatry 2012;25(4):301–6.
7. Siegenthaler E, Munder T, Egger M. Effect of preventive interventions in mentally ill parents on the mental health of the offspring: systematic review and meta-analysis. J Am Acad Child Adolesc Psychiatry 2012;51(1):8–17.
8. Wamboldt MZ, Wamboldt FS. Role of the family in the onset and outcome of childhood disorders: selected research findings. J Am Acad Child Adolesc Psychiatry 2000;39(10):1212–9.
9. Von Sydow K, Retzlaff R, Behar S, et al. The efficacy of systemic therapy for childhood and adolescent externalizing disorders: a systematic review of 47 randomized controlled trials. Fam Process 2013;52(4):576–618.
10. Rickerby ML, Roesler TA, editors. Family-based treatment in child and adolescent psychiatry. Philadelphia: Elsevier; 2015.
11. Weihs K, Fisher L, Baird M. Families, health, and behavior. A section of the commissioned report by the Committee on Health and Behavior: Research, Practice, and Policy Division of Neuroscience and Behavioral Health and Division of Health Promotion and Disease Prevention Institute of Medicine, National Academy of Sciences. Fam Syst Health 2002;20:7–46.
12. Engel GL. The need for a new medical model: a challenge for biomedicine. Science 1977;196:129–36.
13. Anderson LA, Freeman JB, Franklin ME, et al. Family-based treatment of pediatric obsessive-compulsive disorder: clinical considerations and application. Child Adolesc Psychiatric Clin N Am 2015;24(3):535–55.
14. Forsberg S, Lock J. Family-based treatment of child and adolescent eating disorders. Child Adolesc Psychiatric Clin N Am 2015;24(3):617–29.
15. Varni JW, Seid M, Rode CA. The PedsQL: measurement model for the pediatric life inventory. Med Care 1999;37(2):126–39.
16. Varni JW, Sherman SA, Burwinkle TM, et al. The PedsQL family impact module: preliminary reliability and validity. Health Qual Life Outcomes 2004;2(1):55–60.

17. Holahan CJ, Moos RH. The quality of social support: measures of family and work relationships. Br J Clin Psychol 1983;22:157–62.

18. Moos RH. Conceptual and empirical approaches to developing family-based assessment procedures: resolving the case of the family environment scale. Fam Process 1990;29(2):199–208.

19. Calam R, Gregg L, Simpson B, et al. Childhood asthma, behavior problems, and family functioning. J Allergy Clin Immunol 2003;112(3):499–504.

20. Edwards B, Clarke V. The validity of the family relationships index as a screening tool for psychological risk in families of cancer patients. Psychooncology 2005; 14(7):546–54.

21. Birmaher B, Brent DA, Chiappetta L, et al. Psychometric properties of the screen for child anxiety related emotional disorders (SCARED): a replication study. J Am Acad Child Adolesc Psychiatry 1999;38(10):1230–6.

22. Kovacs M. Children's depression inventory (CDI2): technical manual. North Tonawanda (NY): Multi-Health Systems, Inc; 2011.

23. Fairburn CG, Beglin S. Eating disorder examination questionnaire. In: Fairburn CG, editor. Cognitive behavior therapy and eating disorders. New York: Guilford Press; 2008. p. 309–13.

24. Roesler TA, Jenny C. Medical child abuse: beyond Munchausen syndrome by proxy. Elk Grove (IL): American Academy of Pediatrics; 2009.

APPENDIX 1: CLINICAL/RESEARCH MEASURES OF HCPHP

1. Pediatric Quality of Life Inventory (PedsQL) Core 4.0.[15] The PedsQL 4.0 is a 23-item measure of health-related quality of life. Versions exist for parent report as well as child and adolescent (8–18 years) self-report. Responses are provided on a 5-point Likert scale.

2. Pediatric Quality of Life Inventory (PedsQL) Family Impact module 2.0.[16] The PedsQL Family Impact module assesses the impact of pediatric chronic conditions on parents and the family. These 36 items measure parent self-reported physical, emotional, social, and cognitive functioning; communication; and worry. The module also measures parent-reported family daily activities and family relationships. It has been shown to be valid and reliable. Only parents will complete this measure.

3. Illness Beliefs Questionnaire (IBQ). The IBQ was developed by the current research team to assess family beliefs about chronic pediatric illness. It consists of 30 items asked on a 5-point Likert scale. The IBQ has been shown to have convergent validity with other measures and be sensitive to treatment (Nassau JH, Development of an Illness Beliefs Questionnaire for chronic pediatric illness, 2010 [Grant number: R03HD061440]). The IBQ is completed by parents and children 13 or older.

4. Family Relationship Index (FRI).[17] The FRI is a 12-item measure derived from the Family Environment Scale.[18] The FRI is composed of 3 subscales measuring expressiveness (how much family members express feelings directly, 4 items), cohesion (the degree of help, commitment, and support family members provide, 4 items), and conflict (open conflict, anger, and aggression within the family, 4 items). Test-retest reliability and construct validity of the FRI are well established,[18] including for use with families of children with chronic illness.[19,20] The FRI is completed by parents and children 11 years or older.

5. Screen for Child Anxiety-Related Disorders (SCARED).[21] The SCARED is a 41-item symptom inventory of anxiety disorders for children and adolescents 8 years and older that has been shown to be valid and reliable. Both parent-report and self-report versions exist and will be used in this study.

6. Health Care Utilization (HCU). The HCU was developed for program use to assess the frequency with which patients admitted to HCPHP use health care services, as many families use numerous services in attempts to address the significant health care needs of their children. These parent-report items were adapted from the National Health Interview Survey Child Access to Health Care and Utilization module, which assesses health care services utilization. These collect parent-report information of emergency department visits, days hospitalized (both medical and psychiatric), and outpatient visits (both medical and psychiatric) to gather information regarding services provided outside of the Lifespan medical system (LifeChart record). The HCU is completed by parents only.

7. Children's Depression Inventory 2 (CDI-2)–parent report version.[22] The CDI-2 is a 17-item parent-report symptom inventory of children's depressive symptoms for youth ages 7 to 17. The measure has been shown to have strong psychometric properties. Only parents will complete this measure.

8. Eating Disorder Examination–Questionnaire (EDE-Q).[23] The EDE-Q is a self-report measure assessing the features of eating disorders. The psychometric properties of the EDE-Q have been well studied and shown to correspond to clinical interviews for assessment of eating disorders. Only adolescents 13 or older who received the EDE-Q as part of their admission evaluation will complete the EDE-Q as part of their research participation.

Preliminary Outcomes from an Integrated Pediatric Mental Health Outpatient Clinic

CrossMark

Gary R. Maslow, MD, MPH[a],*, Adrienne Banny, PhD[a],
McLean Pollock, PhD, MSW[a], Kristen Stefureac, MSW[a],
Kendra Rosa, MPH[a], Barbara Keith Walter, PhD, MPH[a],
Katherine Hobbs Knutson, MD, MPH[a], Joseph Lucas, PhD[b],
Nicole Heilbron, PhD[a]

KEYWORDS

- Integrated mental health • Emergency department utilization
- Mental health services • Access • Child • Adolescent

KEY POINTS

- Although 1 in 5 children in the United States meet criteria for a diagnosable mental or behavioral disorder, fewer than 20% receive needed mental health services.
- Unmet needs for psychiatric treatment may contribute to increased use of the emergency department (ED) and those with behavioral and psychiatric problems are at an increased risk of ED return.
- Strategies aimed at facilitating continuity of care between ED and outpatient care settings may lower rates of ED visits among pediatric patients.
- This article describes an integrated pediatric evaluation center designed to prevent treatment in the ED by increasing access care for emergent and critical mental health needs.

INTRODUCTION

An estimated 1 in 5 children in the United States meet criteria for a diagnosable psychiatric or behavioral disorder.[1,2] Yet fewer than 20% of these children receive needed mental health services, and even fewer are able to access appropriate, evidence-based care.[3] Limited access to mental health care has been characterized by a decrease in the number of inpatient beds and a scarcity of outpatient resources available for children and adolescents.[4] As a result of this reduced capacity within the

Disclosures: No disclosures.
[a] Department of Psychiatry and Behavioral Sciences, Duke University School of Medicine, 2608 Erwin Road, Suite 300, Durham, NC 27705, USA; [b] Social Science Research Institute, Duke University, Erwin Mill Building, 2024 W. Main Street, Durham, NC 27705, USA
* Corresponding author.
E-mail address: gary.maslow@duke.edu

Child Adolesc Psychiatric Clin N Am 26 (2017) 761–770
http://dx.doi.org/10.1016/j.chc.2017.06.008
1056-4993/17/© 2017 Elsevier Inc. All rights reserved.

childpsych.theclinics.com

Abbreviations

ED   Emergency department
FTE   Full-time equivalent

existing mental health service system, the emergency department (ED) is increasingly used to address pediatric mental health needs.[5–7]

Unmet need for psychiatric treatment may contribute to increased use of the ED for both medical and mental health concerns. Among children and adolescents who present to the ED, those with behavioral and psychiatric problems are at an increased risk of repeated admissions to the ED.[5,8,9] After discharge, up to 36% of children with psychiatric illness return to the ED within 72 hours,[9] and approximately 50% return within 2 months.[10,11] Many presentations among return ED users represent an exacerbation of a chronic psychiatric disorder.[10–12] These patterns of repeated use of the ED, particularly among high-risk children and adolescents with psychiatric conditions, may be related to a variety of factors, including limited or insufficient community mental health resources, lack of insurance coverage, and other barriers to care.

Strategies aimed at facilitating continuity of care between the ED and outpatient care settings may lower rates of ED visits among pediatric patients.[13] Providing patients who are seen in the ED with outpatient appointments before discharge, for example, significantly improves adherence to follow-up care plans, as compared with patients who are given standard discharge instructions.[14–16] Thus, by improving linkages to appropriate mental health services, repeat ED visits may be reduced.

The current article describes an integrated pediatric evaluation center designed to prevent the need for treatment in emergency settings by increasing access to timely and appropriate care for acute mental health needs. The Evaluation Center was developed to address the following goals:

1. Identify youths who could be diverted from the ED by providing clinically informed triage services and enhancing outpatient capacity for urgent assessments; and
2. Integrate mental health care between ED and outpatient care settings in an effort to reduce return ED visits.

METHOD
Evaluation Center Intervention

The Evaluation Center is an outpatient clinic that operates as the primary point of access for pediatric mental health services within a large academic medical center setting. The Evaluation Center is staffed by a multidisciplinary team that includes the following full-time equivalent (FTE) staff: 2.0 FTE licensed clinical social workers, 1.0 FTE licensed practical nurse, 0.4 FTE pediatric psychiatrist, 1.0 FTE nurse practitioner, and 1.0 FTE clinic coordinator. In addition to the permanent staff, the Evaluation Center provides training opportunities for psychiatry fellows and social work interns. The clinic includes an intake room, 2 medical examination rooms, 2 therapy rooms, a financial care counselor office, and a shared workspace for clinicians and the clinic coordinator. Access to translator services (in-person and phone) is available when needed.

The Evaluation Center operates as both a triage center and an outpatient mental health clinic. Referrals for new patient evaluations are received from the pediatric ED, pediatric specialty clinics, pediatric primary care, and the community (eg, community providers, agencies, schools, self-referrals). Consistent with the goal to facilitate continuity of care, patients in the pediatric ED can be discharged directly to the Evaluation Center. Internal, hospital-based referrals are received either by phone, through the electronic health record system, or in the case of urgent referrals, by page to the clinic coordinator. External referrals from the community are triaged primarily by phone. The clinic coordinator manages incoming referrals and determines whether each patient's individual needs can be best met by the Evaluation Center or if triage to a specialty service would be more appropriate (eg, developmental or neuropsychological testing). The clinic coordinator also provides referral information to patients who require linkage to mental health services in their community, either during the initial call or after assessment in the Evaluation Center.

Timely and appropriate referral coordination is facilitated by the use of an interactive referral search tool designed for clinical staff and providers within the hospital system. This database enables clinicians to quickly build personalized lists of community providers for patients. Mental health providers and clinics interested in being added to this database can apply online by completing a provider profile that includes information about types of mental health services provided (eg, assessment, therapy, medication management), populations served, insurance accepted, and capacity for new patients. Once approved, the information may be provided to patients who need referral information for providers in their community. To remain active in the database, participating clinicians are required to log in to their provider profile at least once every 6 months to ensure accurate and current referral information.

Outpatient mental health services provided in the Evaluation Center include assessment, short-term treatment of up to 5 visits, and care coordination. Initial visits are 90 minutes and include 30 minutes to complete intake materials. Specifically, the licensed practical nurse administers and scores self-report and informant-report versions of the DSM-5 Cross Cutting Symptoms measures.[17] The level I screener consists of 25 questions that assess 12 psychiatric domains, including depression, anger, irritability, mania, anxiety, somatic symptoms, inattention, suicidal ideation and behavior, psychosis, sleep disturbance, repetitive thoughts and behaviors, and substance use. Elevated scores on level I symptom domains indicate greater frequency or severity and prompt the administration of level II, symptom-specific measures. The licensed practical nurse assists with the administration of the measures.

After the completion of intake materials, patients meet with a social worker for an initial evaluation. The nurse practitioner or attending psychiatrist is available during these appointments for medication consultation. New patient evaluations may involve a single evaluation completed in 1 day, or an extended evaluation that takes place over the course of multiple sessions (range, 2–5). Patients who receive a single evaluation are appropriately triaged to either internal or community providers who can meet their long-term mental health needs. In the case of extended evaluations, the initial appointment is followed by time to gather collateral information, coordinate care with the referral site, and/or collaborate with other specialists. Follow-up visits also may allow time to provide brief intervention services (ie, psychotherapy, medication management) while coordinating long-term disposition plans. All care involves team-based case management. Accordingly, the multidisciplinary team meets during a regularly scheduled, weekly meeting to develop treatment plans and to coordinate care for complicated cases. Two weeks after discharge from the Evaluation Center, the clinic coordinator conducts follow-up phone calls to ensure that each patient has connected with the appropriate long-term provider. Cases that require continued care coordination are triaged back to the Evaluation Center to consult with a social worker. **Table 1** provides more information related to clinic flow and division of responsibilities.

Table 1
Evaluation center clinic flow

Step in the Clinic Flow	Person Responsible	Key Functions

Referral received
• Internal referral
  ○ Pediatric inpatient
  ○ Pediatric outpatient
  ○ Direct referral from ED
• Self-referral
• Community referral (eg, school system, community agency)
Referral may be via phone, pager (urgent), internal EHR referral (eg, primary care, pediatric specialty clinics)
	LPN	• Screen incoming phone referrals
		  ○ Refer to clinical triage based on phone screen results (eg, safety concerns, complex presenting problem)

	Clinic Coordinator	• Monitor and triage incoming referrals • Coordinate directly with ED to manage urgent referrals • Conduct safety assessments when indicated • Complete phone screens; enter results of phone screen in EHR • Provide coordinated referral for families who will not be scheduled in the Evaluation Center • Liaise with referring providers to confirm status of appointment
Patient arrives at Evaluation Center for appointment	LPN	• Prepare intake materials (eg, screeners, questionnaires) • Room patient, take vitals, medication reconciliation, documentation • Administer and score assessment measures and enter data • Gather any documentation that parent brings (eg, previous evaluations), scan into EHR, file
Evaluation	LCSW	• Liaise with referring providers • Assess/treat patient (psychosocial) • Develop treatment plan and safety plan, if needed • Identify and coordinate with potential long-term providers to ensure availability for new patients • Make recommendations for referral for long-term mental health needs
	MD	• Assess/treat patient (physical examination, psychiatric) • Order laboratory tests • Develop treatment plan and safety plan, if needed • Coordinate with social worker to address psychosocial treatment needs and case management • Make recommendations for referral
Postevaluation coordination and tasks	LPN	• Request records for follow-up • Facilitate follow-up appointments within the Evaluation Center and health system • Manage referrals from Evaluation Center to other specialty clinics (eg, neurology, OT, PT)
	Clinic coordinator	• Contact health system providers and programs and/or community providers and programs to coordinate referral process for long-term follow-up care • Liaise with LCSW and MD regarding patient disposition and treatment plan • Conduct follow-up calls to ensure that patient is connected with community referral

Abbreviations: ED, emergency department; EHR, electronic health record; LCSW, licensed clinical social worker; LPN, licensed practical nurse; OT, occupational therapy; PT, physical therapy.

To ensure prompt access to care for emergent mental health needs, two 1-hour appointment slots are reserved each day for children and adolescents who require urgent assessments, including patients discharged from the ED. Conducted by either a social worker, nurse practitioner, or psychiatrist, these visits focus primarily on safety assessment and safety planning. The goal of safety planning is to lower imminent risk for suicidal behavior by collaboratively generating a written, step-wise list of internal and external coping strategies that the patient can refer to should suicidal thoughts reemerge.[18] Initially developed as a brief intervention for suicidal adults, safety planning interventions have been adapted for use with adolescents and typically include family involvement.[19,20] The main components of the safety plan include:

1. Identification of warning signs (eg, thoughts, emotions, behaviors, situations) that precede suicidal thoughts;
2. Coping strategies that the patient can implement independently (eg, reading, journaling, listening to music, exercise);
3. Specific individuals who can be contacted as a means of distraction from suicidal thoughts;
4. Specific adults who may help to resolve the crisis;
5. Contact information for mental health providers or agencies, including the National Suicidal Prevention Lifeline and webchat; and
6. Restricting access to lethal means.

Patients leave the Evaluation Center with a copy of their safety plan and the clinician includes a copy of the safety plan in the patient's electronic health record. Clinic providers are offered training in safety planning procedures, and weekly team meetings also include time for reviewing clinical procedures, including safety planning.

Review of the Evaluation Center Use and Overview of the Data Analysis Plan

To assess the impact of the Evaluation Center, preliminary data from the 2016 calendar year (January 1, 2016, to December 31, 2016) were reviewed. Data sources include referral and waitlist data gathered by the care management team and use reports for all patients seen by ED and Evaluation Center providers. **Table 2** presents a summary of the demographic characteristics of the patient population who were seen during this period.

In addition, we conducted an analysis using electronic health records from the health system, including data on ED visits and clinic visits. We included all patients with a visit for social work in the interval from September 1, 2015 (when the clinic opened), through January 1, 2017. The date of the baseline social work visit was entered into the analysis and defined as time 0. We presume that ED visit rates are constant (but possibly different) before and after the initiation of care at the Evaluation Center with a possible change in the visit rate at time 0. To avoid cyclical effects corresponding to the days of the week, we aggregated data in 1-week intervals. There is a clear spike in the visit rate around time 0 with 12% of the population visiting the ED at week −1. Because this is a clear violation of our assumption of constant visit rates, data from the 3 weeks before and after the intervention were dropped.

Rates at t weeks after the intervention were computed as the number of visits per observed patient weeks for the population between week 3 and week t. Similarly, rates for the period before intervention were computed as visits per patient week between week $−t$ and week $−3$. Confidence bands were computed from a Poisson model. Observation window for each patient was defined as the time period between the first interaction of any type between the patient and the health system and the last such interaction.

Table 2
Demographic characteristics

	Mean (SD)/Percentage (n)
Evaluation Center patients (n = 641) with completed appointments (n = 1447)	
Visits per patient	2.95 (2.43)
1–2	48% (310)
1–5	81% (521)
Visit provider or type	
New social work	37% (533)
New psychiatry	10% (138)
Returning social work	35% (511)
Returning psychiatry	18% (265)
Age (y)	13.01 (3.84)
Primary diagnosis[a]	
Adjustment disorder	31% (164)
Substance use disorder	1% (5)
Anxiety disorder	14% (74)
Autism spectrum disorder	2% (13)
Attention deficit disorder	24% (125)
Intellectual developmental disorder	3% (14)
Mood disorder	13% (70)
Other disorder	12% (63)
Payor or insurer[b]	
Private insurance	37% (230)
Medicaid (NC)	61% (382)
Other government	2% (16)
Referrals (n = 677 referrals for 641 patients with completed Evaluation Center appointments)	
Via EHR	49% (329)
ED	10% (67)
Primary care	28% (190)
Pediatric subspecialty	22% (72)
Via phone	51% (348)
Business days from scheduling to appointment	13.17 (10.39)
Emergency department patient access (patients discharged, n = 485)	
Patients referred to Evaluation Center	24% (114)
Business days from scheduling to appointment	4.20 (6.28)

Abbreviation: EHR, electronic health record.
[a] Missing information for 113 patients.
[b] Missing information for 13 patients.

RESULTS

During the 2016 calendar year (January 1, 2016, to December 31, 2016), the Evaluation Center team fielded 9717 incoming phone calls for care coordination and triaged 1834 system referrals received through the electronic health record. A total of 1447 visits were completed for 641 patients. The clinic coordinator offered community referrals to callers who were referred for services, but who opted not to be seen in the

Evaluation Center. The most common primary diagnoses were adjustment disorders (31%), attention deficit-hyperactivity disorder (24%), anxiety disorders (14%), and mood disorders (13%; see **Table 2**). Patients ranged in age from 2 to 22 years ($M = 13.01$; $SD = 3.84$).

Of the 1447 completed visits, 46% were intake appointments and 54% were return appointments. By provider type, 72% of visits were completed by a licensed clinical social worker; the remaining 28% of visits were completed by a pediatric psychiatrist. With regard to visit frequency, 81% of patients had 5 or fewer visits and 48% had 1 or 2 visits. The mean number of completed visits was 2.87 ($SD = 1.77$). Patients waited an average of 13 business days ($SD = 10.39$) from the date their appointment was scheduled to the date of their appointment (median, 12 days). Patients referred to the Evaluation Center by the ED waited an average of 4 business days ($SD = 6.28$) from ED discharge to the date of their appointment (median, 2 days).

During the study period, 485 patients who visited the ED were discharged to outpatient services, and 24% of those were referred to the Evaluation Center. Of the total 641 patients with completed visits in the Evaluation Center during the study period, 11% were from the ED. Rates of completion of scheduled initial assessments were slightly lower for the overall group compared with patients referred from the ED, at 57% and 61%, respectively.

The examination of the electronic health record data indicated that, for the 641 patients who had an initial evaluation at the Evaluation Center, there were 333 ED visits in the 30 weeks before this initial Evaluation Center appointment, as compared with 172 ED visits in the 30 weeks after the initial visit. Before the Evaluation Center clinic visit, 93 ED visits were for psychiatric concerns compared with only 51 ED visits for psychiatric concerns after the Evaluation Center visits. **Fig. 1** compares the ED visit rates for this population of patients from before to after the initial visit. This change represents a

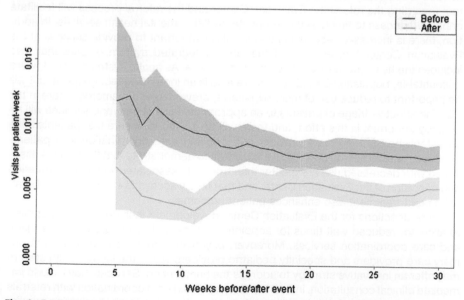

Fig. 1. Emergency department (ED) visit rates. Time is shown on the x-axis with time zero denoting the time of the first social work visit. Green represents ED visit rates per patient week subsequent to that time and red represents visit rates using data before that time.

reduction in the rate of use of the ED for this population of patients after the initial Evaluation Center appointment.

DISCUSSION

The current study examined the use of an innovative outpatient clinic model designed to improve timely access to evidence-based mental health care for children and adolescents and thereby decrease the use of the ED for pediatric psychiatry services. Preliminary results from the first calendar year of operation show that the Evaluation Center provided assessment and short-term treatment services for patients ranging in age from 2 to 22 years and who presented with a wide range of psychiatric, behavioral, and developmental difficulties. In addition to providing direct patient care, the Evaluation Center team served as a hub for coordination of regional referrals for community-based mental health services.

Preliminary results demonstrate that the Evaluation Center contributed to improvements in timely access to psychiatric care, particularly for the system's most urgent and at-risk patients. Specifically, results supported a reduction in use of the ED among patients who completed an initial Evaluation Center appointment with a social worker. As demands for pediatric mental health care in the ED have increased, the Evaluation Center has served as a readily available resource that allows ED providers to more quickly assess, refer, and safely discharge patients with the security of having a coordinated transition of care.

Descriptive data (see **Table 2**) provide a summary of the first full calendar year of clinic operations. Preliminary results inform future prospective studies of effectiveness; however, longitudinal data are needed to examine more thoroughly the impact of the Evaluation Center on use of the ED.

Ongoing attention to increased collaboration and more closely integrated services is needed. Specifically, continued efforts to increase awareness across the hospital system regarding the role of the Evaluation Center and the referral process will facilitate enhanced access to timely and appropriate pediatric mental health services. In addition, there is increased recognition that it will be important to provide services at the Evaluation Center that are part of the larger integrated system of care that also includes the health system, community, and schools. As health systems move toward accountable, population-based care, there also is an increasing recognition that it will be important to reduce use of more expensive, preventable, nonemergent care in the ED. The effective triage of patients to an appropriate level of care and services will be critically important in this effort, and there will be a need to ensure that patients have an established primary care provider and ongoing care coordination in a patient-centered medical home. It will also be important to demonstrate that the savings associated with decreased use are greater than the costs associated with implementation and operation of the Evaluation Center and that timely access to evidence-based evaluation and treatment also enhances patient outcomes.

Future directions for the Evaluation Center development include increased staffing to allow for reduced wait times for appointments, as well as expansion of the triage and care coordination services. Moreover, psychiatric phone consultation with primary care providers and specialty pediatric providers within the larger health system may offer an innovative strategy to address the unmet need. Services may include immediate clinical consultation, in addition to specialized care coordination with referrals to community behavioral health services. Previous research evaluating similar telephone child psychiatry consultation programs support this model as a promising intervention that may facilitate optimal use of specialty care resources.[21,22]

Finally, it will also be important to continue to better understand factors that impact completion rates and to implement innovative, evidence-based strategies to reduce missed appointments, which are common in ambulatory mental health and substance abuse treatment settings.[23,24]

REFERENCES

1. US Department of Health and Human Services. Report of the Surgeon General's Conference on Children's Mental Health: a national action agenda. Washington, DC: US Department of Health and Human Services; 1999.

2. Merikangas KR, He JP, Brody D, et al. Prevalence and treatment of mental disorders among US children in the 2001–2004 NHANES. Pediatrics 2010;125:75–81.

3. Costello EJ, He JP, Sampson NA, et al. Services for adolescents with psychiatric disorders: 12-month data from the National Comorbidity Survey-Adolescent. Psychiatr Serv 2014;65(3):359–66.

4. Dolan MA, Fein JA. Committee on Pediatric Emergency Medicine. Pediatric and adolescent mental health emergencies in the emergency medical services system. Pediatrics 2011;127:e1356–66.

5. Larkin GL, Claassen CA, Emond JA, et al. Trends in US emergency department visits for mental health conditions, 1992 to 2001. Psychiatr Serv 2005;56:671–7.

6. Sheridan DC, Spiro DM, Fu R, et al. Mental health utilization in a pediatric emergency department. Pediatr Emerg Care 2015;31:555–9.

7. Simon AE, Schoendorf KC. Emergency department visits for mental health conditions among US children, 2001-2011. Clin Pediatr (Phila) 2014;53:1359–66.

8. Baillargeon J, Thomas CR, Williams B, et al. Medical emergency department utilization patterns among uninsured patients with psychiatric disorders. Psychiatr Serv 2008;59:808–11.

9. Newton AS, Samina A, Johnson DW, et al. Who comes back? Characteristics and predictors of return to emergency department services for pediatric mental health care. Acad Emerg Med 2010;17:177–86.

10. Alessandrini EA, Lavelle JM, Grenfell SM, et al. Return visits to a pediatric emergency department. Pediatr Emerg Care 2004;20:166–71.

11. Santiago L, Tunik M, Foltin G, et al. Children requiring psychiatric consultation in the pediatric emergency department: epidemiology, resource utilization, and complications. Pediatr Emerg Care 2006;22:85–9.

12. Goldstein AB, Frosch E, Davarya S, et al. Factors associated with a six-month return to emergency services among child and adolescent psychiatric patients. Psychiatr Serv 2007;58:1489–92.

13. Christakis DA, Wright JA, Koepsell TD, et al. Is greater continuity of care associated with less emergency department utilization? Pediatrics 1999;103:738–42.

14. Asarnow JR, Baraff L, Berk M, et al. Effects of an emergency department mental health intervention for linking pediatric suicidal patients to follow-up mental health treatment: a randomized controlled trial. Psychiatr Serv 2011;62:1303–9.

15. Kyriacou DN, Handel D, Stein AC, et al. Factors affecting outpatient follow-up compliance of emergency department patients. J Gen Intern Med 2005;20:938–42.

16. Tran QK, Bayram JD, Boonyasai RT, et al. Pediatric emergency department return: a literature review of risk factors and interventions. Pediatr Emerg Care 2016;32:570–7.

17. Narrow WE, Clarke DE, Kuramoto SJ, et al. DSM-5 field trials in the United States and Canada, part III: development and reliability testing of a cross-cutting symptom assessment for DSM-5. Am J Psychiatry 2013;170:71–82.

18. Stanley B, Brown GK. Safety planning intervention: a brief intervention to mitigate suicide risk. Cogn Behav Pract 2012;19:256–64.

19. Asarnow J, Berk M, Baraff LJ. Family intervention for suicide prevention: a specialized emergency department intervention for suicidal youth. Prof Psychol Res Pract 2009;40:118–25.

20. McManama O'Brien KH, Singer JB, LeCloux M, et al. Acute behavioral interventions and outpatient treatment strategies with suicidal adolescents. Int J Behav Consult Ther 2014;9:19–25.

21. Sarvet B, Gold J, Bostic JQ, et al. Improving access to mental health care for children: the Massachusetts Child Psychiatry Access Project. Pediatrics 2010;126: 1191–200.

22. Hobbs Knutson K, Masek B, Bostic JQ, et al. Clinicians' utilization of child mental health telephone consultation in primary care: findings from Massachusetts. Psychiatr Serv 2014;65:391–4.

23. Molfenter T. Reducing appointment no-shows: going from theory to practice. Subst Use Misuse 2013;48(9):743–9.

24. Gajwai P. Can what we learned about reducing no shows in our clinic work for you? Curr Psychiatry 2014;13(9):13–5, 22-14.

The Emergency Department
Challenges and Opportunities for Suicide Prevention

Joan Rosenbaum Asarnow, PhD*, Kalina Babeva, PhD,
Elizabeth Horstmann, MD

KEYWORDS

- Emergency • Suicide • Self-harm • Pediatric • Adolescent • Guideline
- Integrated care • Hospital

KEY POINTS

- Emergency services can offer life-saving suicide prevention care.
- Brief therapeutic interventions initiated in the emergency department (ED) for youths presenting with suicide/self-harm risk can improve continuity of care and connections with outpatient follow-up treatment, a national suicide prevention objective.
- A care process model and clinical guidance are offered based on current scientific evidence.
- Effective treatment strategies for youth suicide/self-harm prevention are emerging from the scientific literature.
- Increasing availability of these treatments in community settings is crucial for advancing suicide prevention goals.

Disclosure Statement: Dr J.R. Asarnow discloses consulting on quality improvement for depression and suicide prevention. Drs K. Babeva and E. Horstmann have nothing to disclose. Work reported in this article was supported by grants from the National Institute of Mental Health (R01MH112147, R34 MH078082), the United States Substance Abuse and Mental Health Services Administration (U79SM080041), the American Foundation for Suicide Prevention, and Centers for Disease Control (CCR921708). The content is solely the responsibility of the authors and does not necessarily represent the official views of the funding agencies.
David Geffen School of Medicine, Semel Institute for Neuroscience & Human Behavior, University of California, Los Angeles, 300 Medical Plaza, Suite 3310, Los Angeles, CA 90095, USA
* Corresponding author.
E-mail address: jasarnow@mednet.ucla.edu

Child Adolesc Psychiatric Clin N Am 26 (2017) 771–783
http://dx.doi.org/10.1016/j.chc.2017.05.002
1056-4993/17/© 2017 Elsevier Inc. All rights reserved.

childpsych.theclinics.com

Abbreviations	
BH	Behavioral health
CPEP	Comprehensive psychiatric emergency program
ED	Emergency department
ED/FISP	Emergency department/Family Intervention for Suicide Prevention
PES	Psychiatric emergency service
RCT	Randomized, controlled trial
TOC	Teen Options for Change
ZS	Zero Suicide

INTRODUCTION

Suicide is the second leading cause of death among United States youths ages 10 to 24, accounting for nearly 5000 deaths annually, more deaths than any single medical illness in this age group. Despite reductions in other causes of mortality, age-adjusted suicide death rates increased 24% from 1999 through 2014 and exceeded those from motor vehicle accidents among youth ages 10 to 14.[1]

Emergency department (ED) visits offer a window of opportunity to deliver life-saving suicide prevention interventions.[2] Estimates suggest that up to 25% of patients who visit EDs after suicide attempts make another attempt, between 5% and 10% later die by suicide, and a substantial proportion of patients who die by suicide have ED visits during the year before death.[2–4]

This article focuses on the ED as a service delivery site for suicide prevention, and improving access to behavioral health (BH) care more generally. The term behavioral health (BH) is used throughout this article and refers broadly to health promotion related to mental health and substance use/addiction. The article proceeds in 6 sections. First, we discuss the ED as a site for suicide prevention. Second, we examine models for emergency services. Third, we review research on ED screening, therapeutic assessments, and brief interventions. Fourth, we turn to current ED practice guidelines and parameters. Fifth, we consider emergency care processes and offer a care process model of emergency services for suicide and self-harm. Finally, we offer conclusions and suggestions for future directions aimed at optimizing emergency care for the prevention of suicide and self-harm.

THE EMERGENCY DEPARTMENT

EDs provide a safety net in the US health system, owing to federal law (the Emergency Medical Treatment and Labor Act) guaranteeing access to ED care regardless of insurance or ability to pay. Roughly 1.5 million US youth, particularly lower income individuals from underserved populations, receive their primary health care in the ED,[3] and the prevalence of ED visits for BH has increased.[5] Given this increased need for BH treatment within EDs, integrating BH within ED services has potential for suicide prevention in particular, and addressing unmet need for BH care more generally.

Despite the clear need and value of delivering effective BH care in EDs, an Institute of Medicine report suggested that ED care for children and adolescents may be substandard, and shortcomings in training and availability of staff with BH expertise contribute to quality of care problems.[6] The ED setting poses challenges. EDs are often crowded, noisy, lack private space, and youths may be hesitant to honestly discuss sensitive issues with staff they just met. There are other medically and psychiatrically ill patients in the ED, which can be scary and uncomfortable.

The limitations of our health system also create challenges, increased costs, frustration, and lost time for youths and families. Shortages of psychiatric/BH staff and inpatient beds contribute to longer waiting times for BH versus general medical patients, often leading to youths leaving EDs without needed evaluations.[7] Although ED wait and boarding times vary, estimates indicate an average of 6.8 to 34.0 hours,[7] with delays extending from hours to days when patients are waiting for hospital beds. This creates strains on EDs, patients, and families leading to negative experiences and attitudes about BH and psychiatric care.[5]

MODELS OF EMERGENCY PSYCHIATRIC/BEHAVIORAL HEALTH CARE

Table 1 summarizes models of emergency care. These models have generally been established for adults, with little developmental adaptation, although some applications of the mobile crisis response and intensive community-based treatment models have been developed specifically for youth.[8]

The traditional ED consultant model is used in many hospitals. In this approach, when suicide and self-harm risk is identified, a BH specialist, who consults to the ED, is called to do an assessment (now sometimes done using telepsychiatry).[9,10] The BH consultant evaluates safety and imminent risk, followed by triage to appropriate levels of care based on evaluation results.[9] Youths judged to be unsafe for outpatient care or needing further evaluation are generally admitted to inpatient care—either hospitalized on medical units when medical consequences of the suicide attempt or self-harm behavior require intervention, or if available, on psychiatric units when youths are medically stable. When the risk is lower and youths are judged to be safe, patients are discharged home with rapid referral to outpatient care.

Major challenges with the consultant model include shortages of BH consultants and psychiatric hospital beds, inadequate continuity of care, and low rates of follow-up after discharge. With national statistics indicating that roughly one-half of youths presenting to EDs for suicide and self-harm receive no outpatient treatment after discharge,[11–13] improving continuity of care is a national priority (National Strategy for Suicide Prevention, Objective 8.4).[14]

Another model, the dedicated psychiatric emergency service (PES), uses standalone psychiatric EDs, often affiliated with adjacent medical EDs. PES programs offer more extended observation and care (23-hour model) with the goal of stabilizing acute symptoms and avoiding hospitalization when safe and appropriate. Although data are still limited and not fully consistent, a recent demonstration project in Alameda County indicated that a regional PES was associated with a substantially lower average boarding time (1 hour 48 minutes) and an estimated 75% reduction in psychiatric hospitalizations.[7]

Table 1 Models of emergency psychiatric/BH care	
Care Model	**Care Process**
Consultant	BH specialists consult to ED
Psychiatric emergency services	BH service
Comprehensive psychiatric emergency program	BH service, extended care options
Psychiatric urgent care	BH service, walk-in outpatient
Mobile emergency psychiatric services	Emergency BH mobile team
Community-based services	BH team, available 24/7

Abbreviations: BH, behavioral health; ED, emergency department.

Expanding on the PES model, the comprehensive psychiatric emergency program (CPEP) provides more extended observation and care/treatment options. As implemented in New York state, CPEP programs are required to include:

1. Hospital-based crisis intervention services in the ED, including triage, referral, and psychiatric and medical evaluations and assessments;
2. Extended observation beds to provide evaluation, monitoring, and stabilization of acute symptoms for up to 72 hours;
3. Crisis outreach services in the community; and
4. Temporary residential and other required support services for 5 or fewer consecutive days.

State evaluation data suggest that the CPEP model has begun to address targeted quality of care problems and provide a range of treatment alternatives to hospitalization.[15]

Mobile emergency psychiatric services are included in the CPEP model, have been evaluated as a means of responding to psychiatric emergencies, and have shown promise for improving rates of outpatient follow-up care. One randomized, controlled trial (RCT)[16] with an adult CPEP population evaluating follow-up by a CPEP mobile crisis team, compared with clinic referral (similar services offered across programs), found that mobile crisis team patients were significantly more likely to receive an outpatient visit (69.6%), compared with patients in the clinic group (29.6%).[16] Like other data questioning the value of community treatment as usual,[17,18] linkage to treatment was not associated with improvements on measures of clinical or functioning outcomes.

Considerable work has been done on the intensive community based treatment model for youths. Importantly, a large RCT evaluating multisystemic therapy, an intensive home and community-based treatment program, compared with hospitalization for youths presenting with psychiatric emergencies, found advantages for multisystemic therapy on measures of functioning and symptoms, including lower rates of youth-reported self-harm, relative to hospitalization, with lower costs.[19,20] Other intensive community-based treatments that aim to reduce the risk of suicide and self-harm and to minimize hospitalizations have also shown advantages in RCTs, relative to comparator conditions. These community-based treatments include dialectical behavior therapy, delivered as a 4- or 6-month program[21,22]; SAFETY, a 12-week dialectical behavior therapy-informed cognitive-behavioral family treatment designed to be incorporated within emergency services[23]; and a 12-month integrated cognitive–behavioral therapy designed for youths with both suicidality and substance use problems.[24] These interventions include intensive work with the family and youth, and availability for emergency coaching.

The high costs and questionable effectiveness of traditional ED/hospital-based services have stimulated interest in the alternatives to the ED-Consultant model described. More extensive evaluation and rigorously designed demonstration projects are needed.

SCREENING AND BRIEF INTERVENTIONS IN THE EMERGENCY DEPARTMENT

All of the emergency service models begin with risk screening and evaluation. Owing to high acuity and limited resources, the most feasible and efficient approach is to use brief self-report screeners followed by more extensive evaluation for youths with positive screens. Such screeners, like the Ask Suicide-Screening Questions, have shown predictive validity.[25] Adaptive screening algorithms that ask additional questions after positive responses, combined with objective behavioral tasks,[26] could enhance the accuracy and efficiency of screening, allowing more time for therapeutic intervention. Readers are referred elsewhere for more detailed review of screening strategies.[27]

Adding therapeutic components to ED evaluations can mitigate risk, stabilize patients, facilitate triage decisions, and improve continuity of care. Because low rates of follow-up after discharge can make the ED the only point of BH care access, these therapeutic assessments as described elsewhere in this article can offer a "vital link in the suicidal patient's chain of survival."[2]

The specialized emergency room (now ED) and second-generation Family Intervention for Suicide Prevention (ED/FISP)[18,28,29] balance the need for evaluation and treatment using a brief behavioral assessment of imminent risk which evaluates the youth's ability to generate behaviors incompatible with suicide and self-harm, specifically:

1. Recognizing personal strengths and strengths in their social support systems (eg, family);
2. Identifying 3 or more persons from whom to seek support;
3. Discriminating emotional states and identifying suicide and self-harm prompting situations using an "emotional thermometer";
4. Developing a SAFETY plan with concrete steps for safe coping (activities, thoughts, behaviors, and support persons);
5. Committing to using the SAFETY plan versus suicide and self-harm for a specified period.

Thus, the ED/FISP aims to develop and strengthen youths' skills for downregulating suicide and self-harm urges, and mobilize support and feelings of connectedness within the family. The SAFETY plan is shared with parents and caregivers with the goals of facilitating parents' and caregivers' abilities to support the youth in using the safety plan, and support youths in accepting support. Parents and youths are counseled regarding the importance of restricting access to potentially lethal self-harm methods and dangers associated with disinhibition after substance use. The ED/FISP also aims to enhance motivation and commitment to attend follow-up treatment. After discharge, phone contacts are used ($\leq$3 calls) to support linkage to follow-up care, through enhancing motivation and addressing barriers to care. This combination of strong family and youth components enhances youth skills and hopefulness, while also helping parents and caregivers to function like "protective seatbelts" if youths experience intense unbearable emotions and suicidal urges. In an RCT, when compared with usual ED care, the ED/FISP increased the likelihood of receiving outpatient services, with 92% of youths successfully linked to outpatient care. However, linkage to community outpatient treatment "as usual" was not associated with improved clinical outcomes.[18] Alternatively, in 2 trials where the initial ED/FISP was combined with guaranteed access to a structured cognitive–behavioral family intervention, clinical outcomes were improved.[23,28] Indeed, when incorporated as a first in-home session within the SAFETY Program (a cognitive–behavioral family treatment designed to be incorporated within emergency services for youths presenting with suicide attempts and self-harm), the intervention was associated with significantly lower risk of suicide attempts, supporting the benefits of the intervention for protecting against future suicide attempts.[23]

Another therapeutic assessment[17] used a 30-minute cognitive–analytic intervention (with parent involvement when possible) and featured:

1. Construction of a diagram incorporating 3 elements, namely, reciprocal roles, core pain, and maladaptive processes;
2. Identification of a target problem contributing to suicidality;

3. Generating possible "exits" from the problem; and
4. Writing an "understanding letter" that summarizes the diagram and exits.

In an RCT, youth who received the therapeutic assessment were significantly more likely to attend a first outpatient follow-up appointment and at least 4 treatment sessions, than youths receiving usual ED care.[17] However, again, there were no between-group differences in clinical outcomes.

The Compliance Enhancement Intervention[30] is a brief motivational enhancement intervention with youths and parents that includes:

1. Review of treatment expectations/misconceptions;
2. Problem solving treatment barriers;
3. A verbal contract to attend at least 4 outpatient sessions; and
4. Follow-up phone contacts.

After ED discharge, separate phone calls to youths and parents (weeks 1, 2, 4, and 8) assess suicidality, enhance motivation for care, and assist with problem solving treatment barriers. RCT results indicate that at 3 months after discharge, intervention youths attended significantly more treatment sessions than usual care youths, controlling for treatment barriers (eg, insurance coverage, waiting lists).

Similarly, the TeenScreen-ED[31] intervention aims to enhance motivation and address treatment barriers by scheduling an outpatient appointment and sending appointment reminders. RCT results indicate that intervention youths were significantly more likely to attend a mental health appointment by 60 days after discharge relative to comparison youths receiving standard referrals.[31]

Teen Options for Change (TOC),[32] another motivational enhancement intervention, targets adolescents presenting to EDs for nonpsychiatric complaints screening positive for suicide risk. TOC combines personalized feedback on normative risk factors (eg, suicidal ideation, substance use) with identification of youths' values and behavioral goals, and the development of personalized action plans for achieving goals. Follow-up contacts by handwritten note plus phone check-ins during the 5 days after discharge support youths with action plan implementation. In a randomized trial, when compared with usual ED care, TOC youths showed greater reductions in depression at 2 months after discharge; however, groups were similar in rates of BH service use. Here, it is important to note, that unlike the other therapeutic assessments and interventions, TOC emphasized youth outcomes, with less attention to improving rates of post-ED care.

Caring contacts using nondemanding letters and postcards after ED discharge has been emphasized with adults given evidence indicating reduced suicide deaths, suicide attempts, and ED visits.[33,34] However, evaluations with adolescents are limited to 1 study with negative results[35] and the inclusion of a limited number of older adolescents (typically >16 years) in adult samples.

CURRENT GUIDELINES AND PRACTICE PARAMETERS

Practice guidelines, as a representation of evidenced-based practice, have achieved substantial credibility in medicine, are an integral part of emergency medicine, and combined with training can help to improve the quality of care. Guidelines are available online, and a Committee of the American College of Emergency Physicians develops and reviews published guidelines (available at: http://www.acepnow.com/tag/clinical-guidelines/).

Available clinical guidance emphasizes adults. Consensus guidelines for adults were developed by the Suicide Prevention Resource Center (2015) and support clinicians with decisions, initial intervention, and discharge planning (available at: http://www.

sprc.org/resources-programs/caring-adult-patients-suicide-risk-consensus-guide-emergency-departments). A 2016 Clinical Policy article (available at: https://www.acep.org/Clinical—Practice-Management/ACEP-Current-Clinical-Policies/) summarizes evidence on the management of adult suicidal patients.[36]

Recent guidance on suicide and self-harm risk in children and adolescents is limited. The American College of Emergency Physicians practice parameters date from 2001(available at: http://www.jaacap.com/article/S0890-8567(09)60355-5/pdf). Other recommendations and reports focus on ED management of pediatric mental health crises, including 2 clinical reports[37,38] supporting previous joint policy statements of the American Academy of Pediatrics and American College of Emergency Physicians on pediatric mental health emergencies, and one 2015 review including recommendations for youths with suicide and self-harm.[10]

Although these practice guidelines, parameters, and recommendations have differences, they generally emphasize evaluation and assessment of risk levels, triage and management to prevent death and injury, continuity of care, restricting access to dangerous suicide and self-harm methods, and treatment of BH conditions.

Universal screening of all ED patients is controversial. Current Joint Commission on Accreditation of Healthcare Organizations standards require that all patients in psychiatric EDs and patients presenting with psychiatric symptoms to general EDs be screened for suicidality.[39] This standard does not require universal screening for suicidality in medical EDs. Further, the US Preventive Services Task Force's review concluded that current evidence is insufficient to recommend for or against primary care screening for suicide risk (available at: https://www.uspreventiveservicestaskforce.org/).

CARE PROCESS MODEL FOR YOUTHS PRESENTING WITH A RISK FOR SUICIDE AND SELF-HARM

Fig. 1 presents a care process model for youths presenting to ED or emergency services for suicide and self-harm, based on evidence and clinical guidance reviewed. This process begins when patients with suspected suicide and self-harm risk are identified, at which time safety precautions are needed, including close monitoring in a safe setting to prevent suicide and self-harm and/or patients leaving without evaluation. Secondary screening and medical clearance is conducted by ED staff, which may lead ED clinicians to request a psychiatric or BH consultation. The youth and family should be informed about what will be done in the ED in a "collaborative therapeutic assessment and planning process." For child and adolescent patients, it is critical that the evaluation include the youth's condition, characteristics, and environmental risk and protective factors. Because youth may deny and minimize symptoms, sometimes in response to fears that accurate reporting of suicide and self-harm may lead to hospitalization, it is critical to obtain information from parents or caregivers about suicidality and other risk and protective factors. When imminent risk is a concern, the top priority is patient safety. Clinicians may disclose information to protect youths, while following existing laws and regulations set forth in the Health Insurance Portability and Accountability Act. However, collaborating with youths to help them share information or gaining their permission for disclosure can enhance trust and therapeutic interactions. Disclosing information can increase risk by increasing stress or shame in the youth and/or family, requiring careful consideration of potential consequences and protective action as needed.

Clinicians should assess the chain of events leading to presenting suicide and self-harm events, the consequences of the suicide and self-harm event, and identify behaviors, thoughts, and support persons that youths can turn to if he or she experiences

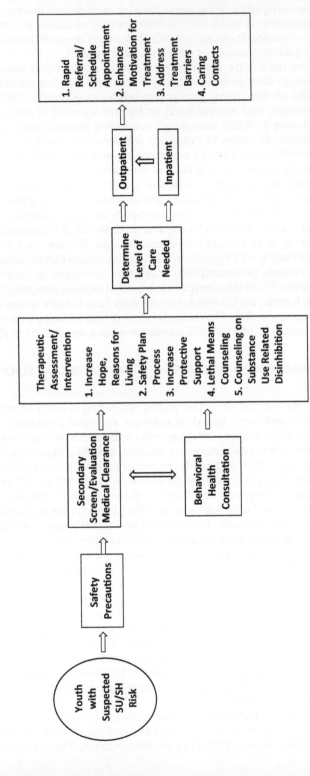

Fig. 1. Care process model for youths presenting with risk for suicide and self-harm (SU/SH). (Courtesy of J. Asarnow, PhD, Los Angeles, CA.)

suicide and self-harm urges again. As in the ED/FISP, and other dialectical behavior therapy and cognitive–behavioral therapy approaches, this assessment can be used to develop a SAFETY plan, practice the plan, obtain a commitment to use the plan, and trouble shoot potential obstacles.[21–23] There are a number of resources to help with SAFETY planning.[40] This differs from a "no suicide contract," which has not been proven effective.[40] Youths' primary care providers and BH providers should be considered as potential support persons, and 24/7 crisis services (eg, National Suicide Prevention Lifeline) should be included. Efforts are needed to enhance protective support, including increasing supportive listening and communication between youths and parents and caregivers, increasing protective monitoring of the youth, counseling parents and youths about the importance of restricting access to dangerous self-harm methods (questions about guns and ammunition should be asked of parents alone to ensure that youth does not learn how to access), and counseling of parents and youths regarding the potential dangers of disinhibition owing to substance use. Work aimed at strengthening motivation to pursue follow-up treatment and addressing barriers to care is important for all youth and families. For youth discharged home, outpatient referral should be facilitated, scheduled before discharge if possible and within the next 7 days (best within 24 hours). Treatment barriers should also be identified and addressed. Postdischarge contact to enhance motivation for care and address treatment barriers have been shown to contribute to increased likelihood of follow-up treatment[17,18,28] and nondemanding caring contacts (eg, calls, postcards, email, texts) can be automated and may improve outcomes.[40]

A critical issue for this process is whether BH care can be integrated within ED workflow patterns. This is important because EDs are often busy, with multiple priorities and limited BH resources.[41,42] Enhanced BH training will provide part of the solution, improving comfort and skill among ED staff and enabling more emergency clinicians to perform initial evaluations, determine the need for consultation, and deliver some brief interventions, as they do for other medical conditions. For instance, when patients come to EDs with chest pain, ED clinicians routinely complete initial risk evaluations and stratifications and, with guidance from consultants, decide on treatment and disposition.[41] A "connected" psychiatric or BH service can provide consultation to ED clinicians (live or through telemedicine), and when needed evaluate patients. There will still be patients that need more thorough psychiatric or BH evaluation and these patients will need to be transferred to facilities that have these resources.

Medical and psychiatric EDs with onsite or colocated BH services can more easily integrate interventions for suicide and self-harm, with BH staff delivering the intervention. This could involve regular ED BH staff, or specialized "suicide prevention crisis teams." Ideally, there is some integration of medical and BH care and communication/collaboration to provide effective care, and clear consistent messages to patients and families.

Finally, the Zero Suicide (ZS; available at: http://zerosuicide.sprc.org/) initiative aims to improve care within health systems, including EDs, to achieve the aspirational goal of ZS within defined health system populations.[41] Grounded in the belief that suicide deaths among individuals receiving care in health and BH systems can be prevented, ZS practices align culture and care to address suicide risk as a threat to health and a health system responsibility. Core elements of zero suicide practices include:

1. A leadership-driven, safety-oriented culture committed to reducing suicide and involving suicide attempt and loss survivors;
2. Systematic identification and evaluation of suicide risk levels;
3. Timely and adequate pathways to care;

4. A competent, confident, and caring workforce;
5. Evidence-based care, including collaborative safety planning, restriction of lethal means, and effective treatment of suicidality;
6. Continued contact and support, especially after acute care; and
7. Data-driven quality improvement (zerosuicide.sprc.com).

This whole system approach has strong potential for addressing many of the problems discussed, like inadequate continuity of care.

SUMMARY

EDs can offer life-saving suicide prevention care, yet hospital-based ED care is at a breaking point and underresourced to serve as a safety net for youth with BH problems.[6] This article reviewed the characteristics of EDs, models of emergency care; ED screening, evaluation, and intervention models; and practice guidelines and parameters. We offered a care process model for youths presenting with suicide and self-harm risk with guidance for clinicians based on current scientific evidence. Although recent service trends are shifting from medical EDs to alternative models that emphasize psychiatric and BH specialty care and community-based services, our care process model can be incorporated within these different models. The trend to community-based emergency services is likely motivated by the high costs of ED and hospital-based care, and accumulating data supporting the advantages of community-based care.[19–24] Nevertheless, there will continue to be youths seen in EDs for suicide and self-harm and other BH problems. It is critical, therefore, that the emergency infrastructure be strengthened through training and building comfort and skill among ED clinicians in evaluating and managing suicidal patients; addressing shortages of psychiatric/BH specialists with child/adolescent expertise; and increasing the availability of effective inpatient and outpatient services. Although effective strategies for youth suicide and self-harm prevention are emerging from the scientific literature, youth suicide rates are not decreasing. It is time to put our knowledge to work and bring evidence-based care to emergency and community services.

REFERENCES

1. Curtin SC, Warner M, Hedegaard H. Increase in suicide in the United States, 1999-2014. NCHS data brief. 2016. Available at: http://www.cdc.gov/nchs/products/databriefs/db241.htm. Accessed April 7, 2017.
2. Larkin GL, Beautrais AL. Emergency departments are underutilized sites for suicide prevention. Crisis 2010;31(1):1–6.
3. Wilson KM, Klein JD. Adolescents who use the emergency department as their usual source of care. Arch Pediatr Adolesc Med 2000;154(4):361–5.
4. Gairin I, House A, Owens D. Attendance at the accident and emergency department in the year before suicide: retrospective study. Br J Psychiatry 2003;183: 28–33.
5. Dolan MA, Fein JA, Committee on Pediatric Emergency Medicine. Pediatric and adolescent mental health emergencies in the emergency medical services system. Pediatrics 2011;127(5):e1356–66.
6. Institute of Medicine, Board on Health Care Services, Committee on the Future of Emergency Care in the United States Health System. Hospital-based emergency care: at the breaking point. Washington, DC: National Academies Press; 2007.

7. Zeller S, Calma N, Stone A. Effects of a dedicated regional psychiatric emergency service on boarding of psychiatric patients in area emergency departments. West J Emerg Med 2014;15(1):1–6.

8. Janssens A, Hayen S, Walraven V, et al. Emergency psychiatric care for children and adolescents: a literature review. Pediatr Emerg Care 2013;29(9):1041–50.

9. Betz ME, Boudreaux ED. Managing suicidal patients in the emergency department. Ann Emerg Med 2016;67(2):276–82.

10. Chun TH, Katz ER, Duffy SJ, et al. Challenges of managing pediatric mental health crises in the emergency department. Child Adolesc Psychiatr Clin N Am 2015;24(1):21–40.

11. Doshi A, Boudreaux ED, Wang N, et al. National study of US emergency department visits for attempted suicide and self-inflicted injury, 1997-2001. Ann Emerg Med 2005;46(4):369–75.

12. Olfson M, Gameroff MJ, Marcus SC, et al. Emergency treatment of young people following deliberate self-harm. Arch Gen Psychiatry 2005;62(10):1122–8.

13. Hughes JL, Anderson NL, Wiblin JL, et al. Predictors and outcomes of psychiatric hospitalization in youth presenting to the emergency department with suicidality. Suicide Life Threat Behav 2016;47:193–204.

14. Office of the Surgeon General, National Action Alliance for Suicide Prevention. 2012 National Strategy for Suicide Prevention: goals and objectives for action. Washington, DC: US Department of Health and Human Services; 2012. Available at: http://nbda.com/articles/industry-overview-2012-free-version-pg34.htm.

15. New York State Office of Mental Health. Annual report to the governor and legislature of New York State on comprehensive psychiatric emergency programs. NYS Office of Mental Health. 2012. Available at: https://www.omh.ny.gov/omhweb/statistics/cpep_annual_report/2012.pdf. Accessed April 7, 2017.

16. Currier GW, Fisher SG, Caine ED. Mobile crisis team intervention to enhance linkage of discharged suicidal emergency department patients to outpatient psychiatric services: a randomized controlled trial. Acad Emerg Med 2010;17(1):36–43.

17. Ougrin D, Zundel T, Ng A, et al. Trial of Therapeutic Assessment in London: randomised controlled trial of Therapeutic Assessment versus standard psychosocial assessment in adolescents presenting with self-harm. Arch Dis Child 2011;96(2): 148–53.

18. Asarnow JR, Baraff LJ, Berk M, et al. An emergency department intervention for linking pediatric suicidal patients to follow-up mental health treatment. Psychiatr Serv 2011;62(11):1303–9.

19. Henggeler SW, Schoenwald SK, Rowland MD, et al. Serious emotional disturbance in children and adolescents: multisystemic therapy. New York: The Guilford Press; 2002. Available at: http://ovidsp.ovid.com/ovidweb.cgi?T=JS&PAGE =reference&D=psyc4&NEWS=N&AN=2002-18214-000.

20. Huey SJ, Henggeler SW, Rowland MD, et al. Multisystemic therapy effects on attempted suicide by youths presenting psychiatric emergencies. J Am Acad Child Adolesc Psychiatry 2004;43(2):183–90.

21. Mehlum L, Tørmoen AJ, Ramberg M, et al. Dialectical behavior therapy for adolescents with repeated suicidal and self-harming behavior: a randomized trial. J Am Acad Child Adolesc Psychiatry 2014;53(10):1082–91.

22. Linehan MM, McCauley E, Berk MS, et al. Dialectical behavior therapy compared to supportive treatment: A randomized controlled trial for adolescents at high risk for suicide. Paper presented at: 50th Annual Convention of the Association for Behavioral and Cognitive Therapies. New York, October 28, 2016.

23. Asarnow JR, Hughes JL, Babeva KN, et al. Cognitive-behavioral family treatment for suicide attempt prevention: a randomized controlled trial. J Am Acad Child Adolesc Psychiatry 2017;56(6):506–14.

24. Esposito-Smythers C, Spirito A, Kahler CW, et al. Treatment of co-occurring substance abuse and suicidality among adolescents: a randomized trial. J Consult Clin Psychol 2011;79(6):728–39.

25. Horowitz LM, Bridge JA, Teach SJ, et al. Ask Suicide-Screening Questions (ASQ): a brief instrument for the pediatric emergency department. Arch Pediatr Adolesc Med 2012;166(12):1170–6.

26. Nock MK, Park JM, Finn CT, et al. Measuring the suicidal mind: implicit cognition predicts suicidal behavior. Psychol Sci 2010;21(4):511–7.

27. Babeva K, Hughes JL, Asarnow J. Emergency department screening for suicide and mental health risk. Curr Psychiatry Rep 2016;18(11):100.

28. Rotheram-Borus MJ, Piacentini J, Cantwell C, et al. The 18-month impact of an emergency room intervention for adolescent female suicide attempters. J Consult Clin Psychol 2000;68(6):1081–93.

29. Asarnow JR, Berk MS, Baraff LJ. Family Intervention for Suicide Prevention: a specialized emergency department intervention for suicidal youths. Prof Psychol Res Pract 2009;40(2):118–25.

30. Spirito A, Boergers J, Donaldson D, et al. An intervention trial to improve adherence to community treatment by adolescents after a suicide attempt. J Am Acad Child Adolesc Psychiatry 2002;41(4):435–42.

31. Grupp-Phelan J, McGuire L, Husky MM, et al. A randomized controlled trial to engage in care of adolescent emergency department patients with mental health problems that increase suicide risk. Pediatr Emerg Care 2012;28(12):1263–8.

32. King CA, Gipson PY, Horwitz AG, et al. Teen Options for Change: an intervention for young emergency patients who screen positive for suicide risk. Psychiatr Serv 2015;66(1):97–100.

33. Motto JA, Bostrom AG. A randomized controlled trial of postcrisis suicide prevention. Psychiatr Serv 2001;52(6):828–33.

34. Carter GL, Clover K, Whyte IM, et al. Postcards from the EDge: 5-year outcomes of a randomised controlled trial for hospital-treated self-poisoning. Br J Psychiatry 2013;202(5):372–80.

35. Robinson J, Yuen HP, Gook S, et al. Can receipt of a regular postcard reduce suicide-related behaviour in young help seekers? A randomized controlled trial. Early Interv Psychiatry 2012;6(2):145–52.

36. American College of Emergency Physicians Clinical Policies Subcommittee. Clinical policy: critical issues in the diagnosis and management of the adult psychiatric patient in the emergency department. Ann Emerg Med 2017;69(4):480–98.

37. Chun TH, Mace SE, Katz ER, American Academy of Pediatrics Committee on Pediatric Emergency Medicine, American College of Emergency Physicians Pediatrics Emergency Medicine Committee. Evaluation and management of children and adolescents with acute mental health or behavioral problems. Part I: common clinical challenges of patients with mental health and/or behavioral emergencies. Pediatrics 2016;138(3):980–9.

38. Chun TH, Mace SE, Katz ER, American Academy of Pediatrics Committee on Pediatric Emergency Medicine, American College of Emergency Physicians Pediatrics Emergency Medicine Committee. Evaluation and management of children with acute mental health or behavioral problems. Part II: recognition of clinically challenging mental health related conditions presenting with medical or uncertain symptoms. Pediatrics 2016;34(3):643–60.

39. Joint Commission on Accreditation of Healthcare Organizations. National patient safety goals. 2015. Available at: http://www.jointcommission.org/assets/1/6/2015_NPSG_HAP.pdf. Accessed April 7, 2017.
40. Capoccia L, Labre M. Caring for adult patients with suicide risk: a consensus-based guide for emergency departments. Suicide Prevention Resource Center; 2015. Available at: http://www.sprc.org/resources-programs/caring-adult-patients-suicide-risk-consensus-guide-emergency-departments. Accessed April 7, 2017.
41. Betz ME, Wintersteen M, Boudreaux ED, et al. Reducing suicide risk: challenges and opportunities in the emergency department. Ann Emerg Med 2016;68(6): 758–65.
42. Baraff LJ, Janowicz N, Asarnow JR. Survey of California emergency departments about practices for management of suicidal patients and resources available for their care. Ann Emerg Med 2006;48(4):452–8.

Integrated Behavioral Health Care in Pediatric Subspecialty Clinics

 CrossMark

Chase Samsel, MD[a,b,c,*], Monique Ribeiro, MD[a,c,d],
Patricia Ibeziako, MD[a,c], David R. DeMaso, MD[a,c]

KEYWORDS

- Integrated care • Health care • Psychosomatic medicine • Pediatric
- Child psychiatry • Comorbidity • Specialty care

KEY POINTS

- Pediatric subspecialty clinic integrated care lags behind primary care.
- Subspecialty care has significant mental health-associated costs and burdens that necessitate integrated behavioral health.
- Child psychiatrists have unique value and skills to colead teams and facilitate treatment in subspecialty care clinics.

INTRODUCTION

With one-fifth of all children and adolescents estimated to have a diagnosable psychiatric disorder,[1] there is an emerging national consensus regarding the importance of providing integrated behavioral health (BH) care in pediatric primary care. These disorders are associated with a disproportionately higher burden of chronic physical disease with accompanying elevated symptom burden, functional impairment, and treatment complexity.[2] It is common for these youths with comorbid BH and physical health conditions to be seen in the subspecialty care setting, which in turn has led to the implementation of models of integrated BH care in pediatric subspecialty clinics.

Disclosure Statement: The authors have no conflicts of interest to disclose.
[a] Department of Psychiatry, 300 Longwood Avenue, Boston Children's Hospital, Boston, MA 02115, USA; [b] Department of Psychosocial Oncology and Palliative Care, Dana-Farber Cancer Institute, 450 Brookline Avenue, SW360A, Boston, MA 02115, USA; [c] Harvard Medical School, 25 Shattuck Street, Boston, MA 02115, USA; [d] Department of Anesthesiology, Perioperative and Pain Medicine, 333 Longwood Avenue, Boston Children's Hospital, Boston, MA 02115, USA
* Corresponding author. Dana-Farber Cancer Institute, 450 Brookline Avenue, SW360A, Boston, MA 02115.
E-mail address: chase.samsel@childrens.harvard.edu

Child Adolesc Psychiatric Clin N Am 26 (2017) 785–794
http://dx.doi.org/10.1016/j.chc.2017.06.004
1056-4993/17/© 2017 Elsevier Inc. All rights reserved.

Abbreviations	
BH	Behavioral health
CAP	Child and adolescent psychiatrist
CF	Cystic fibrosis
NMDA-R	N-methyl-D-aspartate receptor

To date, although the subspecialty literature describes a number of "interdisciplinary" BH programs in a variety of different medical specialty settings, it has not framed (or described) these programs as integrated, despite having the core components of integrated BH care partnerships, namely, consultation, direct service, care coordination, and specialty care provider education.[3] Yet these programs are by no means universal. Although there are similarities between primary and subspecialty care, there are important differences. Compared with primary care providers, subspecialty providers are more likely to consider themselves solely focused on their subspecialty or organ group and are less attuned to responding to mild to moderate psychiatric illnesses.[4] Many patients with chronic physical illnesses tend to identify their subspecialist as their primary care provider with their pediatrician being seen less often, sometimes not for months or even years. These differences may inadvertently place youth at greater risk of having their psychosocial needs inadequately identified.

Integrated BH care in the pediatric subspecialty clinic offers youth with chronic physical illnesses a care setting whereby they are approached from a biopsychosocial perspective as opposed to only an organ system or medical model approach. This article reviews the current status of integrated BH care in six pediatric subspecialty care settings, namely, oncology, palliative care, pain, neuropsychiatry, cystic fibrosis (CF), and transplantation. Although there are many examples of integrated BH, these were selected for their variance, to showcase differences in historical origin (ie, older to newer), service models (eg, embedded to consultative), and robustness of integration (eg, shared decision making to symptom focused).

PEDIATRIC ONCOLOGY

Although survival has vastly improved over the past 20 to 30 years for pediatric oncology patients,[5] the highly distressing treatments and rates of morbidity and mortality have led to the integration of psychiatrists and other BH clinicians embedded in oncology clinics more consistently than other subspecialty settings. It is seen in an evolving integrated field with its own moniker—psychosocial oncology or psychooncology.[6] Pediatric psychosocial oncology is a part of national mission statements, included in decision making bodies such as the Children's Oncology Group, and the benefits of collaborative interdisciplinary work and hospital and medical system support for this integrated care can been seen in national psychosocial standards endorsing integrated psychosocial care.

The Pediatric Psychosocial Standards of Care is an attestation by oncologists, hematologists, and psychosocial oncologists on the importance of providing an integrated BH care model.[7] These standards describe embedded BH care along with the benefits of BH clinicians as coleaders and comanagers of pediatric oncology patients, including specific recommendations for the involvement of child and adolescent psychiatrists (CAPs).[8] Through national credentialing of centers of excellence, which include BH clinicians, these standards will likely reinforce the need for hospitals to include BH integrated care as part of standard care for oncology patients.

Model of Care

The integrated model of psychooncology care aims to provide time-limited, intensive BH support to families. Because most pediatric oncology treatments last 6 to 24 months, this is the time interval most often requiring extensive psychosocial support. Because patients are often high users of inpatient and outpatient treatment, both expected and unexpected, flexibility on the part of BH clinicians to see patients across care settings as consultants and embedded psychosocial oncologists is ideal. Nevertheless, outpatient oncology visits are the more frequent setting of provision of BH services. Depending on the center, significant physical conditions and chemotherapy administrations (eg, bone marrow aspirates in procedure wings, aggressive hydration in chemotherapy bays, and isolation rooms with long treatment administration days) can often be managed in outpatient settings to prevent inpatient hospitalizations, and necessitate more intensive outpatient BH intervention and support.

Shared decision making generally occurs as embedded BH clinicians advocate for patient and family needs, facilitate communication with providers and/or the family, enhance treatment programs and/or provide evidence-based psychotherapy and medication therapies. The BH clinicians commonly assess the following conditions: anxiety and depressive disorders, steroid-induced and chemotherapy-induced mood and psychotic disorders, delirium, sleep disorders, neurocognitive disorders owing to primary oncologic disease and/or oncology treatment, and trauma and stressor-related disorders. Proactive screening, intake, and follow-up of these conditions cooccurring with oncologic diagnosis and treatment phases enable this shared decision making and, as such, psychooncologists are often viewed as part of "the team" more than most other BH integrated clinicians.

PEDIATRIC PALLIATIVE CARE

Growing out of oncology care and now expanding to other subspecialty settings, pediatric palliative care is a rapidly developing specialty focused on the advanced care of patients with life-limiting and life-threatening physical illness.[9,10] This field has led to effective collaborations between palliative care providers and subspecialty clinicians. Palliative care physicians generally include oncologists, intensivists, and/or general pediatricians. Palliative consultations have led to more effective treatment of symptoms such as pain, nausea, dyspnea, anxiety, and depression; heightened psychosocial support for families; and patient-centered advocacy for clear communication with providers and more defined goals of care. Overlapping and variable expertise of palliative care clinicians and CAPs has been described.[10–12]

Model of Care

Close collaboration between CAPs and pediatric palliative care clinicians can be complimentary and collaborative while being mindful of appropriate division of duties.[10,12] However, because the pediatric palliative care delivery structure can also be consultative, their work is often mobile and occurs within other pediatric subspecialty clinics, enabling joint visits with BH clinicians embedded in or consulting to pediatric subspecialty clinics. Pediatric subspecialty providers frequently invite shared decision making from BH and/or pediatric palliative care clinicians for patients with advanced illness when the clinician, patient, and/or their families are experiencing significant physical, psychological, or moral distress.

For example, palliative care consultants and CAPs can use advance directive planning tools such as Voicing My Choices and 5 Wishes to facilitate goals of care discussions for providers and families.[13,14] Advance directives and quality of life discussions are difficult for pediatric subspecialty providers who have grown attached to patients over years and decades, view deaths of patients as a professional failure, experience deaths of patients less frequently than adult providers, and have less expertise in communication than CAPs or other BH clinicians. Palliative care clinicians can also benefit from BH collaboration when especially challenging team dynamics, parent and/or patient personality issues, or severe psychiatric illness may be impeding these discussions.

PEDIATRIC PAIN

Pediatric pain has reached epidemic proportions with an estimated 1.7 million children in the United States alone suffering from moderate to severe persistent pain.[15] Chronic pain is commonly defined as pain persisting for 3 months or more, or beyond the expected period of healing. It has been reported by two-thirds of school-age children in a community sample,[16] with estimates of 5% to 15% of children needing help for their pain and associated problems.[17] Chronic pain is associated with functional, social, and academic impairments, and increased risk for psychopathology frequently presenting as a somatic symptom and related disorder.[18] Disabling chronic pain and its psychiatric comorbidities account for a significant decrease in quality of life.

Multidisciplinary pain rehabilitation is an integrated BH approach to chronic pain that is based on a biopsychosocial model, whereby biological, psychological, individual, social, and environmental factors contribute to and maintain pain symptoms and disability. This approach has the added benefits of better outcomes for medication use, health care use, return to function, and closure of disability claims.[19,20] Selecting the appropriate level of interventions based on individual clinical needs is essential to success, and the evaluation and availability of intermediate integrated care treatment models can prevent the need for higher resource intensive treatment.[21]

Model of Care

The pain rehabilitation model involves an integrated team consisting of a pain physician, BH clinician (often a psychologist), and physical and occupational therapists.[22] CAPs can provide an important consultation role in providing diagnostic assessments, pain neuroscience education, and/or psychopharmacology. As in the other effective subspecialty integrated programs, patients and families are essential partners with the health care providers in identifying strengths and needs, and developing comprehensive and proactive treatment plans that incorporate medical and BH services, adequately meet their needs, and are culturally appropriate. Shared decision making between BH clinicians and pain physicians in this treatment model is critical to success and a perfect fit for child psychiatry leadership in subspecialty teams given their role and skill sets.

Despite evidence for the effectiveness of an integrated pain rehabilitation treatment in chronic pain conditions[23,24] and ideal fit for CAPs, the availability of such programs, particularly those where CAPs are embedded as part the team, remains limited in the United States. To our knowledge, there are fewer than 15 multidisciplinary pain management programs in the country, with only 2 of them having CAPs embedded in the pain team.

NEUROPSYCHIATRY

There has been a recent strengthening of the collaboration between psychiatry and neurology around the paradigm of "neuropsychiatric" disorders.[25] Neuropsychiatrists, who can come from either neurology and/or psychiatry, are trained to comprehensively evaluate and treat patients with complex neurobehavioral problems associated with a range of disorders including in the neurobiological bases and treatment of cognitive, behavioral, and neuropsychiatric manifestations of neurodegenerative diseases, multiple sclerosis, epilepsy, stroke, brain tumors, inflammatory and infectious diseases of the central nervous system, developmental disorders, traumatic brain injury, and other disorders. For instance, the identification of the pediatric autoimmune epileptic encephalopathies, such as anti–N-methyl-D-aspartate receptor (NMDA-R) encephalitis, is an area of increasing scientific interest and clinical need.

Model of Care

The complex presentation of troubling neuropsychiatric disorders such as NMDA-R encephalitis necessitates both neurologic and psychiatric expertise, suggesting an emerging need for collaboration and integrated care within pediatric neurology outpatient and inpatient settings.[26]

That said, the current integrated BH models seen in the neurology subspecialty clinic essentially falls into the use of neuropsychologists working in seizure units and psychologists working in headache clinics. To date, the integration of CAPs lags behind, with referrals being made to specialty psychiatry care settings or inpatient consult–liaison clinicians for occasional outpatient consultation as opposed to providing embedded consultation, treatment, and shared decision making. Robust integration of CAPs likely awaits their further training in the field of pediatric neuropsychiatry.

CYSTIC FIBROSIS

Youth with CF have high rates of depression, anxiety, and nonadherence associated with the well-documented quality of life impairment and life-limiting course. The large International Depression/Anxiety Epidemiologic Study (TIDES) reported elevated rates of depression in 10% of adolescents and 19% of adults; increased symptoms of anxiety were reported in 22% of adolescents and 32% of adults.[27] This led the CF Foundation and the European CF Society, uniquely among subspecialty care settings, to recommend routine screening with Patient Health Questionnaire-9 for depression and Generalized Anxiety Disorder 7 item for anxiety for all patients with CF ages 12 and older, along with offering screening to caregivers of pediatric patients with CF.[28,29]

Model of Care

The CF Foundation's screening algorithm includes psychopharmacologic recommendations based on severity of anxiety and depressive symptoms. Selective serotonin reuptake inhibitors are recommended for moderate levels where psychotherapy has been declined or is not available, and a combination of a selective serotonin reuptake inhibitor and psychotherapy is recommended for severe cases. BH integration has often included BH social workers being embedded in CF clinics and recently an increasing presence of psychologists embedded in or collaborating with CF clinics.

Interestingly, these same studies showed only 6% of the nation's CF centers had a CAP on their team, although 25% of centers reported using psychotropic medications.[30] These findings suggest there is a significant opportunity to integrate and embed CAPs into the CF clinic setting to target need for future research on the efficacy, drug-specific use, and prescribing practices of selective serotonin reuptake inhibitors for patients with CF.

SOLID ORGAN TRANSPLANT PROGRAMS

Cardiac, intestine, liver, lung, and renal transplantation, although options to extend life, are well-documented to be difficult and trying pretransplant and posttransplant experiences.[31] Moreover, the evolution and growth of the field of transplant medicine has intensified the need for BH involvement.

The growth of the field of transplant medicine has been owing to many factors, including greater visibility and presence of organ donation programs, more patients on waitlists as medicine evolves to extend life longer in acute and chronic pediatric illness, and the advancement of immunosuppressant therapies resulting in extended life posttransplantation. This growth has enabled greater consideration of transplanting patients with complex physical, developmental, and/or psychiatric impairments and increased the need for more intense BH interventions and support in kind.[31]

Model of Care

Transplant centers have had integrated BH for years, as the Centers for Medicaid and Medicare Services requires licensed BH clinicians to perform pretransplant psychosocial evaluations before being placed on transplant waitlists. Most centers employ social workers for BH assessment, interventions, and care coordination. Psychologists are increasingly being employed for both BH interventions and research along with a few CAPs. [32] The role for CAPs is persuasive with increasing intensity of transplants resulting in longer posttransplant durations of stay in the intensive care unit, high incidence of delirium, high rates of medical traumatic stress, and substance-induced mood disorders from essential transplant treatments and agents.[33,34]

Large multinational studies have been performed in conjunction with international advocacy and policy work between BH clinicians and pulmonologists that have set up many avenues and opportunities for integrated care.[35] These studies reinforce shared decision making between the medical team and BH clinicians in patient evaluation, management and follow-up. Many integrated care opportunities in nondirect clinical care also exist, as BH transplant clinicians can find many administrative, academic, and programmatic avenues for their involvement in ethics committee meetings, quality improvement work groups, research laboratories, regulatory committees, and listing advisory committees, to name a few.

ROLE OF CHILD AND ADOLESCENT PSYCHIATRISTS

Pediatric subspecialty clinics offer important opportunities for the integration of CAPs into the care of children and adolescents facing complex physical illnesses owing to the prevalence of cooccurring BH and physical health conditions. CAPs have a unique training that combines neuroscience with an understanding about psychological functioning and social roles. In these clinics, CAPs are primed to use their full array of skills as leaders and clinicians, as previously delineated by seminal psychosomatic medicine papers[36–38] to include assessment, pharmacotherapy, short-term psychotherapy, and medical systems support and education. Integrated care allows for better assessment and management of BH in subspecialty clinics, with child psychiatrists helping to develop and implement further risk reduction interventions.

Cost and Resource Use

Improved cost savings and reduced resource use are important driving factors for pediatric integrated care in hospital and health care systems. Although the literature in pediatric subspecialty clinics is limited, inpatient studies have demonstrated reduced durations of stay and reduced patient charges (eg, laboratory tests, studies, or inpatient days) when BH services are involved earlier in pediatric hospitalizations.[39,40] These data combined with convincing cost and resource savings emerging in the primary care integrated BH care literature suggests comprehensive care in pediatric subspecialty clinics could be a similar value addition.[41] Subspecialty clinic integration may provide even further resource savings given the complex impact on total health care use, medical treatment adherence, and family psychosocial functioning, as demonstrated in recent studies.

Health care cost use in a sample of 767 pediatric patients with asthma demonstrated a 51% greater use and cost for patients with depression and with or without anxiety disorders compared with those just with anxiety disorders.[42] These costs were related primarily to laboratory work, radiologic tests, and primary care visits—not mental health or asthma-related expenses. Coordinating care, addressing the mind–body connection, and treating potential psychosomatic illness are valuable additions integrated child psychiatrists can offer this population.

Financial Support

Although there has been an increase over the past decade in pediatric psychosomatic medicine funding for hospital services,[37,38] subspecialty clinic support can be more onerous. This makes integration outside of academic centers and high-revenue subspecialty clinics more difficult, especially because patients with physical and psychiatric comorbidity more frequently miss and reschedule appointments, leading to more care coordination efforts and fewer opportunities for billing. Reducing managed care barriers would be important to facilitate integrated subspecialty care. CAPs are often not on the same insurance panel as subspecialty physicians, so it is important to advocate for both psychiatrist and subspecialty physicians being reimbursed for joint time spent with the child and family as well as for consultative discussion and review of joint cases.

Many traditional outpatient systems that focus on fee-for-service and physician billing alone for pediatric subspecialty payments find it is not a viable approach, because patients need more intense care coordination and there is inadequate reimbursement for care coordination as well as time spent with patients. Value addition negotiations for initiating or increasing integrated care efforts are more persuasive, and they fit better in bundled payment models and accountable care organizations.[4,38] Furthermore, governing body mandates regarding standards of care (eg, transplant, oncology, and CF) that support integration of psychiatry further strengthens the move away from a financial solvency necessity to an organizational, institutional, and accreditation-driven essential needs service.[7,8,28]

Patient and Provider Satisfaction

Families report increased satisfaction when integrated BH services are offered earlier in a medical or surgical hospitalization.[43,44] Pediatric primary care providers have reported increased satisfaction with their delivery of care and job satisfaction when integrated care is introduced into their clinics.[45,46] Long-established adult integrated primary care practices have reported providers negotiating for integrated care presence as one of their top priorities when relocating or renegotiating.[4,47] The reports of increased hospital-supported funding for integrated BH programs represent institutional awareness of better parent-centered care and satisfaction with these models.[38]

SUMMARY

Although integrated BH care models do exist for pediatric subspecialty clinics, there remain significant gaps in their implementation and use analogous to those seen in the pediatric primary care setting despite the importance of providing BH care for youth struggling with disabling cooccurring behavioral and physical conditions. The most integrated services, such as pain and psychosocial oncology, exhibit an ideal of embeddedness and shared decision making that makes the best use of BH and CAP expertise. However, any integration feasible is favorable given the unmet needs of these youth. We support the serious call to action for development and introduction of integrated BH care into pediatric subspecialty clinics as echoed in the pediatric subspecialty literature.[48–51]

REFERENCES

1. Williams J, Klinepeter K, Palmes G, et al. Diagnosis and treatment of behavioral health disorders in pediatric practice. Pediatrics 2004;114(3):601–6.
2. Kline-Simon AH, Weisner C, Sterling S. Point prevalence of co-occurring behavioral health conditions and associated chronic disease burden among adolescents. J Am Acad Child Adolesc Psychiatry 2016;55(5):408–14.
3. DeMaso D, Martini RD, Sulik LR, et al. A guide to building collaborative mental health care partnerships in pediatric primary care. Washington, DC: AACAP Council; 2010. Available at: https://www.aacap.org/App_Themes/AACAP/docs/clinical_practice_center/guide_to_building_collaborative_mental_health_care_partnerships.pdf.
4. Coleman KJ, Magnan S, Neely C, et al. The COMPASS initiative: description of a nationwide collaborative approach to the care of patients with depression and diabetes and/or cardiovascular disease. Gen Hosp Psychiatry 2017;44:69–76.
5. Smith MA, Altekruse SF, Adamson PC, et al. Declining childhood and adolescent cancer mortality. Cancer 2014;120(16):2497–506.
6. Holland JC. History of psycho-oncology: overcoming attitudinal and conceptual barriers. Psychosom Med 2002;64(2):206–21.
7. Wiener L, Kazak AE, Noll RB, et al. Interdisciplinary collaboration in standards of psychosocial care. Pediatr Blood Cancer 2015;62(Suppl 5):S425.
8. Steele AC, Mullins LL, Mullins AJ, et al. Psychosocial interventions and therapeutic support as a standard of care in pediatric oncology. Pediatr Blood Cancer 2015;62(Suppl 5):S585–618.
9. Wolfe J, Klar N, Grier HE, et al. Understanding of prognosis among parents of children who died of cancer: impact on treatment goals and integration of palliative care. JAMA 2000;284(19):2469–75.
10. Buxton D. Child and adolescent psychiatry and palliative care. J Am Acad Child Adolesc Psychiatry 2015;54(10):791–2.
11. Muriel AC, Wolfe J, Block SD. Pediatric palliative care and child psychiatry: a model for enhancing practice and collaboration. J Palliat Med 2016;19(10):1032–8.
12. Samsel C. Integrated care for seriously ill children: the synergy of psychosomatics and palliative care. AACAP News 2016;Vol. 47:210–1.
13. Wiener L, Zadeh S, Battles H, et al. Allowing adolescents and young adults to plan their end-of-life care. Pediatrics 2012;130(5):897–905.
14. Zadeh S, Pao M, Wiener L. Opening end-of-life discussions: how to introduce Voicing My CHOiCES, an advance care planning guide for adolescents and young adults. Palliat Support Care 2015;13(3):591–9.
15. Robins H, Perron V, Heathcote LC, et al. Pain neuroscience education: state of the art and application in pediatrics. Children (Basel) 2016;3(4) [pii:E43].

16. Perquin CW, Hazebroek-Kampschreur AA, Hunfeld JA, et al. Pain in children and adolescents: a common experience. Pain 2000;87(1):51–8.
17. Huguet A, Miro J. The severity of chronic pediatric pain: an epidemiological study. J Pain 2008;9(3):226–36.
18. Cohen LL, Vowles KE, Eccleston C. The impact of adolescent chronic pain on functioning: disentangling the complex role of anxiety. J Pain 2010;11(11): 1039–46.
19. Stanos S. Focused review of interdisciplinary pain rehabilitation programs for chronic pain management. Curr Pain Headache Rep 2012;16(2):147–52.
20. Turk DC. Clinical effectiveness and cost-effectiveness of treatments for patients with chronic pain. Clin J Pain 2002;18(6):355–65.
21. Tegethoff M, Belardi A, Stalujanis E, et al. Comorbidity of mental disorders and chronic pain: chronology of onset in adolescents of a national representative cohort. J Pain 2015;16(10):1054–64.
22. Logan DE, Carpino EA, Chiang G, et al. A day-hospital approach to treatment of pediatric complex regional pain syndrome: initial functional outcomes. Clin J Pain 2012;28(9):766–74.
23. Simons LE, Sieberg CB, Pielech M, et al. What does it take? Comparing intensive rehabilitation to outpatient treatment for children with significant pain-related disability. J Pediatr Psychol 2013;38(2):213–23.
24. Hechler T, Martin A, Blankenburg M, et al. Specialized multimodal outpatient treatment for children with chronic pain: treatment pathways and long-term outcome. Eur J Pain 2011;15(9):976–84.
25. Carson AJ. Introducing a 'neuropsychiatry' special issue: but what does that mean? J Neurol Neurosurg Psychiatr 2014;85(2):121–2.
26. Maneta E, Garcia G. Psychiatric manifestations of anti-NMDA receptor encephalitis: neurobiological underpinnings and differential diagnostic implications. Psychosomatics 2014;55(1):37–44.
27. Quittner AL, Goldbeck L, Abbott J, et al. Prevalence of depression and anxiety in patients with cystic fibrosis and parent caregivers: results of the International Depression Epidemiological Study across nine countries. Thorax 2014;69(12): 1090–7.
28. Quittner AL, Abbott J, Georgiopoulos AM, et al. International Committee on Mental Health in Cystic Fibrosis: Cystic Fibrosis Foundation and European Cystic Fibrosis Society consensus statements for screening and treating depression and anxiety. Thorax 2016;71(1):26–34.
29. Smith BA, Georgiopoulos AM, Quittner AL. Maintaining mental health and function for the long run in cystic fibrosis. Pediatr Pulmonol 2016;51(S44):S71–8.
30. Garcia G, Oliva M, Smith BA. Survey of collaborative mental health providers in cystic fibrosis centers in the United States. Gen Hosp Psychiatry 2015;37(3): 240–4.
31. Cousino MK, Rea KE, Schumacher KR, et al. A systematic review of parent and family functioning in pediatric solid organ transplant populations. Pediatr Transplant 2017;21(3).
32. Skillings JL, Lewandowski AN. Team-based biopsychosocial care in solid organ transplantation. J Clin Psychol Med Settings 2015;22(2-3):113–21.
33. Kemper MJ, Sparta G, Laube GF, et al. Neuropsychologic side-effects of tacrolimus in pediatric renal transplantation. Clin Transplant 2003;17(2):130–4.
34. Smith PJ, Rivelli SK, Waters AM, et al. Delirium affects length of hospital stay after lung transplantation. J Crit Care 2015;30(1):126–9.

35. Smith PJ, Blumenthal JA, Trulock EP, et al. Psychosocial predictors of mortality following lung transplantation. Am J Transplant 2016;16(1):271–7.

36. Bronheim HE, Fulop G, Kunkel EJ, et al. The Academy of Psychosomatic Medicine practice guidelines for psychiatric consultation in the general medical setting. The Academy of Psychosomatic Medicine. Psychosomatics 1998;39(4): S8–30.

37. Shaw RJ, Wamboldt M, Bursch B, et al. Practice patterns in pediatric consultation-liaison psychiatry: a national survey. Psychosomatics 2006;47(1): 43–9.

38. Shaw RJ, Pao M, Holland JE, et al. Practice patterns revisited in pediatric psychosomatic medicine. Psychosomatics 2016;57(6):576–85.

39. Bujoreanu S, White MT, Gerber B, et al. Effect of timing of psychiatry consultation on length of pediatric hospitalization and hospital charges. Hosp Pediatr 2015; 5(5):269–75.

40. Wood R, Wand AP. Quality indicators for a consultation-liaison psychiatry service. Int J Health Care Qual Assur 2014;27(7):633–41.

41. Asarnow JR, Rozenman M, Wiblin J, et al. Integrated medical-behavioral care compared with usual primary care for child and adolescent behavioral health: a meta-analysis. JAMA Pediatr 2015;169(10):929–37.

42. Richardson LP, Russo JE, Lozano P, et al. The effect of comorbid anxiety and depressive disorders on health care utilization and costs among adolescents with asthma. Gen Hosp Psychiatry 2008;30(5):398–406.

43. Kitts RL, Gallagher K, Ibeziako P, et al. Parent and young adult satisfaction with psychiatry consultation services in a children's hospital. Psychosomatics 2013; 54(6):575–84.

44. Lavakumar M, Gastelum ED, Choo TH, et al. Parameters of consultee satisfaction with inpatient academic psychiatric consultation services: a multicenter study. Psychosomatics 2015;56(3):262–7.

45. Greene CA, Ford JD, Ward-Zimmerman B, et al. Strengthening the coordination of pediatric mental health and medical care: piloting a collaborative model for freestanding practices. Child Youth Care Forum 2016;45(5):729–44.

46. Hine JF, Grennan AQ, Menousek KM, et al. Physician satisfaction with integrated behavioral health in pediatric primary care. J Prim Care Community Health 2017; 8(2):89–93.

47. Bentham WD, Ratzliff A, Harrison D, et al. The experience of primary care providers with an integrated mental health care program in safety-net clinics. Fam Community Health 2015;38(2):158–68.

48. Ader J, Stille CJ, Keller D, et al. The medical home and integrated behavioral health: advancing the policy agenda. Pediatrics 2015;135(5):909–17.

49. Plener PL, Molz E, Berger G, et al. Depression, metabolic control, and antidepressant medication in young patients with type 1 diabetes. Pediatr Diabetes 2015;16(1):58–66.

50. Martini R, Hilt R, Marx L, et al. Best principles for integration of child psychiatry into the pediatric health home. Washington, DC: American Academy of Child & Adolescent Psychiatry; 2012. Available at: http://www.aacap.org/App_Themes/AACAP/docs/clinical_practice_center/systems_of_care/best_principles_for_integration_of_child_psychiatry_into_the_pediatric_health_home_2012.pdf. Accessed April 1, 2017.

51. Pediatric Integrated Care. Washington, DC: American Academy of Child & Adolescent Psychiatry. Available at: https://www.integratedcareforkids.org. Accessed April 1, 2017.

Evaluating Integrated Mental Health Care Programs for Children and Youth

CrossMark

Lawrence S. Wissow, MD, MPH[a,*], Jonathan D. Brown, PhD, MHS[b], Robert J. Hilt, MD[c], Barry D. Sarvet, MD[d]

KEYWORDS

- Integrated care • Children • Adolescents • Primary care • Mental health
- Evaluation • Outcomes

KEY POINTS

- Evaluating integrated care programs requires balancing a desire for methodologic rigor and the need to collect data in real time in real world settings.
- Integrated care programs need to adapt and learn on the fly, so that evaluations may best be viewed through the lens of continuous quality improvement rather than evaluations of fixed programs.
- Evaluation plans must be responsive to multiple stakeholders and will likely change over time as programs evolve.
- The ultimate goal of evaluation is to obtain family-reported functional outcome data; World Wide Web–based platforms increasingly make this possible.

INTRODUCTION

Integrated care is widely advocated as a way of providing medical services that are better tailored to patients' needs and as a way of addressing the undersupply or inavailability of specialists.[1,2] In particular, the term integrated care has become short-hand

---

Disclosures: The authors have nothing to disclose.
Supported in part by Substance Abuse and Mental Health Service Administration grant U79SM061259 for the Pediatric Integrated Care Collaborative. The Pediatric Integrated Care Collaborative is a component of the National Child Traumatic Stress Network through the Donald J. Cohen National Child Traumatic Stress Initiative, which encourages collaboration among leaders in child traumatic stress. The role of the funder was solely financial support.

[a] Division of Child and Adolescent Psychiatry, Johns Hopkins School of Medicine, 550 North Broadway, Room 949, Baltimore, MD 21205, USA; [b] Mathematica Policy Research, 1100 1st Street, NE 12th Floor, Washington, DC 20024-2512, USA; [c] Department of Psychiatry and Behavioral Sciences, University of Washington, M/S CPH, PO Box 5371, Seattle, WA 98105, USA; [d] Department of Psychiatry, University of Massachusetts, Medical School at Baystate, 759 Chestnut Street, WG703, Springfield, MA 01199, USA
* Corresponding author.
E-mail address: Lwissow@jhmi.edu

Child Adolesc Psychiatric Clin N Am 26 (2017) 795–814
http://dx.doi.org/10.1016/j.chc.2017.06.005
1056-4993/17/© 2017 Elsevier Inc. All rights reserved.

childpsych.theclinics.com

for attempts to coordinate primary care, mental health, and substance use services in a way that addresses the worldwide lack of access to behavioral health services.

Integration potentially requires considerable investment in restructuring how generalists and specialists work. The investment that may be justified by better health outcomes, avoiding more expensive or risky urgent care, and more efficient use of scarce higher level services. Although integrated care programs may be initiated based on their roots in a particular public health or moral view of how care should be delivered,[3] eventually funders and clinicians need to know that they are effective and in some way produce results that warrant their costs. However, developing a plan to evaluate integrated care is not straightforward.

Evaluating integrated care programs is approached through any number of general implementation science models used to examine complex interventions.[4–6] This literature points out the need to use so-called hybrid study designs to examine how well various aspects of a program are working and the program's overall outcomes.[7] There are many reasons why hybrid designs are important, but for integrated care a primary reason is that an understanding of mechanisms is critical: we care not only about outcomes in the aggregate, but also how and why outcomes may vary for different groups of patients.[8]

Approaches to evaluating integrated care can also be informed by evaluations of other innovations in primary care.[9] Aspects of primary care specifically related to management of chronic illnesses,[10] behavioral counseling,[11] family centeredness,[12] and overall patient experience[13] have also been the subject of assessment efforts and can also be components of integrated care.

In fact, the characteristics of the evaluation literature as it applies to integrated care potentially make it difficult to plan studies in as rigorous or generalizable way as one might like. Nomenclature in the evaluation and health services fields is constantly shifting, making it difficult to find instruments or approaches used for a particular purpose. A recent review of implementation measures[14] found that most (85%) were located through networks of informants and the "gray literature" rather than from peer-reviewed reports. The diversity of instruments reflects true dilemmas and divergences in the purpose of evaluations: evaluators want valid information but also need information that is specific to the programs they are evaluating; evaluators may be interested as much or more in results that lead to a specific program's improvement versus generating generalizable knowledge. Funding cycles may require reporting on outcomes long before measures of meaningful change could be expected. So exactly how evaluation is approached requires first thinking about the evaluation's goals and the nature and stage of development of the program being evaluated.[15]

This article focuses on evaluation approaches to integrated programs targeting children's mental health care. The focus is on programs in which one or more primary care sites seek to improve the mental health care they can provide to the families they serve through collaboration with mental health and community program providers and organizations. In this setting we make several assumptions that guide our discussion of evaluation design and instrument choices. These assumptions, listed next, are subject to change for any particular integrated care program, and may change over time as a particular program evolves from an initial or pilot stage, to being in operation in a single site, to being expanded to new sites:

1. Most integrated care programs take place in real-world practice or policy settings in which rigorous experimental evaluation designs are not possible, either because of the need to initiate the program rapidly at scale[16] or to avoid disruption to existing patient-provider relationships.

2. In these real-world settings it is rarely practical to collect extensive process and outcome measures[17]; funds are usually not available to collect such measures, and they risk posing a burden to patients and creating a barrier to clinical care.
3. The kinds of clinical outcomes expected, although important, may be in statistical terms of small to moderate size, may not be realized immediately, or may result in the reduction in frequency of rare events (emergency room visits, hospitalization, suicides).[18] Thus, sample sizes need to be large and ideally follow-up needs to continue for months to years, especially to capture outcomes related to educational or even workplace success.
4. The most meaningful outcome measures are supplied by families themselves in characterizing their child's symptoms and functioning in key domains (school, family, with peers), but this raises difficulties of finding instruments that might be valid in diverse populations, minimizing burden, assuring high completion rates at multiple time points, and interpreting results in the light of expected disagreements among observers (parents, teachers, youth).[19]
5. Children for the most part live within families who have an enormous influence on their health.[20,21] Thus integrated care for children (compared with programs for adults) must pay particular attention to the needs of parents and other family members in addition to the identified child patient.
6. Most of the interventions used in the primary care setting are at best "evidence-informed" rather than evidence-based.[22] Continuous monitoring of the processes and outcomes of care is needed to drive adjustments to interventions, rather than thinking of them as something fixed that has to be implemented with fidelity.[23,24]
7. Some integrated care programs, such as efforts to improve communication among primary care sites, community agencies, and mental health providers, may not focus on a single disorder and its treatment (eg, as do some adult programs targeting depression); rather, they aim to change the context in which care is provided for a range of disorders.[25] This is particularly important for children, whose emotional and behavior problems are likely to be highly comorbid or not meet criteria for diagnosis.[26] Thus, outcome measures likely have to focus much more on global function than on any specific cluster of symptoms, and impact may vary across sites with different populations if some conditions are more responsive to treatment than others.
8. The programs are dependent for their outcomes on interpersonal factors (relationships among staff members, relationships between staff members and patients) as much as or more so than more readily quantifiable aspects of service delivery, such as counts of the number screens performed or structural aspects, such as having a shared medical record.[27–29]

DEFINING INTEGRATED CARE

Integrated care has been defined in multiple ways[1] and in terms of structural elements (shared records, formal referral mechanisms) and interprofessional relationships.[30] Integrated care shares many elements of the concept of primary care, whose roots go back to the 1930s.[31] Primary care denotes an approach that features coordination among providers caring for the same patient and a long-term personal relationship with a main provider who integrates information across sources.[32] The Chronic Care Model[33,34] formalized several aspects of primary care, specifying functions related to early detection of potentially chronic illnesses, support for generalists' ability to acquire some specialist expertise, ongoing monitoring of patients' status, and increasing closeness of collaboration with specialists if a patient's condition warranted it (often referred to as stepped care). Singer and colleagues[2] make the case that the ultimate purpose of integrated care is to tailor services to individual patient needs and preferences. For any given patient, actions and decisions across providers are co-ordinated to maximize benefit and minimize the chance of harmful or wasteful overlaps in treatment plans. Coordination is grounded in information about the patient that, with consent, is readily shared and mutually evaluated.

Most recently, integrated care has been seen, more strongly than in the past, as moving outside the formal health care system and including links to community-based services that address social determinants of health.[35–37] The principle of "task shifting" some specialty services to generalists,[38] housing specialists within the same clinical space as generalists,[39] screening and referral programs for sub-stance use,[40] mental health telephone consultation services for generalists,[25,41] and the use of community health workers in primary care[42] are all innovations that address parts of a full integrated care model.

AN EVALUATION FRAMEWORK FOR PEDIATRIC INTEGRATED CARE

In this article we use a framework for key domains of integrated care that grew out of the previously mentioned definitions plus the work of teams in a series of learning col-laboratives involving primary care–mental health teams trying to initiate or improve ac-cess to trauma-related services for families with young children.[43] The framework is not exhaustive of all the components of integrated care, but it has proven to be an organizing work that at the outset can seem overwhelming. **Table 1** outlines the do-mains and some possible measurement goals of each. Each domain is discussed in the paragraphs that follow, and in the "What to measure" section.

Inner and Outer Practice Context

Adopting integrated care requires changes in how clinical sites and their teams oper-ate, and delivering integrated care over time requires that individuals within and across teams can work flexibly with each other, mutually solve problems on the fly, and main-tain an empathetic and therapeutic stance toward patients despite unpredictable workloads and emotionally difficult clinical problems.[70] These aspects of workplace culture and climate are important to the uptake of new processes and to the ultimate quality of the care produced.[71,72] They impact patients and staff: patients are more trusting of care when they perceive staff interactions as being more collaborative[73]; they create a safe environment in which patients can move into more mindful states.[74] The larger, outer context in which integration is taking place also influences what is accomplished: how stable is program funding, how worried are providers about pro-ductivity, what support is available for infrastructure needs related to integration.

Changes to Primary Care Structure and Staff Expertise

Integrated care requires changes to how a practice operates and to how individual practice members work.[29] At the overall practice level, the practice may choose to adopt one or more methods of systematically detecting child and family psychosocial problems, or trying to deliver universal preventive interventions. Individual team mem-bers, often primary care providers themselves, may need to acquire new clinical knowledge and skills.[38] The practice may have to invest in initial training and ongoing mechanisms for reinforcing skills and supporting clinical decision-making. In turn, specialists providing this support may need to learn new ways of framing their knowl-edge so that it is best used by primary care providers.[75] Integration programs pose

Table 1
Key domains of integrated child mental health programs, core components, and possible structure and process measures

Domain	Core Components	Possible Areas of Measurement	Examples of Measures
Contextual factors that impact the success of integration	Internal context of practice/clinic	Culture and climate within primary care, specialty, and community partner organizations Assessment of culture as relates to particular aspects of care (ie, trauma-informed care, provision of mental health services) Assessment of climate as relates to staff wellness, work stress, mechanisms for working together; past experience with practice transformation (ie, involvement in patient-centered medical home adoption)	Fallot & Harris assessment tool for trauma-informed care[44] Adaptive reserve[45] AHRQ Team-based Primary Care Measures Database; https://primarycaremeasures.ahrq.gov/team-based-care/
	Context external to individual sites	Financial and organizational support from payers and systems to promote integration Accountability for results related to integrated care Location in mental health workforce shortage area (specific to population served)	Overlap with standards required for Primary Care Medical Home certification
Changes to primary care structures and processes	Whole practice level	Adoption of universal and targeted interventions for prevention case detection, early intervention	COMPASS Primary Health and Behavioral Health Self-Assessment Tool; www.integration.samhsa.gov/operations-administration/assessment-tools#OATI Center for Integrated Health Solutions Framework[46] Patient-Centered Integrated Behavioral Health Care Principles and Tasks Checklist, UW AIMS Center; www.integration.samhsa.gov/AIMS_BHI_Checklist.pdf (and other tools at www.integration.samhsa.gov/operations-administration/assessment-tools) Behavioral Health Capacity Assessment Tool[47] Physical and Behavioral Health Assessment Tool[48] RAND Integration Scale[49] Integrated Practice Assessment Tool http://ipat.valueoptions.com/IPAT/
	Individual provider expertise	Participation in training, use of decision-support mechanisms (eg, consultation lines), confidence in treatment of MH problems, inclusion of MH diagnoses in visits, use of MH-related skills per patient reports or independent assessment	Physician Belief Scale[50] Change in types of consultation questions as integrated care evolves[51]

(continued on next page)

Table 1
(continued)

Domain	Core Components	Possible Areas of Measurement	Examples of Measures
Patient engagement	Participation in program planning	Presence of family members or youth on advisory groups; assessments by participants that family/youth participation is facilitated and meaningful	Medical Home Index[52]
	Patient engagement in own care	Report of therapeutic alliance Reporting of sense of provider-patient centeredness, participatory decision-making, fit of treatment to personal goals Follow-up appointments kept, prescriptions filled and refilled	Session Rating Scales (parent and child)[53,54] Working Alliance Inventory (parent)[55] Treatment Acceptability Rating Scale-Revised[56] Clinically Useful Patient Satisfaction Scale[57]
Social determinants of care	Determination of basic social and developmental needs	Assessment for food, housing insecurity, adequate child care, school readiness or achievement	SWYC,[58] SEEK[59]; see review Chung and coworkers[60] Institute of Medicine Measures of Social and Behavioral Determinants of Health (adults)[61]
	Family-centered care	Use of tools assessing family functioning Assessment of family-centered care (from family perspective)	McMaster GF Family Function Scale[62] Pediatric Integrated Care Scale[63] Family-Centered Care Assessment[12]
	Two- (or multi) generational care	Use of tools assessing parental mental health, substance use, exposure to interpersonal violence Proportion of parents screened; proportion linked to matching services	Edinburg,[64] PHQ-9,[65] AUDIT,[66] SEEK,[59] SWYC[58]
	Linkages to community services and schools	Maintenance of accurate service lists, use of CHWs or others to facilitate linkage; formal arrangements with particular agencies, schools, adult services; proportion of patients successfully linked	Weaver turf-trust collaboration spectrum tool for looking at organizational relationships; http://tamarackcci.ca/blogs/liz-weaver/turf-trust-and-collaboration-spectrum AHRQ clinical-community relationships database for patient-level linkage assessments https://primarycaremeasures.ahrq.gov/clinical-community/

Coordinated, stepped, evidence-based care	Screening and assessment for wellness and mental health problems	Proportion screened, proportion identified as needing services, proportion engaging in services (preventive or indicated)	Screening for clinical depression and follow-up plan[67] Individual tools from **Table 2**
	Adapted treatments available in primary care	Function of colocated providers; caseloads, distribution of types of work (formal and informal consultation, direct care) Range of problems and diagnoses treated	Structural aspects measured by instruments above (eg, COMPASS) SDQ,[68] PSC,[69] PHQ,[65] others (see **Table 2**)
	Information sharing and transfer	Availability of shared medical records, processes for obtaining consent for contact between PCP and specialist; receipt of specialist feedback	Structural aspects measured by instruments above (eg, RAND Integration Scale) Patient Perceptions of Integrated Care http://www.integratedpatientcare.org Consumer Assessment of Healthcare Providers and Systems https://www.ahrq.gov/cahps/surveys-guidance/index.html
	Monitoring of patient outcomes	Presence of dashboard or other mechanism for obtaining and monitoring progress over time	See Zima[67] for National Quality Measures for Child Mental Health Care SDQ Impact Scale,[68] repeat measures with other instruments from **Table 2**

Abbreviations: AHRQ, Agency for Healthcare Research and Quality; AUDIT, Alcohol Use Disorders Identification Test; CHW, community health worker; COMPASS, Care of Mental, Physical and Substance-use Syndromes; MH, mental health; PCP, primary care provider; PHQ, Patient Health Questionnaire; PSC, Pediatric Symptom Checklist; SDQ, Strengths and Difficulties Questionnaire; SEEK, Safe Environment for Every Kid; SWYC, Survey of Well-being of Young Children.

varying challenges to the need to promote (and measure) uptake of new skills and knowledge. Adopting universal screening may allow for little variation in clinicians' work, whereas encouraging use of a new consultant may take considerable marketing.[25]

Patient Engagement

Patient engagement in care is a central tenet of the Chronic Care Model. Treatment of mental health problems, like other potentially long-term problems, requires sustained action and lifestyle changes outside the direct control of health care providers.[34] Patients can report on whether they believe they have developed a working alliance with their providers, and whether they believe that care has been successfully tailored to their needs. Patient involvement in the design of care is also important to the success of integrated care.[76] Patients can give important feedback about features of the primary care setting that facilitate working on psychosocial issues, and on whether proposed methods of care coordination are practical.

Social Determinants of Care

The onset and trajectory of mental health problems are strongly determined by the social and economic circumstances in which people live.[77] For children, families and schools are two main elements of these circumstances. Families provide most of the instrumental and social support that children require, and parental mental health is intimately linked bidirectionally to child mental health.[20,21] The ability of an integrated care system to treat children's mental health problems is severely limited in the absence of mechanisms to help families access services provided by schools, community agencies, and clinical sites where parents may be receiving care.

Coordinated, Stepped, Evidence-Based Care

The ultimate goal of the integrated system, again as articulated by the Chronic Care Model,[33] is to make expert care available to patients as early as possible in their trajectory through the health care system. Evidence-based interventions need to be adapted for delivery in the primary care setting either by primary care providers themselves, other primary care staff, or colocated mental health providers. Mechanisms need to be developed to track improvement in patient function and determine when more intensive efforts at diagnosis or treatment need to be made.[78,79] Clinical and evaluation efforts need to focus on amounts of change that are clinically meaningful from a statistical point of view and from the patient's point of view.[80]

STUDY DESIGNS

Even when integrated care programs are developed from the beginning as research projects, patient-level randomized trials are rarely possible. Patients have ongoing relationships with primary care providers that cannot be disrupted, and providers or practices can usually not develop new interventions for use with only some of their patients. Randomization at the provider, practice, or geographic level (cluster randomization) may be possible but increases sample size requirements and raises the question of what to tell patients about what the system is attempting to do.[81] "Stepped wedge" designs are a form of cluster randomization that attempts to address the further dilemma of wanting all providers to eventually take part in the integrated care system.[82] Stepped wedge designs randomize providers or sites to the order in which they are trained or enter the intervention system, rather than assigning them to an intervention or control arm. Early versions of this approach were known as "wait list control" or parallel cluster studies using just two groups, the initial intervention adopters and those coming later. Stepped wedge trials take the concept further by allowing multiple points of entry as practices come on line in a random order. For clustered and stepped wedge designs, multilevel modeling are used to develop valid estimates of outcomes and impact of key moderators while accounting for clustering and the differing characteristics of providers or sites within each cluster.[83]

The health system context of many integrated care programs frequently makes it difficult or impossible to evaluate them with any form of a truly experimental design. Many evaluations have to use quasiexperimental methods,[84] often only comparing outcomes at multiple time points before and during the roll-out of an integrated care program. Sometimes there may be similar sites or systems that are observed over the same time period and serve as nonequivalent control groups. Time series analyses have been successfully used to examine the impact of screening as a component of integrated care,[85] but have methodologic pitfalls in the absence of control populations being observed over the same time period.[86]

Mixed qualitative and quantitative designs have also been used to evaluate integrated care and other mental health service programs.[37] Qualitative data from focus groups or individual interviews can fill in gaps in the understanding of mechanisms leading to intervention outcomes and can guide judicious use of quantitative data, especially when sample sizes are small and there is considerable risk of misinterpreting trends or potentially random associations found in the exploration of multiple possible outcomes.

LEARNING HEALTH CARE SYSTEMS, THEORIES OF CHANGE, AND "DYNAMIC SUSTAINABILITY"

Many complex interventions are guided by a logic model or "theory of change."[87] These models set out "inputs": partners; resources; target populations; core processes; and then short-, intermediate-, and long-term outcomes (structures that may need to be created, processes that may be observed and patient-level outcomes that may be achieved). **Fig. 1** shows a model for a state-level program supporting uptake of mental health skills by primary care providers. Critics of traditional health services research approaches have argued that these models, no matter how well grounded in prior research, are always approximations[23]; presumed contexts turn out to differ from reality, evidence-based interventions require additional adaptation for the patients actually encountered. Most importantly, evaluation results lag the evolution of the program; they may serve the wider research community but do not arrive in time to help the program refine its operations and improve its impact.

The concepts of "learning health care systems"[88] and Chambers and colleagues'[23] "dynamic sustainability" framework suggest seeing evaluation as an ongoing activity closely related to quality improvement. Measurement of key processes and outcomes is set up so that it is examined at regular intervals, driving adjustments to the logic model. Small subprojects may have to be designed to rapidly collect data informing decisions about procedures that may require changing. As the integrated care project evolves from its initial implementation stage and achieves some level of stability, the balance of data collection may shift from an early focus on verifying assumptions about the population targeted, start-up of key processes, and examining aggregate outcomes to optimizing outcomes across the families involved.[7,15] In particular, programs may want to examine variation in participation or outcome by certain patient characteristics, comparing the characteristics of potentially eligible patients with those who are being served.

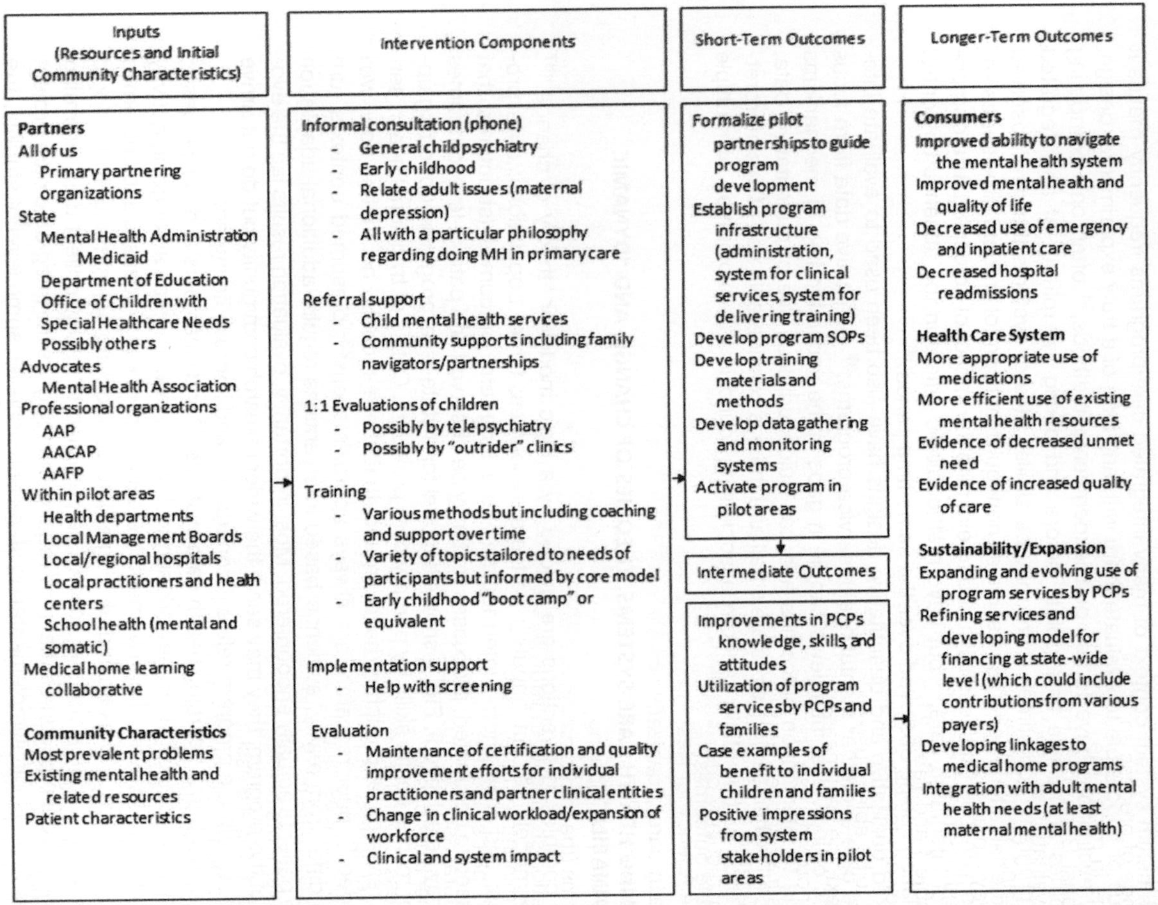

Inputs (Resources and Initial Community Characteristics)

Partners

All of us
- Primary partnering organizations

State
- Mental Health Administration
- Medicaid
- Department of Education
- Office of Children with Special Healthcare Needs
- Possibly others

Advocates
- Mental Health Association

Professional organizations
- AAP
- AACAP
- AAFP

Within pilot areas
- Health departments
- Local Management Boards
- Local/regional hospitals
- Local practitioners and health centers
- School health (mental and somatic)
- Medical home learning collaborative

Community Characteristics
- Most prevalent problems
- Existing mental health and related resources
- Patient characteristics

Intervention Components

Informal consultation (phone)
- General child psychiatry
- Early childhood
- Related adult issues (maternal depression)
- All with a particular philosophy regarding doing MH in primary care

Referral support
- Child mental health services
- Community supports including family navigators/partnerships

1:1 Evaluations of children
- Possibly by tele psychiatry
- Possibly by "outrider" clinics

Training
- Various methods but including coaching and support over time
- Variety of topics tailored to needs of participants but informed by core model
- Early childhood "boot camp" or equivalent

Implementation support
- Help with screening

Evaluation
- Maintenance of certification and quality improvement efforts for individual practitioners and partner clinical entities
- Change in clinical workload/expansion of workforce
- Clinical and system impact

Short-Term Outcomes

- Formalize pilot partnerships to guide program development
- Establish program infrastructure (administration, system for clinical services, system for delivering training)
- Develop program SOPs
- Develop training materials and methods
- Develop data gathering and monitoring systems
- Activate program in pilot areas

Intermediate Outcomes

- Improvements in PCPs knowledge, skills, and attitudes
- Utilization of program services by PCPs and families
- Case examples of benefit to individual children and families
- Positive impressions from system stakeholders in pilot areas

Longer-Term Outcomes

Consumers
- Improved ability to navigate the mental health system
- Improved mental health and quality of life
- Decreased use of emergency and inpatient care
- Decreased hospital readmissions

Health Care System
- More appropriate use of medications
- More efficient use of existing mental health resources
- Evidence of decreased unmet need
- Evidence of increased quality of care

Sustainability/Expansion
- Expanding and evolving use of program services by PCPs
- Refining services and developing model for financing at state-wide level (which could include contributions from various payers)
- Developing linkages to medical home programs
- Integration with adult mental health needs (at least maternal mental health)

Fig. 1. Logic model for telephone consultation process. AACAP, American Academy of Child and Adolescent Psychiatry; AAFP, American Academy of Family Physicians; AAP, American Academy of Pediatrics; MH, mental health; PCP, primary care provider; SOP, standard operating procedures.

WHAT TO MEASURE

Many general frameworks are available to guide the selection of aspects of integrated care that are measured as part of an evaluation. Donabedian's "structure, process, and outcome" framework has been used across a wide range of health care programs.[89] Hoagwood and colleagues'[90] SFCES data framework (Symptoms, Functioning, Consumer perspectives, Environments/context, and Service systems) spans a range of process and clinical outcomes selected with mental health services evaluations in mind. The Substance Abuse and Mental Health Services Administration's National Behavioral Health Quality Framework,[91] work by Brown and coworkers[92] on evaluation of psychotherapy, and guidance from the UK CYIAPT program ("Children and Youth Increasing Access to Psychological Therapies")[17] provide guidance on ways to assess the structure, process, and outcomes of specific mental health interventions that form part of the integrated care program.

Table 1 and Table 2 have examples of potentially practical measures, following our framework for the components of integrated care and the idea that learning systems want to be able to use data to drive program implementation and improvement. In this context, the best measures are those that are either already routinely collected or simple enough to use on a regular basis with little additional investment of effort. Ideally, measures chosen are used to help track the care of individual patients and being aggregated to assess system performance. Measures from the CYIAPT program are particularly brief and were chosen for this purpose.[17]

The Agency for Healthcare Research and Quality defines structures as "feature(s) of a health care organization or clinician related to the capacity to provide high quality health care."[93] In integrated care this may include characteristics of providers (how many are participating, their comfort with particular conditions and treatments) or of systems (the formalization of team meetings or collaborative links, mechanisms for information sharing, or the quality and capacity of community services addressing social determinants of care). In our framework, the outer context in which the integration is taking place and the organizational culture and climate might also be considered structural aspects of care. Markers may include the availability of facilitating funding mechanisms or supports (eg, telephone consultation programs), the presence of staff wellness programs, measures of staff stress and satisfaction, and staff retention or turnover figures. Other factors that might be considered structural could be formalized care sequences relating to roles, communication processes, and collaborations for particular patients. Studies to date have not found a close correlation between structural elements of integrated care systems and outcomes.[27] Some of the tools listed in Table 1 for assessing structure (eg, COMPASS, the Behavioral Health Capacity Assessment Tool) were designed more as checklists in practice transformation projects. In contrast, practice culture and climate have been linked to program uptake and clinical outcomes.[71,72] Many general implementation measures, with reviews, are available without cost at https://societyforimplementationresearchcollaboration.org.

Care processes are observable actions "performed for, on behalf of, or by a patient."[93] Care process measures might include the proportion of children/youth seen in primary care well-visits with a mental health screen performed, the frequency of mental health referrals made, referral success rates (become engaged with a provider), the number of contacts with an integrated care behavioral health provider, or rates of mental health medication prescribing. Programs might want to try to differentiate referrals from care that is managed collaboratively. For a telephone consultation service process measures might include the number of calls received, the proportion of live-connects to a psychiatrist versus call backs, characteristics of the consultations

Table 2
Selected measures for patient and family conditions and outcomes tracking

Instrument	Uses	Comments
Condition-specific		
PROMIS-Anger (http://www.healthmeasures.net/explore-measurement-systems/promis)	Problem classification, change over time, outcomes	Angry mood, negative social cognitions, efforts to control anger Physical aggression not included
PROMIS-Anxiety (http://www.healthmeasures.net/explore-measurement-systems/promis)	Problem classification, change over time, outcomes	Fear, anxious misery, hyperarousal, and somatic symptoms related to arousal
PROMIS-Depression (http://www.healthmeasures.net/explore-measurement-systems/promis)	Problem classification, change over time, outcomes	Negative mood, views of self, social cognition, decreased positive affect and engagement Not somatic symptoms
PROMIS-Peer Relationships (http://www.healthmeasures.net/explore-measurement-systems/promis)	Problem classification, change over time, outcomes	Quality of relationships with friends and other acquaintances
Patient Health Questionnaire-9[65]	Problem classification, change over time, outcomes	Depression
Traumatic Events Screening Inventory for Children (www.ptsd.va.gov/PTSD/professional/assessment/child/index.asp)	Problem classification	Experience of potential traumatic events (injuries, hospitalizations, domestic violence, community violence, disasters, accidents, physical abuse, and sexual abuse)
Revised Children's Anxiety and Depression Scale (http://www.corc.uk.net/outcome-experience-measures/)	Problem classification, change over time, outcomes	Depression, anxiety (several subscales)
How Are Things? (http://www.corc.uk.net/outcome-experience-measures/)	Problem classification, change over time, outcomes	Oppositional-defiant behaviors
Brief Parental Self-Efficacy Scale (http://www.corc.uk.net/outcome-experience-measures/)	Problem classification, change over time	Five positively worded questions about parent confidence in working with child
Overall mental health status and function		
Strengths and Difficulties Questionnaire[68]	Problem classification, change over time, outcomes	Has subscales
Strengths and Difficulties Questionnaire Impact Supplement[68]	Status at baseline, change over time (but not session-by-session), outcomes	Overall function in core social domains

(continued on next page)

Table 2 (continued)		
Instrument	Uses	Comments
Outcome Rating Scales[53,54]	Immediate postsession, very short, meant for repeated measures	Overall function: distress, well-being, social role, overall well-being
Pediatric Symptom Checklist[69]	Status at baseline, change over time (but not session by session), outcomes	General psychosocial screening and functional assessment in the domains of attention, externalizing, and internalizing symptoms
Survey of Well-being of Young Children (www.theswyc.org)	Status at baseline, change over time (but not session-by-session), outcomes	Several age-related versions

(when, how long, which clients), descriptions of consultation advice offered (medication, therapy, referral), provider prescribing patterns, and changes over time.[94] Families' subjective experience of care, and particularly, the extent to which it creates an environment for disclosing emotional and behavioral concerns, might also be considered a process measure.

One important way the evaluation of integrated care programs may differ from other evaluations is that there may be impacts (favorable or not) on processes within multiple systems. Integrated care may be designed to help primary care and specialty care become more efficient. Primary care sites may run more smoothly if they can anticipate and meet the needs of families with complex psychosocial problems; specialty sites may have better rates of attendance if referred families have been better engaged in care and experience a personalized introduction to the specialist. Community services may find that they have a steadier stream of clients. Ideally, evaluations are designed to look for these process impacts across the systems involved, to be able to identify unanticipated consequences of the integration and to find benefits in one system that might offset costs or burdens in another.

Outcomes, "a health state of a patient resulting from health care,"[93] are collected from multiple observers and involve many domains of child and family function. Symptoms and function often diverge, especially among children.[95] Parents, children, and youth can report directly on their own level of function or how well they function together as a family. Families and sometimes school systems may be willing to provide information on educational achievement or attendance.

OBTAINING OUTCOME DATA

One of the most challenging aspects of conducting a meaningful evaluation of an integrated care program is the difficulty of assessing change in symptoms and functioning over time. Although families may return for follow-up care, they may do so at irregular intervals and may not be reassessed in a way that allows for analysis of program impact across patients.

World Wide Web, text, and "smartphone" systems all have the potential for making it possible to contact families systematically and ask them to complete a short instrument. Some of these functions can be embedded in the "patient portals" of electronic medical record systems. An example from adult mental health care is the Treatment Outcome Package, which asks about mental health symptoms and functioning across

12 clinical domains.[96] Providers use this system to email a link to the patient to complete an online questionnaire (which requires 3–5 minutes). The system scores the questionnaire and generates a short report for the provider. Over time, these reports graphically display changes in scores within each domain and benchmark those scores compared with the general nonclinical population. The report alerts the provider if the patient is not making progress as expected and includes a list of suggested treatment practices aimed at improving outcomes. Treatment Outcome Package also generates a section of the report designed to give to the patient as feedback.

A similar approach to serial data collection could be done manually using a secure on-line resource, such as REDCap (www.project-redcap.org). REDCap is widely available at low cost through many universities. It is readily customizable and has several of the instruments in **Table 2** preprogramed into on-line questionnaires that can be presented to families at the time of a visit. REDCap facilitates automated scoring, storage, and aggregation of results, and creation of data sets for analysis. Open Data Kit (www.opendatakit.org) from the University of Washington is a freely available platform for designing questionnaires that can be administered on "smart" devices and uploading data for analysis. It includes more simple "drag and drop" questionnaire creation as well as complex forms that include a variety of forms of data collection. The "Commcare" platform (https://www.commcarehq.org) also allows users to create custom smartphone "apps" that can be used to collect data and communicate with individuals who have installed the application on their phone. Development of the application and piloting with 10 or fewer users is done at no charge; larger numbers of users and HIPAA-compliant data management incur costs. Several other commercial/proprietary systems can perform these functions, including the "patient portals" of electronic medical record systems.

Links to school, insurance, and public record data may also make it possible to ascertain some process and outcome data without actively collecting it from families.[97] For example, Oklahoma, as part of an the ABCD early childhood program, established an Internet portal that linked primary care providers with community agencies involved with developmental assessments and services.[98] The system can track completion of referrals across the different systems responsible for helping children with developmental risks. Medicaid data may be used to identify patients treated by providers participating in integrated care efforts, and to compare them with otherwise similar patients who are seen by nonparticipating providers.[99] Comparisons might include the number and kinds of diagnoses made, prescriptions filled, and emergency or inpatient services used.

SUMMARY

Programs designed to deliver integrated child mental health care represent complex interventions with many similarities to other complex health services programs and to primary care programs and medical home transformations to which they are closely related. Child mental health integration programs, however, have some unique features that may alter the emphasis placed on certain aspects of their evaluation. In addition, perspectives on evaluation of integrated care are changing rapidly, suggesting the need for variations on evaluation approaches that better guide program operations in real time and that place heavier emphasis on collaboration with families and community-based services. Seeing evaluation designs as something that evolves over time as a program matures may make it possible to use designs that are practical and provide the most meaningful outcomes at any given point in the program's evolution.

REFERENCES

1. Peek CJ, the National Integration Academy Council. Lexicon for behavioral health and primary care integration: concepts and definitions developed by expert consensus. AHRQ Publication No.13-IP001-EF. Rockville (MD): Agency for Healthcare Research and Quality; 2013.

2. Singer SJ, Burgers J, Friedberg M, et al. Defining and measuring integrated patient care: promoting the next frontier in health care delivery. Med Care Res Rev 2011;68:112–27.

3. Salmon P, Hall GM. Patient empowerment and control: a psychological discourse in the service of medicine. Soc Sci Med 2003;57:1969–80.

4. Damschroder LJ, Aron DC, Keith RE, et al. Fostering implementation of health services research findings into practice: a consolidated framework for advancing implementation science. Implement Sci 2009;4:50.

5. Campbell NC, Murray E, Darbyshire J, et al. Designing and evaluating complex interventions to improve care. BMJ 2007;334:455–9.

6. Fixsen DL, Naoom SF, Blase KA, et al. Implementation research: a synthesis of the literature (FMHI Publication #231). Tampa (FL): University of South Florida, Louis de la Parte Florida Mental Health Institute, The National Implementation Research Network; 2005.

7. Curran GM, Bauwer M, Mittman B, et al. Effectiveness-implementation hybrid designs. Med Care 2012;50:217–26.

8. Bailey ZD, Krieger N, Agénor M, et al. Structural racism and health inequities in the USA: evidence and interventions. Lancet 2017;389:1453–63.

9. Stange KC, Etz RS, Gullett H, et al. Metrics for assessing improvements in primary health care. Annu Rev Public Health 2014;35:423–42.

10. Lukewich J, Corbin R, VanDenKerkhof EG, et al. Identification, summary and comparison of tools used to measure organizational attributes associated with chronic disease management within primary care settings. J Eval Clin Pract 2014;20:1072–85.

11. Whitlock EP, Orleans CT, Pender N, et al. Evaluating primary care behavioral counseling interventions: an evidence-based approach. Am J Prev Med 2002; 22:267–84.

12. Wells N, Bronhem S, Zyzanski S, et al. Psychometric evaluation of a consumer developed family centered care assessment tool. Matern Child Health J 2015; 19:1899–909.

13. Co JP, Sternberg SB, Homer CJ. Measuring patient and family experiences of health care for children. Acad Pediatr 2011;11(3 Suppl):S59–67.

14. Lewis CC, Fischer S, Weiner BJ, et al. Outcomes for implementation science: an enhanced systematic review of instruments using evidence-based rating criteria. Implement Sci 2015;10:155.

15. Parry GJ, Carson-Stevens A, Luff DF, et al. Recommendations for evaluation of health care improvement initiatives. Acad Pediatr 2013;13(6 Suppl):S23–30.

16. Byatt N, Biebel K, Moore Simas TA, et al. Improving perinatal depression care: the Massachusetts child psychiatry access project for moms. Gen Hosp Psychiatry 2016;40:12–7.

17. Law D, Wolpert M, editors. Guide to using outcomes and feedback tools with children, young people and families. London: Child Outcomes Research Consortium; 2014.

18. Asarnow JR, Rozenman M, Wiblin J, et al. Integrated medical-behavioral care compared with usual primary care for child and adolescent behavioral health: a meta-analysis. JAMA Pediatr 2015;169:929–37.

19. Brown JD, Wissow LS. Disagreement in primary care provider and parent reports of mental health counseling. Pediatrics 2008;122:1204–11.

20. Perrino T, Gonzalez-Soldevilla A, Pantin H, et al. The role of families in adolescent HIV prevention: a review. Clin Child Fam Psychol Rev 2000;3:81–96.

21. Repetti RL, Taylor SE, Seeman TE. Risky families: family social environments and the mental and physical health of offspring. Psychol Bull 2002;128:330–66.

22. Asarnow JR, Kolko DJ, Miranda J, et al. The pediatric patient-centered medical home: innovative models for improving behavioral health. Am Psychol 2017;72: 13–27.

23. Chambers DA, Glasgow RE, Stange KC. The dynamic sustainability framework: addressing the paradox of sustainment amid ongoing change. Implementation Sci 2013;8:117.

24. Garland AF, Bickman L, Chorpita BF. Change what? Identifying quality improvement targets by investigating usual mental health care. Adm Policy Ment Health 2010;37:15–26.

25. Sarvet B, Gold J, Straus JH. Bridging the divide between child psychiatry and primary care: the use of telephone consultation within a population-based collaborative system. Child Adolesc Psychiatr Clin N Am 2011;20:41–53.

26. Briggs-Gowan MJ, Owens PL, Schwab-Stone ME, et al. Persistence of psychiatric disorders in pediatric settings. J Am Acad Child Adolesc Psychiatry 2003;42: 1360–9.

27. Butler M, Kane RL, McAlpine D, et al. Integration of mental health/substance abuse and primary care No. 173 (Prepared by the Minnesota Evidence-based Practice Center under Contract No. 290-02-0009.). AHRQ Publication No. 09-E003. Rockville (MD): Agency for Healthcare Research and Quality; 2008.

28. Brown JD, King MA, Wissow LS. The central role of relationships to trauma-informed integrated care for children and youth. Acad Pediatr 2017 [pii:S1876–2859(17)30015-3]. [Epub ahead of print].

29. Leykum LK, Lanham HJ, Pugh JA, et al. Manifestations and implications of uncertainty for improving healthcare systems: an analysis of observational and interventional studies grounded in complexity science. Implement Sci 2014;9:165.

30. Doherty WJ, McDaniel SH, Baird MA. Five levels of primary care/behavioral healthcare collaboration. Behav Healthc Tomorrow 1996;5:25–7.

31. World Health Organization. A global review of primary health care: emerging messages. Geneva (Switzerland): World Health Organization; 2003.

32. Starfield B. Primary care: balancing health needs, services, and technology. New York: Oxford University Press; 1988.

33. Wagner EH, Austin BT, Von Korff M. Organizing care for patients with chronic illness. Milbank Q 1996;74:511–44.

34. Woltmann E, Grogan-Kaylor A, Perron B, et al. Comparative effectiveness of collaborative chronic care models for mental health conditions across primary, specialty, and behavioral health care settings: systematic review and meta-analysis. Am J Psychiatry 2012;169:790–804.

35. Alley DE, Asomugha CN, Conway PH, et al. Accountable health communities: addressing social needs through Medicare and Medicaid. N Engl J Med 2016;374: 8–11.

36. Beck AF, Tschudy MM, Coker TR, et al. Determinants of health and pediatric primary care practices. Pediatrics 2016;137:1–11.

37. Dowrick C, Bower P, Chew-Graham C, et al. Evaluating a complex model designed to increase access to high quality primary mental health care for under-served groups: a multi-method study. BMC Health Serv Res 2016;16:58.
38. Joshi R, Alim M, Kengne AP, et al. Task shifting for non-communicable disease management in low and middle income countries: a systematic review. PLoS One 2014;9:e103754.
39. McCue Horwitz S, Storfer-Isser A, Kerker BD, et al. Do on-site mental health professionals change pediatricians' responses to children's mental health problems? Acad Pediatr 2016;16:676–83.
40. Levy SJ, Williams JF, Committee on Substance Use and Prevention. Substance use screening, brief intervention, and referral to treatment. Pediatrics 2016; 138(1) [pii:e20161211].
41. Hilt RJ, Barclay RP, Bush J, et al. A statewide child telepsychiatry consult system yields desired health system changes and savings. Telemed J E Health 2015;21: 533–7.
42. Johnson SL, Gunn VL. Community health workers as a component of the health care team. Pediatr Clin North Am 2015;62:1313–28.
43. Dayton L, Agosti J, Bernard-Pearl D, et al. Integrating mental and physical health services using a socio-emotional trauma lens. Curr Probl Pediatr Adolesc Health Care 2016;46:391–401.
44. Brown VB, Harris M, Fallot R. Moving toward trauma-informed practice in addiction treatment: a collaborative model of agency assessment. J Psychoactive Drugs 2013;45:386–93.
45. Jaén CR, Palmer RF. Shorter adaptive reserve measures. Ann Fam Med 2012; 8(Suppl 1):1–2.
46. Heath B, Wise Romero P, Reynolds K. A review and proposed standard framework for levels of integrated healthcare. Washington, DC: SAMHSA-HRSA Center for Integrated Health Solutions; 2013.
47. Lewin Group and Institute for Healthcare Improvement. Behavioral health intergration capacity assessment (BHICA). Falls Church (VA): Institute for Healthcare Improvement; 2014. Available at. http://www.ihi.org/resources/Pages/Tools/BehavioralHealthIntegrationCapacityAssessmentTool.aspx. Accessed April 27, 2017.
48. Pourat N, Hadler MW, Dixon B, et al. One-stop shopping: efforts to integrate physical and behavioral health care in five California community health centers. Policy Brief UCLA Cent Health Policy Res 2015;(PB2015–1):1–11.
49. Scharf DM, Eberhart N, Schmidt-Hackbarth N, et al. Evaluation of the SAMHSA primary and behavioral health care integration (PBHCI) grant program: final report. Rand Health Q 2014;4(3):6.
50. Ashworth CD, Williamson P, Montano D. A scale to measure physician beliefs about psychosocial aspects of patient care. Soc Sci Med 1984;19:1235–8.
51. Cape J, Morris E, Burd M, et al. Complexity of GPs' explanations about mental health problems: development, reliability, and validity of a measure. Br J Gen Pract 2008;56:403–10.
52. Cooley WC, McAllister JW, Sherrieb K, et al. The medical home index: development and validation of a new practice-level measure of implementation of the Medical Home model. Ambul Pediatr 2003;3:173–80.
53. Campbell A, Hemsley S. Outcome rating scale and session rating scale in psychological practice: clinical utility of ultra-brief measures. Clin Psychol 2009;13: 1–9.

54. Wolpert M. CYP IAPT tools: what are they, how were they selected and where can you find them?. In: Law D, Wolpert M, editors. Guide to using outcomes and feedback tools with children, young people and families. London: Child Outcomes Research Consortium; 2014. p. 19–26.

55. Hatcher RL, Gillaspy JA. Development and validation of a revised short version of the Working Alliance. Psychother Res 2006;16:12–5.

56. Reimers TM, Wacker DP, Cooper LJ. Evaluation of the acceptability of treatments for their children's behavioral difficulties: ratings by parents receiving services in an outpatient clinic. Child Fam Behav Ther 1991;13:53–71.

57. Zimmerman M, Gazarian D, Multach M, et al. A clinically useful self-report measure of psychiatric patients' satisfaction with the initial evaluation. Psychiatry Res 2017;252:38–44.

58. Sheldrick RC, Henson BS, Merchant S, et al. The preschool pediatric symptom checklist (PPSC). Development and initial validation of a new social-emotional screening instrument. Acad Pediatr 2013;13:72–80.

59. Dubowitz H, Feigelman S, Lane W, et al. Pediatric primary care to help prevent child maltreatment: the Safe Environment for Every Kid (SEEK) Model. Pediatrics 2009;123:858–64.

60. Chung EK, Siegel BS, Garg A, et al. Screening for social determinants of health among children and families living in poverty: a guide for clinicians. Curr Probl Pediatr Adolesc Health Care 2016;46:135–53.

61. Giuse NB, Koonce TY, Kusnoor SV, et al. Institute of Medicine measures of social and behavioral determinants of health: a feasibility study. Am J Prev Med 2017; 52:199–206.

62. Byles J, Byrne C, Boyle M, et al. Ontario child health study: reliability and validity of the general functioning subscale of the McMaster Family Assessment Device. Fam Process 1988;27:97–104.

63. Ziniel SI, Rosenberg HN, Bach AM, et al. Validation of a parent-reported experience measure of integrated care. Pediatrics 2016;138(6) [pii:e20160676].

64. Venkatesh KK, Kaimal AJ, Castro VM, et al. Improving discrimination in antepartum depression screening using the Edinburgh Postnatal Depression Scale. J Affect Disord 2017;214:1–7.

65. Richardson LP, McCauley E, Grossman DC, et al. Evaluation of the Patient Health Questionnaire-9 item for detecting major depression among adolescents. Pediatrics 2010;126:1117.

66. Harris SK, Louis-Jacques J, Knight JR. Screening and brief intervention for alcohol and other abuse. Adolesc Med State Art Rev 2014;25:126–56.

67. Zima BT, Murphy JM, Scholle SH, et al. National quality measures for child mental health care: background, progress, and next steps. Pediatrics 2013;131(Suppl 1):S38–49.

68. Goodman R. The extended version of the strengths and difficulties questionnaire as a guide to child psychiatric caseness and consequent burden. J Child Psychol Psychiatry 1999;40(5):791–9.

69. Murphy JM, Ichinose C, Hicks RC, et al. Utility of the pediatric symptom checklist as a psychosocial screen to meet the federal early and periodic screening, diagnosis, and treatment (EPSDT) standards: a pilot study. J Pediatr 1996;129:864.

70. Miller WL, McDaniel RR Jr, Crabtree BF, et al. Practice jazz: understanding variation in family practices using complexity science. J Fam Pract 2001;50:872–8.

71. King MA, Wissow LS, Baum RA. The role of organizational context in the implementation of a statewide initiative to integrate mental health services into pediatric primary care. Health Care Manage Rev 2017. [Epub ahead of print].

72. Glisson C, Hemmelgarn A, Green P, et al. Randomized trial of the availability, responsiveness and continuity (ARC) organizational intervention for improving youth outcomes in community mental health programs. J Am Acad Child Adolesc Psychiatry 2013;52:493–500.

73. Becker ER, Roblin DW. Translating primary care practice climate into patient activation: the role of patient trust in physician. Med Care 2008;46:795–805.

74. Marsac ML, Kassam-Adams N, Hildenbrand AK, et al. Implementing a trauma-informed approach in pediatric health care networks. JAMA Pediatr 2016;170:70–7.

75. Sarvet BD, Wegner L. Developing effective child psychiatry collaboration with primary care: leadership and management strategies. Child Adolesc Psychiatr Clin N Am 2010;19:139–48.

76. Dayton L, Buttress A, Agosti J, et al. Practical steps to integrate family voice in organization, policy, planning, and decision making for trauma-informed integrated pediatric care. Curr Probl Pediatr Adolesc Health Care 2016;46:402–10.

77. World Health Organization. What are social determinants of health? Geneva (Switzerland): World Health Organization; 2013. Available at: www.who.int/social_determinants/sdh_definition/en/. Accessed April 27, 2017.

78. Wissow LS, Anthony B, Brown J, et al. A common factors approach to improving the mental health capacity of pediatric primary care. Adm Policy Ment Health 2008;35:305–18.

79. Olin SS, McCord M, Stein RE, et al. Beyond screening: a stepped care pathway for managing postpartum depression in pediatric settings. J Womens Health (Larchmt) 2017. http://dx.doi.org/10.1089/jwh.2016.6089.

80. Fugard A. Understanding uncertainty in mental health questionnaire data. In: Law D, Wolpert M, editors. Guide to using outcomes and feedback tools with children, young people and families. London: Child Outcomes Research Consortium; 2014. p. 77–85.

81. McRae AD, Weijer C, Binik A, et al. When is informed consent required in cluster randomized trials in health research? Trials 2011;12:202.

82. Hemming K, Haines TP, Chilton PJ, et al. The stepped wedge cluster randomized trial: rationale, design, analysis, and reporting. BMJ 2015;350:h391.

83. Imai K, Keele L, Tingley D, et al. Unpacking the black box of causality: learning about causal mechanisms from experimental and observational studies. Am Polit Sci Rev 2011;105:765–89.

84. Campbell DT, Stanley JC. Experimental and quasi-experimental designs for research. Boston: Houghtton Mifflin Company; 1963.

85. Hacker K, Penfold R, Arsenault LN, et al. The impact of the Massachusetts behavioral health child screening policy on service utilization. Psychiatr Serv 2017;68:25–32.

86. Lagarde M. How to do (or not do)… Assessing the impact of a policy change with routine longitudinal data. Health Policy Plan 2012;27:76–83.

87. De Silva MJ, Breuer E, Lee L, et al. Theory of Change: a theory- driven approach to enhance the Medical Research Council's framework for complex interventions. Trials 2014;15:267.

88. Faden RR, Kass NE, Goodman SN, et al. An ethics framework for a learning health care system: a departure from traditional research ethics and clinical ethics. Hastings Center Report Special Report 43 2013;1:S16–27.

89. Donabedian A. The methods and findings of quality assessment and monitoring : an illustrated analysis. Ann Arbor (MI): Health Administration Press; 1985.

90. Hoagwood KE, Jensen PS, Acric MC, et al. Outcome domains in child mental health research since 1996: have they changed and why does it matter? J Am Acad Child Adolesc Psychiatry 2012;12:1241–60.
91. SAMHSA. Available at: https://www.samhsa.gov/data/national-behavioral-health-quality-framework#overview. Accessed April 23, 2017.
92. Brown JD, Scholle SH, Azur M. Strategies for measuring the quality of psychotherapy: a white paper to inform measure development and implementation. Washington, DC: US Department of Health and Human Services, Office of the Assistant Secretary for Planning and Evaluation; 2014. Available at: https://aspe.hhs.gov/report/strategies-measuring-quality-psychotherapy-white-paper-inform-measure-development-and-implementation. Accessed May 1, 2017.
93. AHRQ. Available at: https://www.qualitymeasures.ahrq.gov/help-and about/summaries/domain-definitions. Accessed May 1, 2017.
94. Barclay RP, Penfold RB, Sullivan D, et al. Decrease in statewide antipsychotic prescribing after implementation of child and adolescent psychiatry consultation services. Health Serv Res 2017;52:561–78.
95. Costello EJ, Mustillo S, Erkanli A, et al. Prevalence and development of psychiatric disorders in childhood and adolescence. Arch Gen Psychiatry 2003;60:837–44.
96. Kraus DR. The Treatment Outcome Package (TOP). Integrating Sci Pract 2012;2:43–5.
97. Wilcox HC, Kharrazi H, Wilson RF, et al. Data linkage strategies to advance youth suicide prevention: a systematic review for a National Institutes of Health Pathways to Prevention Workshop. Ann Intern Med 2016;165:779–85.
98. Hinkle L, Hanlon C. Oklahoma's web portal: fostering care coordination between primary care and community service providers. Briefing. Washington, DC: National Academy for State Health Policy; 2012.
99. Kerker BD, Chor KH, Hoagwood KE, et al. Detection and treatment of mental health issues by pediatric PCPs in New York State: an evaluation of Project TEACH. Psychiatr Serv 2015;66:430–3.

Comparing Two Models of Integrated Behavioral Health Programs in Pediatric Primary Care

Miguelina Germán, PhD[a],*, Michael L. Rinke, MD, PhD[b],
Brittany A. Gurney, MA[c], Rachel S. Gross, MD, MS[d],
Diane E. Bloomfield, MD[e], Lauren A. Haliczer, MA[f],
Silvie Colman, PhD[g], Andrew D. Racine, MD, PhD[h],
Rahil D. Briggs, PsyD[i]

KEYWORDS

- Integrated care • Integrated care models • Primary care • Pediatric
- Behavioral health • Satisfaction • Competency

KEY POINTS

- In comparing 2 models of integrated behavioral health in primary care, the model staffed by pediatric psychologists and generalist social workers showed a significant increase in primary care provider referral rates, primary care provider satisfaction with behavioral health services, and some areas of self-reported competency among primary care providers compared with the social work–only model.

Continued

Disclosure Statement: The authors have nothing to disclose.
[a] Department of Pediatrics, Pediatric Behavioral Health Integrated Program (BHIP), Montefiore Medical Center, Albert Einstein College of Medicine, 3411 Wayne Avenue, 8th Floor, Bronx, NY 10467, USA; [b] Department of Pediatrics, Division of Pediatric Hospital Medicine, Montefiore Medical Center, Albert Einstein College of Medicine, 3411 Wayne Avenue, 8th Floor, Bronx, NY 10467, USA; [c] Trauma Informed Care Program (TIC), Behavioral Health Integration Program (BHIP), Department of Pediatrics, Montefiore Medical Group, 3411 Wayne Avenue, 8th Floor, Bronx, NY 10467, USA; [d] Department of Pediatrics, Children's Hospital at Montefiore, Albert Einstein College of Medicine, 3444 Kossuth Avenue, 2nd Floor, Bronx, NY 10467, USA; [e] The Children's Hospital at Montefiore, Albert Einstein College of Medicine, 3444 Kossuth Avenue, Bronx, NY 10467, USA; [f] Department of Psychological and Brain Sciences, University of Massachusetts Amherst, 402 Tobin Hall, 135 Hicks Way, Amherst, MA 01002, USA; [g] Network Performance Group, Montefiore Medical Center, 6 Executive Plaza, Suite 112A, Yonkers, NY 10701, USA; [h] Montefiore Health System, Montefiore Medical Group, Executive Offices, 111 East 210th Street, Bronx, NY 10467, USA; [i] Pediatric Behavioral Health Services, Montefiore Medical Group, 200 Corporate Boulevard South, Suite 175, Yonkers, NY 10701, USA
* Corresponding author.
E-mail address: mgerman@montefiore.org

Child Adolesc Psychiatric Clin N Am 26 (2017) 815–828
http://dx.doi.org/10.1016/j.chc.2017.06.009
childpsych.theclinics.com

Continued

- At sites staffed with pediatric psychiatrists in addition to psychologists, primary care providers reported feeling more competent managing school-age and adolescent attention deficit hyperactivity disorder compared with primary care providers in sites without pediatric psychiatrists and psychologists.
- Hiring behavioral health staff with specific training in pediatric evidence-informed mental health treatments may be a critical variable in increasing referral rates and primary care providers satisfaction and competency.

INTRODUCTION

As providers in mental health, we are beginning to coalesce around the practice innovation of integrated behavioral health in primary care practices that treat children. We do so in response to various assumptions: first, most adult mental health illnesses have their roots in childhood.[1] Second, the primary care setting is almost universally accessed by children in the United States.[2] Third, when pediatric primary care providers (PCPs) attempt to refer patients to mental health services in the community, only 20% follow through on these referrals.[3] These facts support the assertion that medical and behavioral health services should be integrated into one setting. Indeed, a recent meta-analysis of 31 randomized controlled trials (RCTs) comparing integrated behavioral health models of any kind with usual care concluded that such integration efforts leads to significant improvements in the mental health of children and adolescents.[4] However, to the best of our knowledge, no published studies have evaluated the effects of different types of integrated models on pediatric primary care staff's behavior or knowledge.

Adult Behavioral Health Integrated Care Models

In the adult literature, the collaborative care model has emerged as the most evidence-based approach to treating depression and anxiety within the primary care setting.[5] More than 50 RCTs have been published showing the efficacy of this model.[5] In adult primary care, the collaborative care model is well defined and consists of a PCP, a consulting psychiatrist, and a behavioral health care manager (typically a master's-level clinician).[6] The PCP is responsible for conducting the initial assessment and starting the adult patient on medication; the psychiatrist consults with the PCP and care manager on the treatment plan but does not treat patients directly, and the care manager offers evidence-based therapy, typically problem-solving therapy (PST) for 6 to 10 sessions.[7] These multidisciplinary teams meet regularly to discuss patient care and provide consultation, and the goal of these programs is to screen the population and provide treatment on a broad scale.

Translating Adult Models of Integrated Care to Pediatric Populations

In medicine and mental health, many innovative models that target adults are eventually translated or adapted for pediatric populations. However, program designers need to consider important differences between adult and pediatric patient populations when developing collaborative care models. First, best-practice guidelines for children with depression and anxiety state that the first-line treatment should be a course of therapy to be followed by psychotropic medication only if the child is not responding to therapy.[8] Second, the behavioral health care specialist will need expertise in differential assessment of pediatric mental health disorders because there is a level of diagnostic complexity with children that requires specialized training, such as the ability to conduct differential diagnoses among learning disabilities, attention deficit hyperactivity disorder (ADHD), and trauma, particularly in young children.[9] In addition, the behavioral health care manager will need expertise in multiple evidence-based treatments if the program is intended to treat a variety of mental health problems. To date, there is no single evidence-based treatment that can treat pediatric depression, anxiety, attention, disruptive, and trauma disorders, which are the most common presenting mental health problems for children and adolescents.[10,11]

Regarding medication, most psychotropic medications are not approved by the US Food and Drug Administration (FDA) for pediatric patients with the exception of stimulants, fluoxetine, and escitalopram.[12] Even with FDA approval, many parents, who are the gatekeepers to their children's treatment, are reluctant to start their children on these types of medications,[13,14] particularly after the FDA published a black box warning on antidepressants being associated with an increase in suicidality among adolescents.[15] For these reasons, PCPs who treat children and adolescents may be more reluctant to prescribe these medications compared with those who treat adults. Given these differences, pediatric integrative care models in primary care may require different workflows and potentially different types of providers. These realities have implications for the role of the PCP and the pediatric psychiatrist and the level of knowledge and expertise needed in the behavioral health care manager compared with adult models.

Design, Staffing, and Treatment Considerations in Pediatric Behavioral Health Integrated Models

Given the differences outlined above between the adult and pediatric patient population and primary care environments, PCPs who treat children can screen and identify patients who need behavioral health services, but some may want or need assistance from the behavioral health specialist to diagnose the specific mental health illness.[16] Additionally, PCPs may require more training and consultation to develop competency and comfort in prescribing psychotropic medications, as they generally receive only 2 months of training in treating behavioral health illnesses (during a 3-year residency program), and surveys indicate pediatricians find this training to be inadequate.[17,18] Pediatric psychiatrists may need to see patients directly to start them on medication and then transition the patient to the PCP for medication maintenance.

On the pediatric side, there have been 5 RCTs published on the collaborative care model, 3 of which targeted depressed adolescents and 2 of which targeted behavior problems such as anxiety, ADHD, and oppositional defiant disorder of younger children (age 5–12 years). Two studies did not include a pediatric psychiatrist on the collaborative care team; however, all teams included the PCP, and the backgrounds of the care managers were more diverse than in adult models (master's-level and doctoral-level clinicians). In their review of integrated care programs that treat children, Asarnow and colleagues[4] found these programs to have a medium-to-large effect size compared with other models. Stancin[19] recently declared that integrated behavioral health in primary care settings that treat children needs to move beyond debating *why* this approach to care should be prevalent and shift to studying *how* best to design, staff, and evaluate different models of integrated care.

Therefore, we sought to fill this gap by comparing 2 integrated behavioral health practice models of how to design, staff, and treat behavioral health problems in pediatric and family medicine primary care practices. The 2 practice models, both designed to bring behavioral health services into primary care settings that treat pediatric patients, differed in the following domains and are described in detail in the methods section:

- Training background of behavioral health specialists
- Types of behavioral health referrals accepted by behavioral health specialists
- Types of behavioral health problems treated by the behavioral health specialists within the practice
- Availability of specific, evidence-informed treatments for pediatric depression, anxiety, trauma, and attentional/disruptive problems for pediatric patients within primary care
- Consultation available to PCPs regarding pediatric psychotropic medications and medication management
- Training/educational activities for PCPs and practice staff regarding assessment of behavioral health problems.

This study sought to examine feasibility measures across the 2 types of integrated models, the Generalist Behavioral Health (GBH) model versus the Behavioral Health Integrated (BHIP) model. We hypothesized that psychologists in the BHIP model would receive a higher percentage of pediatric behavioral health referrals compared with the social workers in the GBH model. We also hypothesized that BHIP model PCPs would report higher levels of satisfaction and competency regarding addressing behavioral health issues in their patients than GBH model PCPs.

METHODS
Study Design

The authors conducted a prospective, natural experiment (coinciding with the sequential rollout of a new program) comparing 2 models of behavioral health integration in 13 primary care sites in the Bronx, NY. Before this rollout, 13 primary care sites practiced a model of behavioral health integration staffed with generalist social workers (some of the practices had licensed master social work credentials and others had licensed clinical social work credentials). All 13 sites conducted universal behavioral health screening of all children (ages 6 and older) using the Pediatric Symptom Checklist-17[20] during the child's annual health maintenance visit.

Between September 2014 and February 2015, the first 6 months of our new program implementation, 8 of the 13 primary care sites received a new model of integrated care, continuing with generalist social workers but with the addition of integrated pediatric psychologists with expertise in diagnosing and treating ADHD, anxiety, conduct, depression, and trauma. Four of the 8 practices also received an integrated pediatric psychiatrist. This new model was called the *Pediatric Behavioral Health Integrated Program* (BHIP). This natural experiment enabled the comparison of the GBH model to the BHIP model during this 6-month period. Sites that received the BHIP model were chosen based on office space availability, and control sites were chosen to ensure a matched design regarding percentage of patients served receiving Medicaid (5 sites in the treatment group and 5 sites in the control group each had >70% Medicaid patients). The findings presented here focus on feasibility measures, including referral rates to behavioral health, PCP self-reported competency and satisfaction regarding behavioral health management, and PCP views on the importance of using a validated screening tool for evaluating pediatric mental health problems. This study was approved by the Montefiore Medical Center Institutional Review Board.

Study Sample

Our study sample included 2 groups: (1) pediatric patients ages 6 to 18 years old and (2) pediatric PCPs, nurses, and front desk staff from the 13 pediatric primary care sites. For the group of pediatric patients, we included all pediatric patients who attended at least 1 health maintenance visit at one of the 13 study sites between September 2014 and February 2015. This cohort of patients was identified using the electronic medical record (EMR) system. There were no exclusion criteria. The provider sample included all PCPs, nurses, and front desk staff from the 13 study sites.

Two Models of Care

Generalist behavioral health provider model

In this model, the mental health clinician was a generalist social worker. The social workers accepted referrals from PCPs for both pediatric and adult patients spanning a wide range of behavioral health problems and concrete needs (eg, housing). They were also available to provide crisis interventions and conduct suicide risk assessments. In addition to their social work graduate experience, they all received-on-the job training in Problem Solving Therapy (PST).[7] PST is a step-by-step process in which the therapist guides the patient in the practice of evaluating and generating solutions for life problems.[21] Of note, there is a substantial literature supporting the efficacy of PST to treat adult depression and adult physical health problems (see meta-analysis review of 39 RCTs by Malouff and colleagues).[21] However, this same meta-analysis found only 3 of 39 studies that examined a pediatric sample. PST has some evidence to treat adolescent depression, suicidal ideation, and conduct/substance problems.[22,23] The GBH model social workers were trained to provide PST for a maximum of 12 to 14 sessions, help the patient manage any related concrete needs, and, for those patients who required more long-term therapy, refer them to community mental health sites. The only option for PCPs who wanted to refer pediatric patients for treatment within their primary care setting for behavioral health issues was to refer to the social workers.

Pediatric behavioral health integrated program

In the BHIP model, a pediatric psychologist was added to each of the sites that previously only had a generalist social worker. The pediatric psychologists accepted referrals from PCPs for patients (ages 6 through 18 or 21 years, depending on when the pediatric practice transitioned patients to adult medicine) and advertised the practice model as providing specific, evidence-informed therapies for ADHD, anxiety, depression, trauma, and disruptive disorders. The pediatric psychologists were trained in evidence-informed modularized approaches to treat these presenting problems (see Briggs and colleagues, 2016).[24] Pediatric psychiatrists provided consultation and education to PCPs to improve their competence and confidence in managing patients with ADHD through either small-group discussions or one-on-one consultation. In addition, the psychiatrists were responsible for initiating psychotropic interventions for pediatric patients and, when appropriate, working to ultimately transfer the case to the PCP for long-term medication management. The BHIP team also specified what they could *not* provide (eg, treatment for autism spectrum disorder, treatment for patients with serious and persistent mental illness, and comprehensive academic evaluations). The role of the previously existing generalist social worker had to be negotiated within each practice with the addition of these psychologists and psychiatrists with expertise in pediatric behavioral health. Social workers at 2 BHIP sites elected to focus exclusively on their adult patients, and no longer accept any pediatric referrals. Social workers at the other 6 BHIP sites requested to be able to continue to treat adolescent patients but not younger children. These decisions were made in collaboration with supervisors and reflected any additional evidence-based training that the social worker had received. In all practices, it was made clear that social workers had expertise, at a minimum, in providing PST, crisis intervention, concrete services, and connecting families with community mental health referrals. Depending on the site (as described above), PCPs who wanted to refer pediatric patients for treatment within their primary care setting for behavioral health issues could either refer to the social worker or pediatric psychologist.

Data Collection

The primary outcome of this study compared the percentage of patients referred to social workers in the GBH sites versus the clinical psychologists in the BHIP sites. We also compared provider satisfaction and competency between the 2 models.

Referrals

The number of referrals (including demographics on gender, race/ethnicity, and health insurance) was collected through the EMR. A query of the EMR found all patients ages 6 to 21 referred to the social workers in GBH sites or the psychologists in BHIP sites between September 2014 and February 2015. It should be noted that referrals did not come directly to psychiatrists and instead were directed to psychologists. Research assistants cleaned and double checked the data pulled from the EMR. A separate query of the EMR identified the number of health maintenance visits for patients (6–21 years) at the different sites, and these numbers were aggregated for the 2 models (BHIP vs GBH).

Satisfaction and competency

Self-reported satisfaction and competency with behavioral health services at the GBH and BHIP sites was assessed using questionnaires administered through Survey Monkey. The survey asked about provider satisfaction regarding mental health services for their patients and their job overall and provider competency with behavioral care of pediatric patients. Primary care providers' satisfaction was assessed using a series of questions adapted from a survey used in the Child and Adolescent Psychiatry for Primary Care.[25] These questions were:

Please indicate how satisfied you are with the following, as it pertains to your school age and adolescent patients only:

- Time it takes to find mental health providers
- Availability of mental health appointments for my patients
- Ease of referring a patient for mental health appointments
- Feedback from mental health providers about my patients
- Mental health care received by my patients
- My job as a pediatrician as it relates to the mental health needs of pediatric patients

Nurses and front desk staff were asked 1 general satisfaction question regarding their role in helping families access behavioral health services: Please indicate how satisfied you are with your ability to help a family access pediatric mental health services. A 4-point Likert response scale was used ranging from *not at all satisfied* to *extremely satisfied*.

Competency was assessed by asking PCPs to indicate how competent they felt addressing the following issues in both school-aged children (6–11 years) and in adolescents (12–18 years): ADHD, depression, anxiety, trauma, providing behavioral advice (eg, time out, reward systems), suicidal ideation, and next steps to take after a patient has a positive mental health screen. A 4-point Likert response scale was used ranging from *not at all competent* to *very competent*. Full survey questionnaires are available on request.

Importance of screening with validated tools

PCPs in both the GBH and BHIP sites were asked a single question regarding screening: how important do you think it is that a validated screening tool is used to evaluate for pediatric mental health problems at each well-child visit? PCP response choices ranged from *very important*; *important but do not typically have enough time*; and *not important, my own surveillance and evaluation is sufficient*. Nurse response choices were *very important, somewhat important, or not at all important*.

Analytical Plan

The data were analyzed by using SPSS v 23.0 (SPSS Inc, Chicago, Illinois). Descriptive statistics were performed to describe the study sites, rates of referrals, competency and satisfaction rates, importance of screening, and time spent managing behavioral health of the whole sample. Patient demographics for the 2 models were compared using χ^2 tests. Referral rates were calculated by dividing the number of referrals by the total number of patients who attended a health maintenance visit during the study period and were analyzed using a χ^2 test. To examine differences in satisfaction scores across the program models, independent sample *t* tests were used. Independent sample *t* tests were also used to compare mean scores on PCP self-reported competency items. Chi square tests were used to compare ratings on the perceived importance of using a validated screening tool between the 2 models.

RESULTS

Site variables are listed in **Table 1**. Demographics (age, gender, race/ethnicity, and health insurance) of the referred patient samples for the 2 models are listed

Table 1
Site demographics between the 2 models

Model	% Medicaid or Self-Pay	# of Patients Age 6–18	# of PCPs (Attendings)	# of PCPs (Residents)	# of Nurses and Front Desk Staff
BHIP					
Site A	13	5144	7	0[a]	17
Site B	74	1032	5	0[a]	10
Site C	74	4727	15	36	23
Site D	79	4313	10	12	9
Site E	78	5440	21	38	45
Site F	7	3080	4	0[a]	11
Site G	64	491	4	0[a]	5
Site H	82	1008	5	0[a]	8
GBH					
Site I	85	1880	21	15	42
Site J	9	3296	5	0[a]	13
Site K	78	1190	2	0[a]	10
Site L	76	1787	2	0[a]	14
Site M	67	1264	11	17	18

[a] Nonteaching practices.

in **Table 2** along with the practice staff respondent demographics. Of note, only 1 of 44 PCP responses from the BHIP practices came from a site that did not have an integrated psychiatrist.

Referral Rates

Fig. 1 depicts the referral rates between the 2 models.

Self-reported Satisfaction

Mean scores on all satisfaction items were significantly different between the GBH and BHIP practices, favoring the BHIP model. PCPs in BHIP practices reported higher levels of satisfaction in the time, availability, and ease in finding behavioral health services for their patients, in receiving feedback from the behavioral health providers about their patients, in the quality of care received by their patients, and their own job satisfaction as it related to the mental health needs of their patients ($P<.05$ for all) (**Fig. 2**).

Table 2
Sample demographics

	Model		P Value
	BHIP	GBH	
Patient sample			
Demographics			
Age in years, mean (SD)	11.75 (3.85)	12.01 (3.79)	NS
% Female	49.1	50.9	NS
% Race/ethnicity			
Hispanic	37.1	44.4	NS
Black	29.9	20.5	<.05
White	4.4	0.0	<.05
Other	19.6	22.8	NS
Unknown	9.1	12.3	NS
% Insurance			
Medicaid	65.3	81.3	<.05
Commercial	30.8	15.8	<.05
Self-pay	2.1	2.3	NS
Unknown	1.7	0.6	NS
Provider/staff sample:			
Total PCPs sent the survey	161	81	—
Total PCP respondents (%)	44	23	—
MD (attending)	28	16	—
MD (resident)	8	4	—
Nurse practitioner	0	1	—
Unknown	8	2	—
Total nurses/front desk staff sent the survey	126	81	—
Total nurses/front desk staff respondents (%)	32 (25.4)	27 (33.3)	—

Abbreviations: MD, medical doctor; NS, not significant.

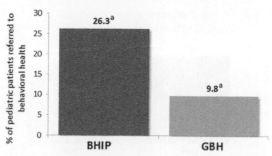

Fig. 1. Referral rates to behavioral health compared between the 2 models. [a] P<.05; BHIP model had 1164 referrals out of 4425 health maintenance visits. GBH model had 171 referrals out of 1748 health maintenance visits.

Nurses and front desk staff were also asked to indicate level of satisfaction with their ability to help a family access pediatric mental health services. No differences were found for nurses and front desk staff between the 2 models (Fig. 3).

Self-reported Competency

PCPs in the BHIP versus GBH practices reported feeling more competent managing school-age and adolescent ADHD compared with PCPs in the GBH practices (P<.05). Similarly, the BHIP PCPs felt more competent in the next steps to take after patients tested positive on a behavioral health screen for their school-age and adolescent patients (P<.05). No differences were found in PCPs' self-reported competency to address anxiety, depression, trauma, suicidal ideation, or provide behavioral advice (Figs. 4 and 5).

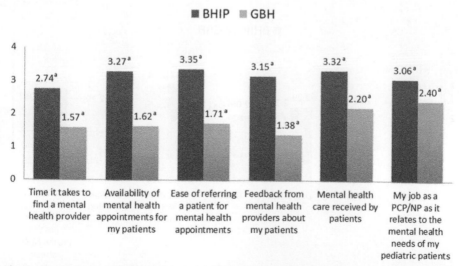

Fig. 2. Mean scores of PCP satisfaction with behavioral health services compared between the 2 models. PCPs were given the following instructions: Please indicate how satisfied you are with the following as it pertains to your school-age and adolescent patients only. Scale ranges from 1 = not at all satisfied, 2 = slightly satisfied, 3 = moderately satisfied, 4 = extremely satisfied. [a] P<.05. NP, nurse practitioner.

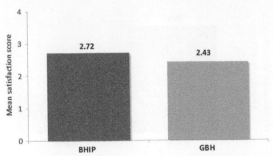

Fig. 3. Mean scores of nurse/front desk staff self-reported satisfaction with their ability to help a family access behavioral health services compared between the 2 models. Nurses and front desk staff were given the following instructions: Please indicate how satisfied you are with your ability to help a family access pediatric mental health services. Scale ranges from 1 = not at all satisfied, 2 = slightly satisfied, 3 = moderately satisfied, 4 = extremely satisfied. Differences not significant at *P*>.05.

Importance of Screening with Validated Tools

Results were not statistically significant between the 2 models for neither PCPs nor nurses and front desk staff in rating the importance of using a validated screening tool (**Table 3**).

DISCUSSION

The findings from this study suggest that a BHIP model staffed by pediatric psychologists and psychiatrists can be feasibly implemented in a large urban primary care network and improves referral rates to pediatric mental health practitioners, PCP-reported satisfaction with mental health services, and PCP self-reported competence

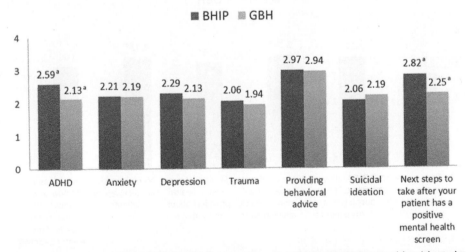

Fig. 4. Mean scores of PCP self-reported competency in addressing behavioral health problems for 6- to 11-year old patients compared between the 2 models. PCPs were given the following instructions: Please indicate how competent you feel addressing the following issues in a school-age child (6–11 years). Scale ranges from 1 = not at all, 2 = somewhat, 3 = competent, 4 = very competent. [a] *P*<.05.

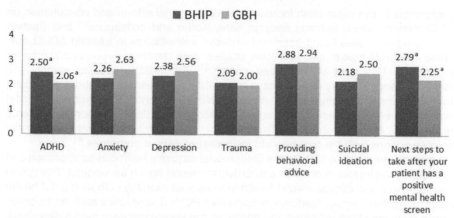

Fig. 5. Mean scores of PCP self-reported competency in addressing behavioral health problems for 12- to 18-year-old patients compared between the 2 models. PCPs were given the following instructions: Please indicate how competent you feel addressing the following issues in an adolescent (12–18 years). Scale ranges from 1 = not at all, 2 = somewhat, 3 = competent, 4 = very competent. [a] $P<.05$.

managing school-age and adolescent ADHD. The BHIP model was seen by providers as improving access to and quality of mental health care. This study is one of the first to address the impact of a BHIP model on the comprehensive mental health needs of children and adolescents in pediatric primary care sites.

Prior studies implementing integrated behavioral health models have focused on specific disease states (eg, depression)[26] or age groups (eg, children 12–18 years old).[27] These studies, when collated in a meta-analysis, suggest significant benefit from integrated behavioral health models over standard care models, especially when targeting symptoms or specific disease states.[4] Although this study did not expressly investigate patient outcomes, it did identify benefits in self-reported PCP satisfaction and competence around ADHD management for all age groups. It is not surprising that PCPs felt increased competence in ADHD management, as the

Table 3
Ratings of perceived importance of using a validated screening tool to evaluate pediatric mental health problems at each well-child visit

	Model			
	BHIP	GBH	X^2	P Value
PCP ratings (%)				
Very important	13 (29.5)	5 (21.7)	4.311	NS
Important, but do not typically have enough time	22 (50.0)	13 (56.5)	—	NS
Not important; my own surveillance and evaluation is sufficient	1 (2.3)	3 (13.0)	—	NS
Other	8 (18.2)	2 (8.7)	—	NS
Nurse/front desk staff ratings (%)				
Very important	20 (74.1)	21 (87.5)	1.453	NS
Somewhat important	7 (25.9)	3 (12.5)	—	NS
Not at all important	0 (0)	0 (0)	—	NS

Abbreviation: NS, not significant.

psychiatrists in the clinic often focused their educational efforts and consultation on ADHD-related topics. Echoing findings here, Kolko and colleagues[28] and Epstein and colleagues[29] also found improved provider self-efficacy in treating ADHD outcomes in a BHIP-type model, and other studies have identified strong provider satisfaction with this type of integrated care.[27,30] As multiple studies identify the inadequate access many children have to mental health services[31] and the difficulty providers have in engaging youth in mental health treatment,[32] this short-term model can both increase early access and engage patients immediately as soon as problems are identified. As prior publications illustrate, it will continue to be important to identify the interventions with the highest yield for pediatric patient outcomes.[4]

Successful implementations of the BHIP model require a team-based approach and significant investments in clinician and provider mental health awareness. This group of researchers and clinical mental health leaders met monthly with all mental health practitioners, held regular feedback session with PCPs and practice staff, and worked hard to increase standardization and fidelity to the short-term care model described. Anecdotal reports from mental health clinicians suggest that the coordination of mental and physical health, creating a true medical home for patients, was beneficial for both practitioners and patients. Future work could compare the reduction of mental health practitioner and PCP burnout when this team-based approach is applied.

Limitations of this study include the variability in which the BHIP model was applied across sites given the personal decision of some social workers to continue or not continue to treat pediatric patients and the addition of psychiatrists to some teams and not others. The authors feel the success in increasing referral rates in the BHIP model speaks to the strength of this team-based approach despite variations in exact implementation methodology. This finding echoes those of prior research suggesting that various collaborative care models also contribute to improved patient care.[4] Measurement bias, nonresponse bias, and social desirability bias are always a risk in all self-report survey studies, and we attempted to minimize these biases by having providers complete anonymous surveys. Sites were not randomly assigned to BHIP or GBH, and clear differences exist between the site populations who were referred to mental health practitioners in each group, as a greater percentage of the BHIP referral patients identified their race/ethnicity as black or white and had commercial insurance. Given the increasing evidence that the BHIP model was beneficial to patient care, we believed it was not appropriate to withhold that model from 50% of sites for an extended period and therefore did not choose to perform strict randomization. Additionally, randomization of 13 sites may have led to unbalanced confounders in each group because of the small number of sites involved. Finally, this study did not examine patient outcomes, as that was beyond the scope. Prior findings suggest BHIP's efficacy to improve patient outcomes.[4]

BHIP shows appreciable benefit over a GBH model in terms of mental health referral rates and provider reports of competence and satisfaction. Although future work can focus on patient symptom outcomes, we suggest that increased focus on testing the benefits of different pediatric team models and pediatric treatment models to enhance both patient access to mental health and provider satisfaction and competence with mental health are needed.

REFERENCES

1. Kessler RC, Berglund P, Demler O, et al. Lifetime prevalence and age-of-onset distributions of DSM-IV disorders in the national comorbidity survey replication. Arch Gen Psychiatry 2005;62(6):593.

2. Chevarley F. Statistical brief #12: Children's access to necessary health care. 2001. Available at: https://meps.ahrq.gov/data_files/publications/st12/stat12.shtml. Accessed March 3, 2017.

3. Radovic A, Reynolds K, McCauley HL, et al. Parents' role in adolescent depression care: primary care provider perspectives. J Pediatr 2015;167(4):911–8.

4. Asarnow JR, Rozenman M, Wiblin J, et al. Integrated medical-behavioral care compared with usual primary care for child and adolescent behavioral health. JAMA Pediatr 2015;169(10):929.

5. Woltmann E, Grogan-Kaylor A, Perron B, et al. Comparative effectiveness of collaborative chronic care models for mental health conditions across primary, specialty, and behavioral health care settings: systematic review and meta-analysis. Am J Psychiatry 2012;169(8):790–804.

6. Team structure. Available at: https://aims.uw.edu/collaborative-care/team-structure. Accessed March 3, 2017.

7. PST certification. Available at: https://aims.uw.edu/care-partners/content/pst-certification. Accessed March 3, 2017.

8. Walkup J. Practice parameter on the use of Psychotropic medication in children and adolescents. J Am Acad Child Adolesc Psychiatry 2009;48(9):961–73.

9. Brown NM, Brown SN, Briggs RD, et al. Associations between adverse childhood experiences and ADHD diagnosis and severity. Acad Pediatr 2017;17(4):349–55.

10. Merikangas K, He J, Brody D, et al. Prevalence and treatment of mental disorders among US children in the 2001-2004 NHANES. Pediatrics 2010;125(1):75–81.

11. Merikangas K, He J, Burstein M, et al. Lifetime prevalence of mental disorders in U.S. adolescents: results from the national comorbidity survey replication–adolescent supplement (NCS-A). J Am Acad Child Adolesc Psychiatry 2010; 49(10):980–9.

12. Hieber R. Toolbox: psychotropic medications approved in children and adolescents. Ment Health Clinician 2013;2(11):344–6.

13. The MTA Cooperative Group. A 14-Month Randomized clinical trial of treatment strategies for attention-deficit/Hyperactivity disorder. Arch Gen Psychiatry 1999; 56(12):1073.

14. Asarnow JR, Jaycox LH, Duan N, et al. Effectiveness of a quality improvement intervention for adolescent depression in primary care clinics. JAMA 2005; 293(3):311–9.

15. Richmond TK, Rosen DS. The treatment of adolescent depression in the era of the black box warning. Curr Opin Pediatr 2005;17(4):466–72.

16. Heneghan A, Garner A, Storfer-Isser A, et al. Pediatricians role in providing mental health care for children and adolescents: do pediatricians and child and adolescent psychiatrists agree? J Dev Behav Pediatr 2008;29(4):262–9.

17. Williams J. Diagnosis and treatment of behavioral health disorders in pediatric practice. Pediatrics 2004;114(3):601–6.

18. Stein R, Horwitz S, Storfer-Isser A, et al. Do pediatricians think they are responsible for identification and management of child mental health problems? Results of the AAP Periodic Survey. Ambul Pediatr 2008;8(1):11–7.

19. Stancin T. Commentary: integrated pediatric primary care: moving from why to how. J Pediatr Psychol 2016;41(10):1161–4.

20. Gardner W, Murphy M, Childs G, et al. The PSC-17: a brief pediatric symptom checklist with psychosocial problem subscales. A report from PROS and ASPN. Ambul Child Health 1999;5(3):225–36.

21. Malouff J, Thorsteinsson E, Schutte N. The efficacy of problem solving therapy in reducing mental and physical health problems: a meta-analysis. Clin Psychol Rev 2007;27(1):46–57.

22. Eskin M, Ertekin K, Demir H. Efficacy of a problem-solving therapy for depression and suicide potential in adolescents and young adults. Cogn Ther Res 2008; 32(2):227–45.

23. Azrin NH, Donohue B, Teichner GA, et al. A controlled evaluation and description of individual-cognitive problem solving and family-behavior therapies in dually-diagnosed conduct-disordered and substance-dependent youth. J Child Adolesc Substance Abuse 2001;11(1):1–43.

24. Briggs RD, German M, Schrag Hershberg R, et al. Integrated pediatric behavioral health: implications for training and intervention models. Prof Psychol Res Pract 2016;47(4):312–9.

25. CAP PC NY | Child and Adolescent Psychiatry for Primary Care. CAP PC NY. 2017. Available at: http://www.cappcny.org/home/. Accessed March 17, 2017.

26. Asarnow JR, Jaycox LH, Tang L, et al. Long-term benefits of short-term quality improvement interventions for depressed youths in primary care. Am J Psychiatry 2009;166(9):1002–10.

27. Richardson L, McCauley E, Katon W. Collaborative care for adolescent depression: a pilot study. Gen Hosp Psychiatry 2009;31(1):36–45.

28. Kolko DJ, Campo J, Kilbourne AM, et al. Collaborative care outcomes for pediatric behavioral health problems: a cluster randomized trial. Pediatrics 2014;133(4): e981–92.

29. Epstein JN, Rabiner D, Johnson DE, et al. Improving attention-deficit/hyperactivity disorder treatment outcomes through use of a collaborative consultation treatment service by community-based Pediatricians. Arch Pediatr Adolesc Med 2007;161(9):835.

30. Pidano AE, Kimmelblatt CA, Neace WP. Behavioral health in the pediatric primary care setting: needs, barriers, and implications for psychologists. Psychol Serv 2011;8(3):151–65.

31. Rickwood D, Deane FP, Wilson CJ, et al. Young people's help-seeking for mental health problems. Adv Ment Health 2005;4(3):218–51.

32. Garety PA, Craig TK, Done G, et al. Specialized care for early psychosis: symptoms, social functioning and patient satisfaction: randomized controlled trial. Br J Psychiatry 2006;188(1):37–45.

Payment for Integrated Care

Challenges and Opportunities

Katherine Hobbs Knutson, MD, MPH

KEYWORDS

- Healthcare payment • Integrated care • Child and adolescent psychiatry
- Health services

KEY POINTS

- Currently, there are multiple barriers to payment for integrated behavioral and physical health care.
- Capitated payment models hold promise for supporting integrated care.
- Examples of national models of innovative payment systems for integrated care are described.

INTRODUCTION

The importance of integrated care for individuals with behavioral health disorders is well established. For the adult population, those with serious and persistent mental illness have an estimated 20-year decreased life expectancy, often because of comorbid chronic physical health conditions such as cardiovascular disease.[1] By addressing these behavioral and physical health disorders in tandem, improved health and functional outcomes may be realized. Adults with high utilization of high-cost health services such as emergency and inpatient care often have comorbid behavioral health disorders.[1] Often these individuals are unable, or unwilling, to receive treatment in the behavioral health specialty arena.[1] Thus, by bringing behavioral health treatment into settings in which they do receive care—such as primary care—these individuals may be more likely to engage in treatment.

For children and youth (hereafter called *youth*), limited access to behavioral health specialists is the key driver for integrated care. As opposed to adults, a relatively low proportion of youth have comorbid behavioral health and physical medical conditions.[2] Given the low prevalence, integrating care for the purpose of addressing youths' combined behavioral and physical health conditions may be good clinical

Disclosures: None.
Department of Psychiatry, Duke University School of Medicine, 2608 Erwin Road, Suite 300, Durham, NC 27705, USA
E-mail address: Katherine.hobbsknutson@duke.edu

Child Adolesc Psychiatric Clin N Am 26 (2017) 829–838
http://dx.doi.org/10.1016/j.chc.2017.06.010
childpsych.theclinics.com

practice but it is of limited utility from a population perspective. However, of the 13% to 40% of youth in the United States with a mental health disorder,[3] more than 60% go without treatment.[4] For those who do receive treatment, most access care outside of specialty mental health arena, such as in primary care or educational settings.[4] There is a longstanding shortage of specialty behavioral health providers for youth that is unlikely to change in the near future.[5] Therefore, reorganizing the service delivery system—through such interventions as integrating behavioral and physical health care—is vital for improving access on a population level.

As there is almost universal access to pediatric primary care in the United States,[6] through integrated care, we may bring behavioral health treatment into a setting in which youth are likely to present. Youth and their families usually feel comfortable with their primary care providers (PCPs), and often they have relationships with these providers that started at birth.[7] Families may choose primary care practices that are conveniently located close to home, school, or parents' work. Thus, logistic issues related to attending behavioral health appointments may be overcome. Currently, many youth receive their total behavioral health treatment from their PCPs.[4,8] Thus, from a work force perspective, by supporting PCPs to continue delivering the front line of behavioral health care for youth with mild-to-moderate disorders, we may reserve specialty resources for those youth with severe and complex conditions, those who Child and Adolescent Psychiatrists are uniquely trained to treat.

Despite the clear advantages of integrated behavioral health and primary care,[9] funding mechanisms to support these services are lacking.[6,7] As many health systems are transitioning to value-based payment arrangements, they are caught in a difficult position of trying to deliver integrated care in a largely fee-for-service payment environment. For reasons that will be discussed in this article, providing integrated services within a fee-for-service payment structure is challenging, if not impossible. Alternative payment arrangements, including capitation, hold promise for supporting integrated health care delivery systems nationally. These different payment structures and examples of innovative methods that have been successful in multiple health systems are described.

CHALLENGES RELATED TO PAYMENT FOR INTEGRATED CARE

Almost all integrated care models call for team-based care.[6,10] For example, in collaborative care models, trained case or care managers work alongside pediatric PCPs to provide first-line behavioral health treatment and coordinate behavioral and physical health services.[9] A cornerstone of the patient-centered medical home is team meetings, or *huddles*, supporting multidisciplinary treatment planning.[11] Along the integrated care continuum, communication between specialties is essential.[10] In many fee-for-service systems, however, this coordination and communication among treatment providers and service types is minimally reimbursed, if at all.[6,7] Therefore, many health systems and primary care clinics have substantial difficulty financially supporting staff to execute care coordination tasks. Thus, although care coordination is a central component of integrated care, it is often neglected in fee-for-service payment arrangements.

Another major hurdle to providing integrated care are Medicaid-based prohibitions on reimbursement for health services provided on the same day, so called same-day billing.[6,12] The Medicare program and several state Medicaid programs have removed these restrictions, but they remain in several locations as a measure to protect against redundant payment for services. These restrictions may disproportionately affect low-income individuals such as Medicaid recipients, as they may have particular difficulty with transportation and other logistic issues related to attending health care appointments on separate days.[12] By limiting providers' ability to bill for services performed by different specialists on the same day, delivering a multidisciplinary team-based approach to health care is almost impossible.

Separating payment for physical versus behavioral health through insurance carve-outs complicate, if not prohibit, integration.[6,7] Although the landscape is changing, in many locations physical health providers are not reimbursed for claims submitted with behavioral health diagnoses, creating a major hurdle for these providers to engage in integrated care.[6] Separating physical and behavioral health payment also creates a competitive system in which cost shifting may occur. For example, patients who present repeatedly for physical illness that is driven by an underlying behavioral health problem often are the financial responsibility of the physical health payor. In these cases, the behavioral health payor does not have an incentive to engage in the management of these patients who clearly span both spheres. Separate payment systems create logistical barriers to integration at the practice level, as separate payment contracts, regulations, and reimbursement processes exist artificially for health conditions that are inextricably linked.[7]

In some cases, providing integrated care within a fee-for-service payment arrangement is possible, especially when same-day billing is permitted. For example, the salary of a collocated behavioral health specialist can be supported by revenue gained from patient visits, if the volume of patients with behavioral health disorders in the practice is sufficient.[13] In the community setting, however, given that an estimated 13% to 40% of youth in the general population has a behavioral health disorder,[3] small primary care practices may have too few patients to command sufficient revenue to support an on-site specialty provider. Even in medical specialty clinics within hospitals, in which the proportion of youth with comorbid physical and behavioral health conditions may be higher, because of high overhead costs and the lower reimbursement for behavioral health compared with physical health services, it can be difficult to financially support a collocated specialty provider.[13] The inadequate behavioral health specialty work force creates an additional barrier, making collocation impossible in many areas. To address these issues, specialty behavioral health providers may span several associated clinical sites, either in person or by telehealth. To be effective, these multisite arrangements require substantial care coordination that may be supported by the clinical site or insurance payors or may often go unfunded.

VALUE-BASED PURCHASING HOLDS PROMISE FOR INTEGRATED CARE

Value-based purchasing is a collective term referring to payment for health services that is intended to reward quality and health outcomes as opposed to the volume of billed visits. There are many types of value-based purchasing arrangements, each with varying levels of incentives for quality, financial performance, or reduction in waste. As shown in **Fig. 1**, as payment models move away from fee-for-service in the lower left corner toward capitation in the upper right corner, there are increasing incentives to improve quality and lower the cost of care for individual providers (x axis) and groups of providers such as health systems (y axis). Today, many health systems have multiple payment contracts spanning the continuum from fee-for-service to capitation.

Currently, the most popular value-based payment arrangement is pay-for-performance,[14] in which health care providers receive financial rewards for showing positive health outcomes for their attributed patient population. Pay-for-performance arrangements often exist within a fee-for-service system, and they help incentivize quality in addition to volume. Capitated, or global, payments are another example of value-based

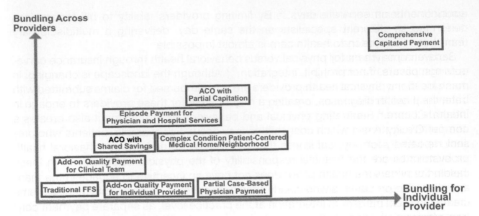

Fig. 1. Starting with traditional fee-for-service, examples of value-based purchasing arrangements with increasing incentives for improving quality and reducing the cost of care. (*From* McClellan M, Patel K, Latts L, et al. Implementing value-based insurance products: a collaborative approach to Health care transformation. The Brookings Institute Health Policy Issue Brief, 2015. Available at: https://www.brookings.edu/wp-content/uploads/2016/07/061615-Health-Policy-Brief-VBIP.pdf. Accessed May 17, 2017; with permission.)

payments that are the subject of this article. In capitated payment arrangements, health systems or clinics (hereafter called *providers*) are allotted a set amount of money to support their patients' total health services during a specified period. For example, for each member of its attributed population, providers may be given a single payment on a monthly basis for all of the health services delivered. This payment is often called a *per-member per-month* or *pmpm* rate. The pmpm rate is usually adjusted for existing health conditions; that is, providers may receive a higher pmpm rate for individuals with complex health problems.

In such capitated arrangements, providers may have varying levels of potential savings and risk, also called *insurance risk*. If the provider delivers all of the health care at a cost that is lower than the pmpm rate, then it may keep a portion of the savings. Similarly, if the cost of health services is greater than the pmpm rate, then the provider may be required to pay for a portion of the loss. Providers that assume insurance risk are incentivized to improve efficiency, as they stand to reap financial benefits by lowering the cost of care. Given growing evidence for improved efficiency of coordinated care delivery systems,[11] such as integrated behavioral and physical health services,[15] providers may adopt such service delivery models when they enter into value-based payment arrangements.

Clearly, there are other perverse incentives of capitated payment models, such as providers choosing only healthy patients or delivering inadequate health services. By choosing healthy patients, likely fewer health services will be required, thus maximizing savings for the provider. Also, by delivering few or inadequate health services, providers may reap better savings. Mature capitated systems address these negative incentives in several ways. For one, providers have various restrictions prohibiting them from denying patients who are assigned or elect to be part of their attributed population. In practice, most patients are attributed to provider systems according to where they receive primary care or who they define as their primary care provider. Although providers may not be allowed to keep patients from enrolling, they can use other tactics such as expanding selectively into geographic regions populated by younger or healthier individuals. Because patients tend to choose primary care practices in close proximity to their home or work, by being selective in their geographic footprint, providers may maximize the likelihood of attracting a healthier population.

To overcome the risk of providers delivering inadequate health services to maximize savings, payors may monitor population health outcomes. For example, for a provider to share in any savings realized by delivering services at a cost less than the pmpm rate, the provider may be required to show maintenance or improvement of population health. Common measures of population health are defined by the National Committee for Quality Assurance Healthcare Effectiveness Data and Information Set and include items such as hemoglobin A1c levels less than 8% for diabetic individuals or systolic blood pressure less than 140 mm Hg for hypertensive individuals.[16] By holding providers responsible for population health and the cost of care, the incentives are aligned to provide effective treatment in a more efficient manner. Again, integrated care is one example of a service delivery model that may improve health outcomes and efficiency.[15] Thus, integrated care models may be supported by health systems that enter into these capitated and other value-based payment arrangements.

NATIONAL EXAMPLES OF CAPITATED PAYMENT ARRANGEMENTS SUPPORTING INTEGRATED CARE FOR YOUTH
Health Homes: New York State

Health Homes were developed as an amendment to the Social Security Act added through the Patient Protection and Affordable Care Act section 2703. States have the option of developing Health Home services through their state Medicaid plans. The purpose of Health Homes is to integrate physical, behavioral health, and community-based support services for adults and children with at least 2 chronic health conditions.[17] Health Home components include comprehensive care management, care coordination, coordination specific to transitions between health care settings, individual and family support, referral to community and social support services, and incorporation of information technology into health services.[17] There are various types of providers for Health Home services, including designated providers such as community mental health centers, a team of behavioral health care professionals, and/or a multidisciplinary health care team.[17] Through integrated delivery of health services, Health Homes may improve efficiency, quality, and patient and family satisfaction, specifically for youth with serious emotional disturbance (SED).

There is interest in tailoring the Health Home model for youth with SED.[17] These youth differ from adults with serious mental illness in several ways. For example, many adults with serious mental illness have chronic disease courses and comorbid physical health problems. However, as youth progress through development, they may have episodic, as opposed to chronic, courses of illness. They also are less likely to have comorbid physical health problems compared with adults.[2] By definition, the care for youth with SED involves families and caregivers and multiple systems including education, health care, and possibly child protective services and juvenile justice. Because the presentation and treatment of behavioral health disorders differ substantially between adults and youth, Health Homes should be specifically tailored to meet the unique needs of each group.

Given evidence for effectiveness and the widespread adoption of the wraparound care model for youth with SED,[18] adaptation of the wraparound model of care for incorporation into state Health Home programs has been proposed.[17] Many of the principles of Health Homes are shared with the wraparound care model, including the inclusion of community-based supports, care coordination, and a family-centered approach.[17] The wraparound care model does not explicitly include physical health services, but measures may be taken to integrate these services for the purposes of designing a Health Home for youth. Given that many states already have the infrastructure to support the wraparound model of care, transitioning this infrastructure to support Health Homes may be appropriate.[17]

The New York state Health Home program is supported by a capitated payment structure.[19] The Health Home program was launched in 2012, and since that time, the state has worked to tailor the program for youth with SED.[20] Specifically, the state has focused on expanding case management services to include health care providers and community support services from the multiple systems serving youth, including education, child protective services, and juvenile justice.[20] The state proposed expanding the list of chronic conditions addressed through Health Homes to make it more relevant to youth by including overweight/obesity, respiratory disease such as asthma, and trauma-related disorders, in addition to those already covered such as substance abuse disorders, mental health disorders, cardiovascular disease, and metabolic disease.[20] New York state has worked to coordinate the Health Home program with other existing service programs such as Early Intervention, the special education system, and the wraparound system of care.[20] Measuring and monitoring health outcomes is a core component of any Health Home program, and New York state has additionally incorporated a structured measure of youth function.[20] Through the focus on integration of behavioral and physical health services and coordination with community-based systems of care, the New York state Health Home model may provide improved quality and efficiency of services. The capitated payment structure, with monitoring of health outcomes, supports the design and delivery of this model of care.

Blended and Braided Funding Streams: Wraparound Milwaukee

To create a capitated payment structure, states may consider combining funding from multiple sources. When funds are blended, they are pooled together, with their sources being indistinguishable.[21] Braided funding streams remain separate with separate accounting, but they are coordinated at the point of service delivery to meet a specific health or social need.[21] For example, given that youth with SED are often served by multiple systems, through blending or braiding, states could combine funding for Medicaid, child protective services, juvenile justice, and education.[22] States also could create joint funding streams with Medicaid and other federal sources such as Substance Abuse and Mental Health Services Administration state block grants or Health Resources and Services Administration Services for Children with Special Healthcare Needs grants.[22] These joint funding sources could be managed by a centralized governing body. From this centralized funding source, capitated payments supporting the total health-related services could be provided for enrollees while monitoring health outcomes over time. Thus, redundancies that exist when payments and systems remain separate could be overcome, potentially realizing cross-sector integration and coordination of care.

Wraparound Milwaukee is one such program that has blended funding from multiple sources to support the wraparound model of care for youth with SED.[18] Wraparound Milwaukee combines public funding from the Medicaid, Child Protective Services, juvenile justice, and mental health systems.[18] These pooled funds are administered by a managed care entity housed at the county Behavioral Health Division.[23] Wraparound Milwaukee is intended to serve youth with SED who are identified by juvenile justice or Child Protective Services to be at imminent risk of treatment or placement in an out-of-home setting.[23] The program has repeatedly shown widespread acceptance by patients and families, clinical and functional improvements for enrollees, and reduction in costs.[23] Such braided and blended funding mechanisms create a type of capitated structure to allow for coordination of care across service providers and delivery systems. Building on this example, incorporating funding for physical health would support integrated networks addressing the total health needs of youth.

Creating Capitation Within Fee-For-Service: The Montefiore Health System

While serving its predominantly low-income and medically vulnerable population in the Bronx, New York, the Montefiore Health System has maintained a favorable financial position with positive total and operating margins.[24] The financial stability of the Montefiore Health System is in part owing to innovative programs that address social determinants of health, chronic disease management, and support for patients with high health care costs.[24] Recognizing the substantial positive impact on health of providing behavioral health services early in life, the Montefiore pediatric primary care community clinics have collocated behavioral health specialty providers.[25] Montefiore has been successful in aggressively transforming the care delivery system, with a focus on coordination across settings and disease states. It has done so within a largely fee-for-service environment.

In 1995, the Montefiore Health System established an Integrated Provider Association (IPA) that included the medical center and physicians.[24] Through the IPA, Montefiore created a capitated payment system, accepting insurance risk for a portion of its patient population. In 1996, Montefiore developed a Care Management Company to manage the insurance risk for the IPA, process insurance claims, and provide care management services for its enrolled patients, many of whom had a high burden of chronic medical conditions and social determinants of health.[24] In 2010, only one-third of patients in the Montefiore Health System were enrolled in the Care Management Company, with the rest insured by other payors.[24] However, the clinical programs and care coordination established by the Care Management Company resulted in improved efficiency across the system. In 2014, given this track record of success, Montefiore was awarded a Health Care Innovation Award from the Center for Medicare and Medicaid Services to expand on its integrated behavioral health and primary care program for adults and children, supported by a capitated payment arrangement.

The Montefiore example highlights the incentives for health systems to invest in more efficient care delivery methods, such as integrated care, when they enroll in value-based payment arrangements. It has been estimated that in 2015, greater than 50% of total payor and provider contracts were fee-for-service, but by 2020 this proportion would decrease to approximately 24% to 32%, replaced largely by pay-for-performance and capitated arrangements.[14] During this transition, while still maintaining most fee-for-service contracts, providers may begin to offer integrated care by embedding behavioral health specialty providers in medical settings that serve a large volume of patients. Then as the tide changes toward a greater proportion of value-based arrangements, these providers will be poised to expand on these initial investments, potentially tipping the scale toward improved population health and reduced cost of care as the Montefiore Health System has demonstrated.

Patient-Centered Medical Home: Colorado

The Patient-Centered Medical Home (PCMH) is a model of primary care focused on coordination across providers, care delivery settings, and health-related systems.[26] The pillars of the PCMH for youth include care that is accessible in terms of geography and payment and is family centered, continuous, coordinated, comprehensive, compassionate, and culturally competent.[27] Integration of behavioral health services into primary care is included as a key component of the PCMH described by the Agency for Healthcare Research and Quality.[26] Capitated payment structures are needed to support the multidisciplinary nature of the PCMH model, given its major focus on coordination of care.

In 2007, Colorado passed Chapter 346 to increase access to PCMH for children. In 2009, Colorado launched a 3-year pilot of a statewide multiple payor arrangement supporting the PCMH.[28] The pilot included 15 primary care sites that were certified PCMH by the National Committee for Quality Assurance. These primary care sites were paid a capitated monthly rate and pay-for-performance incentives in a fee-for-service structure. Quality metrics included outcomes related to diabetes, depression screening, and tobacco counseling. Compared with non-PCMH practices, after 2 years, the PCMH pilot programs showed significant reductions in emergency department utilization and costs, but performance on quality measures was mixed.[28] Although capitated payment models are necessary to support the care coordination and multidisciplinary approach of the PCMH, the effects of this model of service delivery remains under investigation. Multiple states and health systems are pursuing PCMH designation for youth, and so research into the clinical and cost effectiveness is ongoing.

SUMMARY AND FUTURE DIRECTIONS

Integration of behavioral and physical health services is widely supported in the medical and health care financing communities. Integrated care for youth may be specifically helpful for improving access to behavioral health services, especially given the national limited supply of pediatric behavioral health specialists. By integrating behavioral health services in medical settings, youth and their families may be more likely to access care, and many of the logistic barriers associated with treatment provided in separate settings may be overcome.

A multidisciplinary team approach to care and robust care coordination services are primary components of almost all integrated care models. Given that these services have limited reimbursement in a fee-for-service payment arrangement, integrating care in this environment is almost impossible. Furthermore, because of Medicaid-based restrictions on same-day billing for health services, a team-based approach to care is severely limited. However, capitated models hold promise for supporting integrated behavioral and physical health services. In capitated payment systems, providers have incentives to improve the efficiency of health care by maintaining or improving quality at a lower cost. Given improvement in quality and decreased use of high-cost health services associated with integrated care models, providers may adopt these systems when they enter into value-based payment arrangements.

There are multiple promising programs nationally that have built integrated services through creative capitated payment systems. With further research and development of these programs, we may refine the infrastructure and payment methods required to support these modes of care delivery. A major current threat is the difficulty in identifying the appropriate capitated rate to account for the total cost of care while incentivizing efficiency. Further, methods for adjusting these capitated payments to capture varying levels of complexity of the attributed patient population are in development. We need further research on appropriate health outcome measures to ensure that patients are indeed maintaining or improving health despite lower costs of care. As we move forward toward wider dissemination of integrated health care systems, continued research and refinement of the financial models to support implementation are vital for sustainability.

REFERENCES

1. Gerrity M, Zoller E, Pinson N, et al. Integrating primary care into behavioral health settings: What works for individuals with serious mental illness. 2014. Available at: http://www.milbank.org/uploads/documents/papers/Integrating-Primary-Care-Report.pdf. Accessed April 14, 2017.

2. Pires S, Grimes KE, Allen K, et al. Faces of medicaid: examining children's behavioral health service utilization and expenditures. 2013. Available at: http://www.chcs.org/media/Faces-of-Medicaid_Examining-Childrens-Behavioral-Health-Service-Utilization-and-Expenditures1.pdf. Accessed October 21, 2014.

3. Merikangas KR, He JP, Brody D, et al. Prevalence and treatment of mental disorders among US children in the 2001-2004 NHANES. Pediatrics 2010;125(1): 75–81.

4. Costello EJ, He JP, Sampson NA, et al. Services for adolescents with psychiatric disorders: 12-month data from the National Comorbidity Survey-Adolescent. Psychiatr Serv 2014;65(3):359–66.

5. Thomas CR, Holzer CE. The continuing shortage of child and adolescent psychiatrists. J Am Acad Child Adolesc Psychiatry 2006;45(9):1023–31.

6. Tyler ET, Hulkower RL, Kaminski JW. Behavioral health integration in pediatric primary care: considerations and opportunities for policymakers, planners, and providers. 2017. Available at: https://www.milbank.org/wp-content/uploads/2017/03/MMF_BHI_REPORT_FINAL.pdf. Accessed April 14, 2017.

7. American Academy of Child and Adolescent Psychiatry Committee on Health Care Access and Economics Task Force on Mental Health. Improving mental health services in primary care: reducing administrative and financial barriers to access and collaboration. Pediatrics 2009;123(4):1248–51.

8. American Academy of Pediatrics Committee on Psychosocial Aspects of Child and Family Health. The new morbidity revisited: a renewed commitment to the psychosocial aspects of pediatric care. Pediatrics 2001;108(5):1227–30.

9. Asarnow JR, Rozenman M, Wiblin J, et al. Integrated medical-behavioral care compared with usual primary care for child and adolescent behavioral health: a meta-analysis. JAMA Pediatr 2015;169(10):929–37.

10. Collins C, Hewson DL, Munger R, et al. Evolving models of behavioral health integration in primary care. 2010. Available at: http://www.milbank.org/uploads/documents/10430EvolvingCare/EvolvingCare.pdf. Accessed May 17, 2017.

11. National Committee for Quality Assurance. Benefits of NCQA patient-centered medical home recognition; 2016. Available at: http://www.ncqa.org/Portals/0/Programs/Recognition/PCMH/NCQA1005-1016_PCMH%20Evidence_Web.pdf. Accessed July 30, 2017.

12. Roby DH, Jones EE. Limits on same-day billing in Medicaid hinders integration of behavioral health into the medical home model. Psychol Serv 2016;13(1):110–9.

13. Weiss M, Schwartz BJ. Lessons learned from a colocation model using psychiatrists in urban primary care settings. J Prim Care Community Health 2013;4(3): 228–34.

14. McKesson Corporation. The state of value-based reimbursement and the transition from volume to value in 2014. 2014. Available at: http://mhsinfo.mckesson.com/rs/mckessonhealthsolutions/images/MHS-2014-Signature-Research-White-Paper.pdf. Accessed February 15, 2016.

15. Vogel ME, Kanzler KE, Aikens JE, et al. Integration of behavioral health and primary care: current knowledge and future directions. J Behav Med 2017;40(1): 69–84.

16. National Committee for Quality Assurance. Available at: http://www.ncqa.org/homepage. Accessed April 14, 2017.

17. Pires S. Customizing health homes for children with serious behavioral health challenges. 2013. Available at: http://www.chcs.org/media/Customizing_Health_Homes_for_Children_with_Serious_BH_Challenges_-_SPires.pdf. Accessed May 17, 2017.

18. Simons D, Pires SA, Hendricks T, et al. Intensive care coordination using high-quality wraparound for children with serious behavioral health needs: State and community profiles. 2014. Available at: http://www.chcs.org/media/ICC-Wraparound-State-and-Community-Profiles1.pdf. Accessed September 30, 2015.

19. New York State Health Home SPA for Individuals with Chronic Behavioral and Medical Health Conditions. 2012. Available at: https://www.medicaid.gov/state-resource-center/medicaid-state-technical-assistance/health-homes-technical-assistance/downloads/new-york-spa-12-11.pdf. Accessed April 14, 2017.

20. Health Home application to serve children. 2014. Available at: https://www.health.ny.gov/health_care/medicaid/program/medicaid_health_homes/docs/hh_serving_children_app_part_l.pdf. Accessed April 14, 2017.

21. Stroul BA, Pires SA, Armstrong MI, et al. Effective financing strategies for systems of care: examples from the field – a resource compendium for financing systems of care. 2nd edition (RTC study 3: financing structures and strategies to sup-port effective systems of care, FMHI pub. #235-03). Tampa (FL): University of South Florida, Louis de la Parte Florida Mental Health Institute (FMHI), Research and Training Center for Children's Mental Health; 2009.

22. SAMHSA-HRSA Center for Integrated Health Solutions. Integrating behavioral health and primary care for children and youth. 2013. Available at: http://www.integration.samhsa.gov/integrated-care-models/Overview_CIHS_Integrated_Care_Systems_for_Children.pdf. Accessed October 29, 2014.

23. Wraparound Milwaukee: one child, one plan. Available at: http://wraparoundmke.com/. Accessed July 30, 2017.

24. Chase D. Montefiore Medical Center: integrated care delivery for vulnerable populations. The Commonwealth Fund. 2010. p. 53. Available at: http://www.commonwealthfund.org/~/media/Files/Publications/CaseStudy/2010/Oct/1448_Chase_Montefiore_Med_Ctr_case_study_v2.pdf. Accessed May 16, 2017.

25. Pediatric integrated care: The montefiore experience. Available at: http://www.nhmh.org/page35.html. Accessed May 17, 2017.

26. Agency for Healthcare Research and Quality. Patient Centered Medical Home Resource Center. Available at: http://pcmh.ahrq.gov/. Accessed May 17, 2014.

27. National Center for Medical Home Implementation. Available at: https://medicalhomeinfo.aap.org/Pages/default.aspx. Accessed April 14, 2017.

28. Rosenthal MB, Alidina S, Friedberg MW, et al. A difference-in-difference analysis of changes in quality, utilization and cost following the Colorado multi-payer patient-centered medical home pilot. J Gen Intern Med 2016;31(3):289–96.

Essential Elements of a Collaborative Mental Health Training Program for Primary Care

Lisa L. Giles, MD[a,b], D. Richard Martini, MD[a,b],*

KEYWORDS

- Collaborative • Mental health • Training program • Primary care

KEY POINTS

- Training primary care provider (PCPs) in the provision of mental health care requires an understanding of what services to prescribe, and how best to deliver high-quality care to the greatest number of patients.
- Mental health integration creates a patient- and family-centered approach to team-based care that provides evidence based treatments targeting specific populations with identifiable and measurable outcomes.
- Collaborative mental health training provides the knowledge and skills needed to address the behavioral and mental health needs of children and adolescents in primary care.

INTRODUCTION

Primary care provides most of pediatric mental health services given the limited availability of specialists.[1] An additional challenge for the primary care provider (PCP) is the patient with comorbid psychiatric and physical illness, including chronic disorders like neurologic disease, diabetes, cancer, recurrent physical pain, obesity, and physical inactivity. The interaction of these disorders is bidirectional, where patients and families make poor decisions around compliance and lifestyle choices that subsequently complicate their medical prognosis.[2–4] Training PCPs in the provision of mental health

Disclosure Statement: Not applicable.
[a] Primary Children's Hospital, 100 North Mario Capecchi Drive, Salt Lake City, UT 841113, USA;
[b] Division of Pediatric Psychiatry and Behavioral Health, Department of Pediatrics, University of Utah School of Medicine, 100 North Mario Capecchi Drive, Salt Lake City, UT 841113, USA
* Corresponding author. Primary Children's Hospital, 100 North Mario Capecchi Drive, Salt Lake City, UT 84113.
E-mail address: richard.martini@hsc.utah.edu

Child Adolesc Psychiatric Clin N Am 26 (2017) 839–850
http://dx.doi.org/10.1016/j.chc.2017.06.012
1056-4993/17/© 2017 Elsevier Inc. All rights reserved.

childpsych.theclinics.com

Abbreviation	
PCP	Primary care provider

care requires an understanding of not only what services to prescribe, but how best to deliver high-quality care to the greatest number of patients. PCPs should be able to discriminate among various program options and decide how best to incorporate mental health integration into their practice, given available resources and the needs of their patient population. There are, however, fundamental components and principles of collaborative care that provide the structure necessary for program success, and that should be a part of any training program for primary care practitioners.

LEARNING THE BASIC PRINCIPLES OF MENTAL HEALTH INTEGRATION IN PRIMARY CARE PRACTICE

Mental health integration creates a patient- and family-centered approach to team-based care that provides evidence based treatments targeting specific populations with identifiable and measurable outcomes. Care is personalized to the needs of the child with an emphasis on informing the relationship between the caregiver and the patient. Some of this care is based on information sharing and a focus on self-care management. Measures of quality and cost should be included in the process along with an array of choices for care that reflects the nature and severity of the mental illness. Reimbursement should be aligned with outcomes so that practitioners are rewarded for providing incentives for wellness and maintain patients at the least restrictive level of care. Specialty care is accessible to patients and families either through local mental health professionals or through available resources in tertiary care. The goal is the creation of an integrated network that includes community resources as well as larger components of a health care system.[5,6] In collaborative care, treatment is defined by evidence-based practices, meaning that patients are offered treatments for psychiatric disorders that are either based on research evidence or commonly accepted clinical practice. Collaborative care is among the only integrative psychiatric care models with data demonstrating its effectiveness because of the standardization of these clinical processes.[7]

DEFINING ACCOUNTABILITY FOR QUALITY AND CLINICAL OUTCOMES

The process requires the identification of leaders within the practice who will define the scope of clinical service and identify champions within that practice who will advocate for and coordinate patient care. The goal is the creation of a collaborative care team that provides clinical direction to the program. Protocols are developed for frequently occurring and emergent situations, including school failure, suicidal ideation, substance abuse, psychiatric emergencies, and comorbid physical and psychiatric illness.

RECOGNIZING THE DIFFERENCE BETWEEN CONSULTATION, COLOCATION, AND COLLABORATIVE CARE

In consultation, the psychiatrist provides a diagnostic or treatment recommendation away from the primary care site and may only have direct contact with the patient in the office after a referral from the PCP. The limitation of the model is that there will never be enough available psychiatrists or mental health professionals to sufficiently cover patients who need services. PCPs are also detached from the consultation process and may feel that they are referring their patients into a system separate from their practice. Consultations typically involve complete assessments by the psychiatrist and emphasize communication and the development of working relationships with PCPs.[8] Consultations work best for single cases that are acute and require immediate attention, but do not address the ongoing mental health needs of a primary care practice. Colocation brings the mental health professional's practice into the primary care site with greater opportunities for interaction with the PCP, improved communication through shared medical records, and an ability to move patients between clinicians.[9] However, the process shifts the challenges of access to psychiatry into the primary care practice. Patient slots quickly fill and there is limited availability for follow-up appointments. Interactions between the psychiatrist and PCP are based primarily on individual cases and the separation between primary and mental health practices allows for little communication on patient and family compliance with recommendations. Colocation is challenging if not impossible in rural practices, where few mental health professionals are available. Collaborative care focuses on the caseload in the primary care practice, and creates a system that supports patients and families through the availability of a care manager. PCPs receive input on behavioral health problems within days rather than months and refer only the most challenging patients for psychiatric assessment. The psychiatrist meets regularly with the case manager and with members of the primary care practice to review difficult patients and provide continuing education. Through this process, the psychiatrist contributes to the care of multiple patients in a day, rather than the few who would be scheduled for assessments. Over time, the PCP and the clinic staff become more comfortable managing mental health issues and are able to make adjustments in care when patients are not improving, and initiate care for children and adolescents with more complicated behavioral or mood problems.[10] With greater involvement in the provision of mental health services through collaborative care, the care manager and PCP become familiar with resources in the community including special education, speech and language services, substance abuse treatment, physical and occupational therapy, and individual and family therapy.

UNDERSTANDING THE ROLES OF THE COLLABORATIVE CARE TEAM

The process begins by assessing the demand, and the specific tasks that must be accomplished, including the level of support required by the PCP, for collaborative care to succeed. This process requires a review of current resources and an understanding of the workflow in the practice. The characteristics of the population served and the capabilities of the practice to provide mental health interventions determine the clinical role of the PCP and the need for access to therapists in the community.

Primary Care Clinician

The primary care clinician is typically overextended by her clinical practice and questions whether to become involved in the delivery of mental health services. The preference historically has been to refer to behavioral health and struggle with limited access. In a collaborative model, the PCP manages all aspects of patient care, including prevention and screening, early identification and intervention for common mental health problems, and psychopharmacologic treatment for some of these disorders.[11,12] The PCP makes adjustments in care in consultation with the care manager, psychiatrist, and additional mental health providers.

Consulting Mental Health Professional

The consulting mental health professional meets regularly with the PCP and care coordinator to review cases followed in the practice, and by doing so to gradually increases the skills of the PCP in diagnosing and treating psychiatric illness. Psychiatric consultation should follow an identified procedure that includes presentation, time for questions, and recommendations with the understanding that the PCP is responsible for the outcome. As the PCP becomes more competent in the identification of mental illness and the provision of care, referrals to the consulting mental health professional became more complicated and more appropriate for a tertiary mental health provider. The consulting mental health professional should also support the PCP in the care of complex patients who are not improving or who present in crisis. Short-term psychotherapeutic interventions can also be delivered in the primary care practice through direct patient contact, telepsychiatry, or by phone.[13,14] Sessions are typically limited in number and focus on simple treatments, including problem solving techniques and behavioral interventions.[15]

Care Coordinator

The care coordinator within a primary care practice can be a mental health practitioner, a member of the administrative staff, or a parent who participated in collaborative care and is available to guide the patient and family through the process.[16] The care coordinator introduces the patient and family to the practice of collaborative care, educates them on the roles of the PCP and the mental health providers, and acts to facilitate their engagement in assessment and treatment. She or he also works with the PCP to ensure an adequate flow of patients into the practice and a balance between initial assessments and follow-up appointments. Outcome data are essential for program success and the care coordinator ensures that information is collected and tracked systematically. Collaborative care can be complicated when attempting to provide mental health services and monitoring compliance in a rural location, while arranging consultation from a tertiary care center miles away. Psychopharmacologic treatment, for example, requires access to medications, a role for the PCP when prescribing these drugs, and a plan to monitor the patient's and family's compliance with the regimen. The care coordinator should be familiar with the range of mental health services offered locally, including specialty care and substance abuse, and be prepared to provide counseling even in a supportive role.

Tertiary Mental Health Services

An integrated mental health care system in any primary care practice has limitations based on the skills of the clinicians and the practical challenges of the setting. Caring for young patients with comorbid psychiatric disorders including dual diagnoses, and with serious mental illness like psychosis and reactive attachment disorders requires access to a tertiary behavioral health care system, preferably through the consulting mental health professional.[17] These patients are not lost to the PCP, however, and through the collaborative care relationship are returned to their communities when stable enough to be managed in primary care.

IDENTIFYING OUTCOME MEASURES TO DETERMINE PROGRAM SUCCESS

Implement a plan to ensure fidelity to the collaborative care model by including periodic reviews among PCP, clinical staff, case manager, and consulting psychiatrist. The program supports the ability of the PCP to identify and treat mental health problems in the context of changes in typical practice patterns, includes outcome measures in the process, and works to ensure access to medical records across providers.[18–20] A clinical work flow is defined for the practice and includes the number of encounters per day, the typical range of medical, psychiatric, and social problems, and relative frequency of acute and chronic problems. The collaborative care program monitors the frequency of patient assessment and subsequent follow-up to determine whether patients have access and opportunities for treatment change and improvement. Expectations are created for each practice based on the number of contacts per patient per month that are considered appropriate and the percentage of patients who should meet this requirement. Contacts may be in person, by phone, or through telepsychiatry, and standardized assessment scales are included in the information gathering process.

UNDERSTANDING REFERRAL PATTERNS TO THE CONSULTING MENTAL HEALTH PROFESSIONAL

Referral patterns to the consulting mental health professional should be reviewed regularly with specific targets identifying the number of patients per day, productivity expectations in the PCP clinic, rates of compliance with appointments among specific patient populations, and the availability of scheduled time for consultation and education. Referral rates for psychiatric consultation should be established with patients who are treated by the PCP and not improving over a 3- to 6-month period. Consultations include exchanges that encourage case formulation and enables the practice to review compliance and effective implementation. Population-based efforts that identify a group of patients with a specific diagnosis for study or that examine services for patients under a contract for care can effectively track outcomes in collaborative care.[21] Electronic medical records make this easier and it is important to incorporate program expectations into documentation templates and to identify those disorders that will be followed in the primary care practice.[22]

Treatment success in collaborative care practices is measured as an indicator of program effectiveness, particularly in comparison with those sites without the intervention.[23] A patient registry creates a data summary including identifying information, working diagnosis, current presentation, safety issues, medications, and disposition along with a summary of treatment history including contacts and referrals. Standardized symptom measures (Youth Outcome Questionnaire, Patient Health Questionnaire-9) are used during follow-up appointments to determine the patient's progress and the need for treatment changes. Targets for point improvement are set by the program as well as the percentage of patients expected to reach that target. Medical conditions can also be monitored using laboratory or physiologic measures in conjunction with patient symptoms and function as indicators of outcome.

ADDRESSING THE FINANCIAL INCENTIVES AND DISINCENTIVES FOR COLLABORATIVE CARE

The Centers for Medicare and Medicaid Services recently announced a payment structure for patients with mental health conditions who are participating in a collaborative system. It allows for the reimbursement of the activities of a behavioral health care manager both at the time of an initial assessment and in subsequent follow-up appointments.[24] This structure may serve as an incentive for third-party payers to support mental health integration in primary care. Population-based studies that examine collaborative care in the treatment of depression alone and with comorbid physical illness demonstrate cost savings. Intermountain Healthcare showed how a relatively small investment in mental health integration can yield significant savings for insurance providers in a large health care system.[25]

TEACHING MENTAL HEALTH COMPETENCIES IN THE PRIMARY CARE SETTING

Another essential element of a collaborative mental health training program is providing the knowledge and skills needed to address the behavioral and mental health needs of children and adolescents in primary care settings. The American Academy of Pediatrics has published competencies requisite for providing mental health services in pediatric primary care settings.[12] These mental health competencies are built on the unique strengths of PCPs and the opportunities inherent in the primary care setting. As listed in **Box 1**, these competencies (many of which come from the American Academy of Pediatrics' recommendation) include 3 main sections, namely, a focus on mental health anticipatory guidance, assessment, and treatment approaches.

Competencies of Mental Health Anticipatory Guidance

In addition to learning the more traditional concepts of mental health assessment, diagnosis, and treatment, there is also a need for competencies in psychosocial screening, recognizing developmental variations, and overall promoting resiliency in children. PCPs, who already have longitudinal relationships with children and their families are experts with anticipatory guidance and understand common behavioral problems in the context of a child's developmental and environment. PCPs can recognize behavioral challenges that are variants of normal development and offer appropriate reassurance or suggest additional interventions if needed.[12] PCPs can counsel parents to prevent behavioral and mental health problems and promote physical and emotional wellness.[26]

Box 1
Mental health competencies for primary care providers

Mental health anticipatory guidance
  Recognize behavioral challenges in the context of normal development
  Integrate psychosocial updates into all visits
  Appropriate screening for psychosocial distress, adverse childhood experiences, and mental health problems
  Promote resilience in children and their families

Assessment
  Recognize and assess various behavioral difficulties
  Assess severity of suicidal thinking and actions
  Differentiate normal behavioral variants, mental health disorders, and physical conditions with mental health manifestations
  Use evidence based-tools and apply criteria from the *Diagnostic and Statistical Manual of Mental Disorders* to diagnoses specific psychiatric disorders

Treatment and monitoring
  Initiate crisis and treatment plans
  Educate families on initial steps of treatment and referral if indicated
  Understand when to refer for crisis, therapy, and/or psychiatry
  Describe role of psychotherapy in treatment
  Initiate brief supportive therapeutic interventions if indicated
  Initiate evidence-based psychopharmacology if indicated
  Monitor clinical improvement and effects of interventions

Data from Committee on Psychosocial Aspects of Child and Family Health and Task Force on Mental Health. Policy statement–the future of pediatrics: mental health competencies for pediatric primary care. Pediatrics 2009;124(1):410–21.

The primary care setting is the ideal place to screen and elicit psychosocial concerns and exposure to adverse childhood experiences.[12] Obtaining a psychosocial update can be integrated into all primary care settings, setting the stage for important discussion around the entire child, mind, body, and environment. There are a number of useful screening tools available that screen for adverse childhood experiences, psychosocial distress in general, or more specific mental health problems.[27–29] Using validated tools, such as the Pediatric Symptom Checklist for broad screening and the Patient Health Questionnaire-9 for depression screening in adolescents, helps to increase the early recognition of mental health challenges.[29–31]

PCPs also are valuable in finding ways to support and help families in strengthening resiliency. Resiliency can be increased through reinforcing child and family strengths and counseling families in healthy lifestyles.[32] Much of what already happens in primary care involves education that promotes resiliency, including counseling families regarding nutrition, exercise, play, limiting screen time, healthy sleep habits, family time, and stress management skills.[12] PCPs can elicit strengths as well as challenges in adolescents and families, facilitate youth to derive their own solutions, and offer youth and parents positive coping strategies.[33] Improving resilience helps to minimize the impact of adverse childhood experiences and mental illness on families.

Competencies of Assessment

PCPs have the unique opportunity to positively influence the clinical outcome of youth with emerging behavioral problems, whether or not they meet strict criteria from the *Diagnostic and Statistical Manual of Mental Disorders* for a disorder. PCPs should be comfortable with assessing attachment and communication concerns, avoidant behaviors, aggressive or oppositional behaviors, withdrawal concerns, academic difficulties, and exposure to trauma or loss.[12] With the appropriate knowledge and skill set, PCPs can have a positive effect on overall outcome and functioning, even when problems do not meet strict criteria for a diagnosis or the diagnosis is still unknown.[12,34]

Most pediatricians and even pediatric residents report comfort level with diagnosing and managing attention deficit hyperactivity disorder.[35] With appropriate training, PCPs can expand their capacity to effectively care for other commonly occurring pediatric mental health problems. PCPs can be educated on the growing evidence base to aid in the assessment and identification of anxiety, depression, and substance abuse.[36–41] Additionally, evidence-based tools that can aid PCPs in assessing the severity of suicidal thinking or behaviors and other urgent mental health concerns.[42–44]

Competencies of Treatment and Monitoring

By appropriately assessing and diagnosing mental health conditions early, PCPs have a unique opportunity to educate children and families about self-management strategies and offer first-line treatments. Treatment plans, including crisis plans if indicated, can be implemented, either alone or in collaboration with mental health professionals. PCPs should understand when to refer for therapy, psychiatric consultation, or an urgent crisis evaluation.[12]

When indicated, PCPs should feel comfortable initiating brief supportive therapeutic interventions, including motivational interviewing, and aspects of cognitive–behavioral therapy, supportive therapy, and solution-focused therapy.[12,45,46] PCPs can apply these skills to increase patient's optimism and willingness to work toward improvement, in addition to symptom management and reducing family conflict. Knowledge of these skills also helps PCPs to prepare a family to better understand why they are being referred to a mental health professional and to have a better understanding of the purpose of therapy.

PCPs should also feel comfortable initiating evidence-based pharmacologic interventions when indicated for youth suffering from impairing attention deficit hyperactivity disorder, anxiety, and depression.[12,47,48] With the appropriate training, PCPs should feel comfortable prescribing simulant and nonstimulant medications along with selective serotonin reuptake inhibitors. Additionally, they should have knowledge of indications and side effects of commonly used non–selective serotonin reuptake inhibitor antidepressant medication, mood stabilizers, and antipsychotic medications.[49] Whether providing direct care or referral, PCPs are in a unique position to provide ongoing monitoring and applying chronic care principles to youth with mental health disorders.

VARIOUS METHODS OF TRAINING PRIMARY CARE PROVIDERS FOR MENTAL HEALTH INTEGRATIONS

Teaching these proposed mental health competencies can be accomplished through multiple different education approaches for both residents and experienced clinicians. More information is needed to determine which of these approaches will lead to improved outcomes.

Historically, there is little evidence that residency training prepares pediatricians to care for mental health concerns. Although pediatric and other primary care residents are increasingly being exposed to mental health experiences during training, in a recent survey from the American Academy of Pediatrics, 65% of the responding pediatricians indicated they lacked training in the treatment of children and adolescents with mental health concerns.[50] A 2014 survey of pediatric residency directors found that the majority of pediatric training programs did not emphasize mental health training and were unaware of the published mental health competencies for pediatricians developed by the American Academy of Pediatrics.[51] A growing numbers of residency programs have added additional didactics in mental health assessment and treatment and offer child psychiatry electives. In a recent article in *Pediatrics*, McMillan and colleagues[26] call for increasing the behavioral and mental health curriculum in pediatric residencies.

In addition to a more robust curriculum, there is also the need for collaborative training models, thus teaching both the knowledge competencies and the skill-based collaborative competencies. Colocation of pediatric and child psychology trainees already exist in some primary care settings, enhancing the training of both groups of trainees.[52] Models that train residents in practices that integrate mental health providers and have behavioral and mental health specialists available as educators are desirable.[26,51,53] There are opportunities for academic generalists to collaborate with mental health specialists to co-precept continuity clinics or partner to conduct inpatient rounds.[12]

Experienced PCPs may be more likely to benefit from approaches that build on skills they already have.[12] PCPs can increase their mental health knowledge and skills through continuing education opportunities, ranging from hour-long local educational opportunities to self-directed learning from resources available from the American Academy of Pediatrics, the American Academy of Child and Adolescent Psychiatry, and other national agencies. Additionally, clinicians can work toward maintenance of certification in enhancing mental health competencies by monitoring their mental health care in quality improvement projects. Systems that develop pay-for-performance and quality indicators for employees for health plans or employees can incentivize appropriate mental health treatment in the primary care setting.[12]

Several groups have developed comprehensive trainings to prepare primary care professionals (and mental health specialists) for their roles in collaborative practice.[6,54] These programs can offer certificate programs signifying the enhanced learning that has occurred. Typically, they use a combination of on-line training, in-person discussions, and ongoing collaborative problem solving opportunities.

A powerful educational strategy is the learning that occurs through a PCPs relationship with mental health specialists—the authentic collaboration in the assessment and management of children in their mutual care and regular exchange of information. Whether the collaboration involves a statewide network, practice-specific model, or something in between, and whether it involves telephone or video consultation or an embedded member of the clinic, the relationship becomes a driving force for shared learning. Some collaborative relationships involve a formal didactic component or collaborative office rounds in addition to the shared management of patients.

SUMMARY

These success of mental health integration in primary care is based on creating an environment that encourages collaboration and supports appropriate care for patients and families while offering a full range of services. Training programs for primary care practitioners should include sessions on how to build and maintain such a practice along with information on basic mental health competencies.

REFERENCES

1. Cunningham PJ. Beyond Parity: primary care physicians' perspectives on access to mental health care. Health Aff 2009;28(3):490–501.
2. American Academy of Child and Adolescent Psychiatry, practice parameter for the psychiatric assessment and management of physically ill children and adolescents. J Am Acad Child Adolesc 2009;48:213–33.
3. Knight AM, Vickery ME, Muscal E, et al, CARRA Investigators. Identifying targets for improving mental healthcare of adolescents with systemic lupus erythematosus: perspectives from pediatric rheumatology clinicians in the United States and Canada. J Rheumatol 2016;43(6):1136–45.
4. Ducat L, Rubenstein A, Philipson LH, et al. A review of the mental health issues of diabetes conference. Diabetes Care 2015;38(2):333–8.
5. American Academy of Child and Adolescent Psychiatry Committee on Health Care Access and Economics Task Force on Mental Health. Improving mental health services in primary care: reducing administrative and financial barriers to access and collaboration. Pediatrics 2009;123(4):1248–51.
6. REACH's Patient-Centered Mental Health in Pediatric Primary Care (PPP). Available at: www.thereachinstitute.org/services/for-primary-care-practioners. Accessed March 8, 2017.
7. Asarnow JR, Rozenman M, Wiblin J, et al. Integrated medical-behavioral care compared with usual primary care for child and adolescent behavioral health: a meta-analysis. JAMA Pediatr 2015;169(10):929–37.
8. Katon W, Unutzer J. Consultation psychiatry in the medical home and accountable care organizations: achieving the triple aim. Gen Hosp Psychiatry 2011; 33(4):305–10.
9. Hacker K, Goldstein J, Link D, et al. Pediatric provider processes for behavioral health screening, decision making, and referral in sites with colocated mental health services. J Dev Behav Pediatr 2013;34(9):680–7.

10. Kolko DJ, Campo J, Kilbourne AM, et al. Doctor-office collaborative care for pediatric behavioral problems: a preliminary clinical trial. Arch Pediatr Adolesc Med 2012;166(3):224–31.

11. Olson AL, Kelleher KJ, Kemper KJ, et al. Primary care pediatricians' roles and perceived responsibilities in the identification and management of depression in children and adolescents. Ambul Pediatr 2001;1(2):91–8.

12. Committee on Psychosocial Aspects of Child and Family Health and Task Force on Mental Health. Policy statement–The future of pediatrics: mental health competencies for pediatric primary care. Pediatrics 2009;124(1):410–21.

13. Hilty DM, Yellowlees PM. Collaborative mental health services using multiple technologies: the new way to practice and a new standard of practice? J Am Acad Child Adolesc Psychiatry 2015;54(4):245–6.

14. Goldstein F, Myers K. Telemental health: a new collaboration for pediatricians and child psychiatrists. Pediatr Ann 2014;43(2):79–84.

15. Kroenke K, Unutzer J. Closing the false divide: sustainable approaches to integrating mental health services into primary care. J Gen Intern Med 2017;32(4):404–10.

16. Asarnow JR, Jaycox LH, Tang L, et al. Long-term benefits of short-term quality improvement interventions for depressed youths in primary care. Am J Psychiatry 2009;166(9):1002–10.

17. Aupont O, Doerfler L, Connor DF, et al. A collaborative care model to improve access to pediatric mental health services. Adm Policy Ment Health 2013;40(4):264–73.

18. Zatzick D, Russo J, Lord SP, et al. Collaborative care intervention targeting violence risk behaviors, substance use, and posttraumatic stress and depressive symptoms in injured adolescents: a randomized clinical trial. JAMA Pediatr 2014;168(6):532–9.

19. Williams SB, O'Connor EA, Eder M, et al. Screening for child and adolescent depression in primary care settings: a systematic evidence review for the US preventive services task force. Pediatrics 2009;123(4):e716–35.

20. Wissow LS, Brown J, Fothergill KE, et al. Universal mental health screening in pediatric primary care: a systematic review. J Am Acad Child Adolesc Psychiatry 2013;52(11):1134–47.

21. Fallucco EM, Bejarano CM, Kozikowski CB, et al. Long-term effects of primary care provider training in screening, assessment, and treatment of adolescent depression. J Adolesc Health 2015;56(2):S97.

22. Hagan JH. Discerning Bright Futures of electronic health records. Pediatr Ann 2008;37(3):173–9.

23. Goldman ML, Spaeth-Rublee B, Nowels AD, et al. Quality measures at the interface of behavioral health and primary care. Curr Psychiatry Rep 2016;18:39.

24. Press MJ, Howe R, Schoenbaum M, et al. Medicare payment for behavioral health integration. N Engl J Med 2017;376:405–7.

25. Reiss-Brennan B, Brunisholz KD, Dredge C, et al. Association of integrated team-based care with health care quality, utilization, and cost. JAMA 2016;316(8):826–34.

26. McMillan JA, Land M Jr, Leslie LK. Pediatric residency education and the behavioral and mental health crisis: a call to action. Pediatrics 2017;139(1) [pii: e20162141].

27. Weitzman C, Wegner L, Section on Developmental and Behavioral Pediatrics. Promoting optimal development: screening for behavioral and emotional problems. Pediatrics 2015;135(2):384–95.

28. Chung EK, Siegel BS, Garg A, et al. Screening for social determinants of health among children and families living in poverty: a guide for clinicians. Curr Probl Pediatr Adolesc Health Care 2016;46(5):135–53.

29. Murphy JM, Bergmann P, Chiang C, et al. The PSC-17: subscale scores, reliability, and factor structure in a new national sample. Pediatrics 2016;138(3) [pii:e20160038].

30. Siu AL, US Preventive Services Task Force. Screening for depression in children and adolescents: US preventive services task force recommendation statement. Pediatrics 2016;137(3):e20154467.

31. Richardson LP, McCauley E, Grossman DC, et al. Evaluation of the Patient Health Questionnaire-9 Item for detecting major depression among adolescents. Pediatrics 2010;126(6):1117–23.

32. Taliaferro LA, Borowsky IW. Beyond prevention: promoting healthy youth development in primary care. Am J Public Health 2012;102(Suppl 3):S317–21.

33. Ginsburg KR, Carlson EC. Resilience in action: an evidence-informed, theoretically driven approach to building strengths in an office-based setting. Adolesc Med State Art Rev 2011;22(3):458–81, xi.

34. Wissow LS, Gadomski A, Roter D, et al. Improving child and parent mental health in primary care: a cluster-randomized trial of communication skills training. Pediatrics 2008;121(2):266–75.

35. Stein RE, Horwitz SM, Storfer-Isser A, et al. Do pediatricians think they are responsible for identification and management of child mental health problems? Results of the AAP periodic survey. Ambul Pediatr 2008;8(1):11–7.

36. Connolly SD, Bernstein GA, Work Group on Quality Issues. Practice parameter for the assessment and treatment of children and adolescents with anxiety disorders. J Am Acad Child Adolesc Psychiatry 2007;46(2):267–83.

37. Siegel RS, Dickstein DP. Anxiety in adolescents: update on its diagnosis and treatment for primary care providers. Adolesc Health Med Ther 2012;3:1–16.

38. Zuckerbrot RA, Cheung AH, Jensen PS, et al, GLAD-PC Steering Group. Guidelines for adolescent depression in primary care (GLAD-PC): I. Identification, assessment, and initial management. Pediatrics 2007;120(5):e1299–312.

39. Cheung AH, Kozloff N, Sacks D. Pediatric depression: an evidence-based update on treatment interventions. Curr Psychiatry Rep 2013;15(8):381.

40. Harrop E, Catalano RF. Evidence-based prevention for adolescent substance use. Child Adolesc Psychiatr Clin N Am 2016;25(3):387–410.

41. Beaton A, Shubkin CD, Chapman S. Addressing substance misuse in adolescents: a review of the literature on the screening, brief intervention, and referral to treatment model. Curr Opin Pediatr 2016;28(2):258–65.

42. Shain BN, American Academy of Pediatrics Committee on Adolescence. Suicide and suicide attempts in adolescents. Pediatrics 2007;120(3):669–76.

43. Posner K, Brown GK, Stanley B, et al. The Columbia-Suicide Severity Rating Scale: initial validity and internal consistency findings from three multisite studies with adolescents and adults. Am J Psychiatry 2011;168(12):1266–77.

44. Horowitz LM, Bridge JA, Teach SJ, et al. Ask Suicide-Screening Questions (ASQ): a brief instrument for the pediatric emergency department. Arch Pediatr Adolesc Med 2012;166(12):1170–6.

45. Keeley RD, Brody DS, Engel M, et al. Motivational interviewing improves depression outcome in primary care: a cluster randomized trial. J Consult Clin Psychol 2016;84(11):993–1007.

46. Klar H, Coleman WL. Brief solution-focused strategies for behavioral pediatrics. Pediatr Clin North Am 1995;42(1):131–41.

47. Subcommittee on Attention-Deficit/Hyperactivity Disorder, Steering Committee on Quality Improvement and Management. ADHD: clinical practice guideline for the diagnosis, evaluation, and treatment of attention-deficit/hyperactivity disorder in children and adolescents. Pediatrics 2011;128(5):1007–22.

48. Cheung AH, Zuckerbrot RA, Jensen PS, et al. Guidelines for adolescent depression in primary care (GLAD-PC): II. Treatment and ongoing management. Pediatrics 2007;120(5):e1313–26.

49. Giles LL, Martini DR. Challenges and promises of pediatric psychopharmacology. Acad Pediatr 2016;16(6):508–18.

50. Horwitz SM, Storfer-Isser A, Kerker BD, et al. Barriers to the identification and management of psychosocial problems: changes from 2004 to 2013. Acad Pediatr 2015;15(6):613–20.

51. Green C, Hampton E, Ward MJ, et al. The current and ideal state of mental health training: pediatric program director perspectives. Acad Pediatr 2014;14(5): 526–32.

52. Pisani AR, leRoux P, Siegel DM. Educating residents in behavioral health care and collaboration: integrated clinical training of pediatric residents and psychology fellows. Acad Med 2011;86(2):166–73.

53. Bunik M, Talmi A, Stafford B, et al. Integrating mental health services in primary care continuity clinics: a national CORNET study. Acad Pediatr 2013;13(6):551–7.

54. AIMS Center. Advancing integrated mental health solutions. Available at: https:// aims.uw.edu/resource-library. Accessed April 7, 2017.

The Basic Science of Behavior Change and Its Application to Pediatric Providers

 CrossMark

Allison R. Love, PhD[a], Peter S. Jensen, MD[b,c],*, Lisa Khan, Ed.M.[d], Tiffany West Brandt, PhD[a], James Jaccard, PhD[e]

KEYWORDS

- Medical provider training • Continuing medical education • Pediatric primary care
- Integrated health care • Behavior change • Self-efficacy • Normative beliefs
- Expected values

KEY POINTS

- Pediatric primary care providers (PPCPs) are the front line for early identification and treatment of youth mental health disorders, particularly in underserved communities in which specialty services are not readily available.

Continued

Disclosure: P.S. Jensen is Professor of Psychiatry, Department of Psychiatry, University of Arkansas for Medical Sciences; President and CEO of The Resource for Advancing Children's Health (REACH) Institute, a nonprofit 501c3 organization; and receives book royalties from Guilford Press, Random House, and the American Psychiatric Association Press, Inc. L. Khan is Director of the Patient-Centered Mental Health in Pediatric Primary Care (PPP) program, developed and delivered by The REACH Institute. The authors A.R. Love, T.W. Brandt, and J. Jaccard have nothing to disclose. Additional information: Present and past Steering Committee members of the PPP program who have participated in developing and implementing this program include Larry Amsel, MD; Diane Bloomfield, MD; Gabrielle Carlson, MD; M. Lynn Crismon, PharmD; Cathryn Galanter, MD; Harlan Gephart, MD; Larry Greenhill, MD; Peter S. Jensen, MD; Christopher Kratocvhil, MD; Danielle Laraque, MD; Laurel Leslie, MD; Rachel Lynch, MD; Elena Mann, MD; Suzanne Reiss, MD; Mark Riddle, MD; Lisa Hunter Romanelli, PhD; Martin Stein, MD; Ruth E.K. Stein, MD, Lynn Wegner, MD; Mark Wolraich, MD; Rachel Zuckerbrot, MD.

[a] Psychiatric Research Institute, University of Arkansas for Medical Sciences, 4301 West Markham Street, Slot 654, Little Rock, AR 72205, USA; [b] Child and Adolescent Psychiatry, Psychiatric Research Institute, University of Arkansas for Medical Sciences, 4301 West Markham Street, Slot 654, Little Rock, AR 72205, USA; [c] The Resource for Advancing Children's Health (REACH) Institute, 404 5th Avenue, 3rd Floor, New York, NY 10018, USA; [d] Patient-Centered Mental Health in Pediatric Primary Care Program, The REACH Institute, 404 5th Avenue, 3rd Floor, New York, NY 10018, USA; [e] Silver School of Social Work, New York University, 1 Washington Square North, New York, NY 10003, USA

* Corresponding author. Child and Adolescent Psychiatry, Psychiatric Research Institute, University of Arkansas for Medical Sciences, 4301 West Markham Street, Slot 654, Little Rock, AR 72205.
E-mail address: psjensen@uams.edu

Child Adolesc Psychiatric Clin N Am 26 (2017) 851–874
http://dx.doi.org/10.1016/j.chc.2017.06.011
childpsych.theclinics.com

Continued

- To enhance their willingness and ability to fill this role, PPCPs need intensive training and ongoing coaching support in applying guidelines for screening, diagnosing, and treating pediatric mental health conditions.
- Traditional continuing medical education and/or performance incentive strategies are inadequate for changing provider practice behavior. Targeted, dynamic training programs that combine multiple educational techniques can be effective, but are cumbersome and lack guiding theoretic frameworks.
- The theories and methods from behavioral change science, communication science, and adult learning offer powerful strategies for developing effective training programs that produce sustained practice changes, but are rarely applied to physician continuing education programs.
- This article describes a training program grounded in behavioral science research designed to increase PPCPs' ability, commitment, and persistence in implementing practice behavior changes so as to deliver high-quality mental health services within primary care.

INTRODUCTION

As the health care system moves toward integrated behavioral health care models, primary care providers are increasingly expected to know how to recognize and address mental health problems in their practices.[1–3] Pediatric primary care providers (PPCPs) are well positioned to have a substantial positive impact on child behavioral health because they can provide early detection and intervention services for children who might otherwise remain unidentified or untreated until they are more impaired. PPCPs are also an important port of entry to the children's mental health care system by referring families for specialty assessment and treatment when indicated, and supporting these services through encouragement and accountability discussions with the families at follow-up visits. The value of PPCPs is particularly salient in underserved communities, in which the availability of psychosocial and psychiatric services is limited and the PPCPs may be the only providers servicing the mental health needs of children in the local area.

Provider Education Programs Do Not Reliably Produce Practice Behavior Change

For PPCPs, an integrated behavioral health care approach includes performing practice behaviors such as administering and interpreting screening measures, developing diagnostic formulations, creating a comprehensive treatment plan, prescribing psychiatric medications, and coordinating care with specialty mental health providers. However, PPCPs receive little training in assessing and managing children's mental health disorders during residency.[4] Therefore, practicing PPCPs necessarily need additional education, training, and support to change their practices and meet these new demands. However, few effective teaching programs have been developed and/or widely disseminated thus far.[5] There are a small number of online learning modules for PPCPs to learn these skills on their own time, but there are limited data to predict which clinicians may enroll in online learning, how many complete such programs, and to what extent enrollees have applied the information in practice. Time-limited, unidirectional learning approaches have been found to have little or no impact on practitioner behavior change.[6,7] This finding is not surprising given that, in order for this approach to succeed, learners must initiate the interaction with the information, comprehend the new material, and engage in novel practice behaviors, all without the benefit of support and feedback. However, traditional continuing medical education (CME) routinely uses ineffective so-called hit-and-run learning strategies such as didactic lectures[6,7] or distributing printed educational materials.[5,8] In order to design more effective medical education courses, it is important to identify educational strategies and theory-based frameworks that offer the greatest possibilities for impact in changing providers' practice behavior.

Systematic reviews of continuing educational strategies have aided in the identification of strategies that have variable, or contingent, impacts on provider behavior; those that have consistently positive but small effects; and approaches with a medium or moderate impact. CME methods shown to have variable impact, depending on variables such as length of learning program and size or nature of the professional audience, include the use of local opinion leaders (ie, influential people who try to persuade providers to follow evidence-based practice guidelines),[5,9] audit and feedback (ie, performance is measured and compared with standards or targets),[10] and tailored interventions (ie, assessing determinants of practice and potential barriers, then creating a customized intervention plan).[11] Some medical education strategies that show consistently positive but limited effectiveness in changing provider behavior include educational outreach efforts (ie, trained representatives visit clinicians face to face to advise them on practice changes),[12] reminders (eg, delivered via computer systems or on paper),[13,14] and e-learning strategies.[15] Interactive educational interventions and/or those that combined multiple strategies into 1 multifaceted intervention (eg, educational meetings that use active teaching methods, audit and feedback, reminders), show the greatest impact on provider behavior change.[5–7,16] Health care systems that opt for 1-time trainings rarely experience practice change gains, whereas systems that invest in interactive trainings and create a learning community that supports the provider to make positive practice changes are more likely to realize benefits such as improved patient outcomes or cost savings.[17]

Although research suggests there may be a cumulative positive impact on clinician practice behavior from using multiple learning strategies concurrently, there is no clear theoretic or empirical framework to drive decisions about which strategies to choose and how to combine them. There is a need for theory-driven training methods that are consistently effective at increasing PPCPs' commitment and follow-through to engage in new practice behaviors. Basic science frameworks for human behavior and behavior change in fields such as social psychology, communication, and adult learning have been successfully applied to develop interventions focused on changing patient health behaviors. However, these frameworks have rarely been applied to provider practice behaviors,[18] despite the wealth of theory-driven education strategies that might be applied to providers to reliably increase their uptake and adoption of best new practices. In addition, provider intervention frameworks that are grounded in theoretic models lend themselves to systematic evaluation and improvement. When training programs do not have the desired impact or effectiveness, the models can be used to develop a hypothesis about sources of interference and guide subsequent changes that, in turn, can be evaluated and refined. This article describes 3 theoretic frameworks and their application to an interactive, integrated training program for PPCPs on identifying, assessing, and managing mental health concerns in children, delivered since 2006 to more than 2200 PPCPs by The Resource for Advancing Children's Health (REACH) Institute, a nonprofit provider training and practice change organization.

Behavioral Science Theories and Principles Can Be Incorporated into Provider Education Programs

Behavioral decision theory

Understanding factors that influence behavior and behavior change is the first step to designing an effective program or intervention. Four decades of basic science research across multiple fields of study were synthesized to identify 8 key determinants of behavior and behavior change.[19] Jaccard and colleagues[20] summarized these 8 factors, along with 2 additional factors from their own research, in an integrated conceptual framework that is now known as behavioral decision theory (BDT).[21] When considering behavioral performance, note that the target outcome could be a single practice behavior (eg, inquiring about suicidal thoughts with every patient), a category of behaviors (eg, identifying mental health symptoms in primary care patients), or a goal (eg, improving patient health outcomes). For the purposes of this article, the term behavior performance is used to refer collectively to any of these 3 types of outcomes. However, it is vital to identify the individual behaviors that comprise a category or are in service of reaching a particular goal when conducting behavioral analysis research.[19]

BDT organizes behavioral decision making into 2 sequences. These 2 sequences are linked by a central variable, known as behavioral intention (BI), which has been defined as "a person's subjective probability that he will perform some behavior."[22] The strength of a person's motivation or intention to perform a behavior is the single best predictor of whether or not a behavior will be performed.[18] If a person does not intend to engage in the target behavior, it is unlikely to occur. Therefore, the use of educational strategies specifically designed to strengthen providers' BI by targeting 1 or more of these predictive factors may increase the likelihood that a practice recommendation is later implemented. The first BDT sequence (**Fig. 1**A) represents 5 variables that have an immediate impact on the strength and direction of BI. Although not an exhaustive list of all possible determinants of BI, these 5 represent the most robust, the most immediate, and the most predictive factors described in the empirical literature.[19–21]

First, beliefs and expectancies refers to an individual's perceptions of the anticipated advantages and disadvantages associated with a given behavior. Bandura[23] described this as a belief or expectancy that the outcome of the behavior is more desirable than undesirable. Without a belief that the behavior will yield a desirable

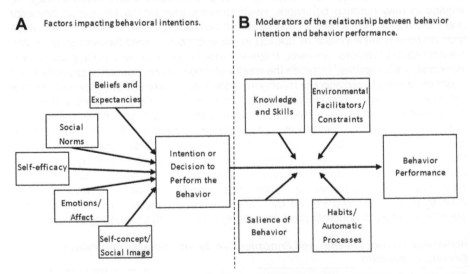

Fig. 1. Model of the key components of behavioral decision making. (*Adapted from* Jaccard J. The prevention of problem behaviors in adolescents and young adults: Perspectives on theory and practice. J Soc Social Work Res 2016;7(4):597; with permission.)

outcome, it is unlikely that the person will intend to perform it. For example, a PPCP who expects that selective serotonin reuptake inhibitors (SSRIs) are likely to improve a depressed adolescent's symptoms with few or no side effects is more willing to prescribe them than a provider who believes that SSRIs increase youth risk of suicidal ideation or self-harm behavior.

Second, BI is influenced by perceived social norms, and strengthened when there is a positive appraisal of the benefits of the behavior because people important to the individual endorse it. For example, A PPCP's intent to follow a new guideline or begin performing an unfamiliar procedure may be strengthened if national experts and/or practice colleagues approve of this behavior.

A third predictor of BI, self-efficacy, refers to individuals' self-appraisal of their ability to perform the target behavior successfully whether they think they are capable of doing the behavior that will lead to the desirable outcome. There are multiple sources of information that inform or influence people's expected self-efficacy.[23] Direct, hands-on experiences are the most influential in self-efficacy appraisals because they are based on personal mastery. Vicarious experiences, such as witnessing a colleague effectively performing the new behavior, can also be influential, although their impact is moderated by factors such as how closely the learner identifies with the person modeling the behavior.

Fourth, emotions and affect describe people's emotional reaction to the anticipation or experience of performing the behavior. For example, a strong negative emotional reaction may reduce the likelihood of behavioral performance (feeling guilty prescribing a child a medication that causes side effects), whereas a positive reaction increases the likelihood (finding it rewarding to hear that a patient is doing better in school after starting the medication that was prescribed).

Another variable shown to predict the strength of BI is self-concept/image. This variable refers to the degree to which the target behavior is congruent or incongruent with the individual's self-imposed standards and/or the social image the individual wishes to project. For example, PPCPs who take pride in staying up to date on the research and recently learn of a new guideline they are not currently using may say to themselves, "I'm a good doctor and I want to change my practice behavior so I am delivering state-of-the-art care." The positive or negative self-evaluation, in turn, provides an incentive to initiate and/or persist in a behavior until the goal or standard is reached.[23]

The first BDT sequence describes 5 variables that affect the strength and direction of BI. However, even with a strong positive intention, other factors can affect the behavioral outcome. The second BDT sequence (see **Fig. 1**, part B) describes 4 factors that may facilitate or hinder behavioral performance even when a strong positive BI is present. Most importantly, the individual must have sufficient knowledge and skill to perform the intended behavior, and there must be the presence of sufficient facilitators and/or the absence of notable constraints in the environment for the behavior to occur. Fishbein and colleagues[19] argue that BI, knowledge/skill, and appropriate environmental conditions are the necessary and sufficient ingredients for behavioral performance to occur. In addition, Jaccard and colleagues[20] argue that the behavior must also be salient enough for the person to remember to perform it, and preexisting habits or automatic processes must not interfere with execution of the new behavior.

As noted by Jaccard,[21] the unidirectional arrows in **Fig. 1** suggest a simple additive effect of each determinant on BI or actual behavior when, in reality, the relationship is complex. The weighted influence of each variable differs across behaviors, individuals, time, and contexts. Furthermore, the relationships among these factors may be reciprocating or bidirectional. Most notably, when an individual attempts to perform the target behavior, the resulting outcome provides direct experience and information that feeds back into both the BI and behavioral performance sequences. For example, expecting and addressing obstacles to performing a new behavior may enhance self-efficacy and lead to a positive emotional experience, whereas an unsuccessful attempt may decrease self-efficacy and increase negative outcome beliefs. The impact of failure or success on any given attempt depends on the timing of outcome (eg, early or late in the learning trajectory) and the total pattern of experiences (eg, proportion of success to failures relative to the number of attempts).[23]

Systematically addressing the first sequence's 5 variables (expectancies, norms, self-efficacy, emotions, and/or self-image) within a PPCP training program might strengthen the learner's BI. However, as noted earlier, there is frequently a gap between BI and the eventual performance of a behavior even when the individual's BI is strong. To address this gap, behavior scientists have identified effective cognitive strategies for (1) framing behavioral goals by imagining the benefits of a desired future and then potential obstacles present in the current reality (termed mental contrasting) and (2) forming a planned response and visualizing its use when confronted with the anticipated obstacles (termed implementation intention).[24] Mental contrasting increases the salience of the target behavior, influences commitment to realizing the future goal, and primes people to take action to overcome obstacles. Implementation intentions create a prospective memory and individual plan to address anticipated obstacles to successfully performing the intended behavior, thereby automatizing the planned reaction. Research has shown that coupling these 2 cognitive strategies to create a personalized behavioral goal attainment plan increases the likelihood that BI will translate into successful behavioral performance.[24]

As noted earlier, knowledge and skill are important factors moderating the relationship between BI and behavior performance. Research on adult learning principles provides rich resources for effective curriculum design and educational techniques to optimize knowledge acquisition and retention. A brief review is given next.

Adult learning and education principles

Adult learning and education research is important to the development of effective training interventions because it offers practical strategies to facilitate participant learning.[25] Although there is no widely accepted overarching theory of adult education, there is widespread agreement on the essential principles and specific methods that should guide effective adult education efforts.[25(pp74,75)] Part of this agreement is grounded in the recognition that learning as an adult is different than learning as a child and, therefore, different methods must be used to teach adult learners (andragogy) as opposed to children (pedagogy). According to Knowles and colleagues,[25] effective adult learning methods differ from typical pedagogical teaching methods in at least 9 key areas, respectively:

1. Learner preparation (helping learners develop reasonable expectations vs minimal/none)
2. Learning climate (warm, supportive, and democratic vs authoritarian and evaluative)
3. Curriculum planning (extensive learner input and feedback vs little to none)
4. Assessment of individuals' learning needs and goals (constructed by learners with teachers' input vs teacher driven)
5. Setting course objectives (mutually negotiated between teachers and learners vs teacher driven)

6. Designing learning plans (sequenced by learner readiness vs logic of subject matter)
7. Teaching/learning methods (active involvement, and skill-based practice vs rote memory)
8. Learning and teaching techniques (experiential and hands-on with ongoing feedback, vs didactic)
9. Evaluation of learning (mutual rediagnosis of learning needs and program effectiveness vs teacher-developed testing).

Another area of difference includes the degree of attention paid to the physical environment, such that any obstacles that might interfere with learning (eg, room temperature, auditory distractions, hunger, poor lighting, seating configuration) are carefully addressed.[25,26]

Attention must also be given to the educators guiding the learning. Adult educational information is best presented by educators who are considered to be facilitators or coaches partnering with adult learners to help them master new knowledge and skills. Furthermore, adult educators must strengthen learners' motivation (or BI) to apply new skills and behaviors in life settings and situations by inspiring (rather than requiring) them to implement new behaviors (eg, by sharing success stories of the new practices being implemented). For example, identifying and managing pediatric depression is highly relevant to the clinical demands PPCPs face each day; therefore, an effective educator should provide information and examples that address why it is important for PPCPs to know how to effectively address this mental health problem within their clinical settings. Moreover, educators must create a safe learning environment that respects learners' preexisting knowledge, opinions, and beliefs, while using methods that open learners' minds to new information and correct potential biases or misinformation. In addition, it is important for educators to accept that adult learners bring with them life experience, which means that the learners may have areas of expertise that the educator does not. Thus, the educator must be willing to also be a learner.

Cognitive neuroscience research applications
Over the last decade, educators have become increasingly interested in applying cognitive and social neuroscience to adult educational methods. Relevant research findings support many of the principles and practices of andragogy noted earlier, and also expand on them with 3 important neuroscience meta-findings [25]:

1. Emotions play a critical role in learning. Positive emotions such as humor, warmth, and a personal sense of safety within the learning context can enhance learning and memory, whereas negative emotions such as anxiety, uncertainty, and fear can interfere. As such, strategies like so-called ice breakers to create warmer relationships among strangers are often used to establish an emotionally secure learning environment.[26,27] Likewise, information delivered within an emotional context (eg, surprise, humor, suspense) are better retained than "dry" facts.
2. Learning is more effective when it builds on existing knowledge. Retention and recall are enhanced when new material scaffolds on the learner's preexisting experiences rather than providing large amounts of novel information that lacks relevance or relation to prior bases of knowledge.
3. Stimulating inquiry primes learning. Information that is delivered through teaching techniques that stimulate learners' need to know (eg, prompting the audience with a rhetorical question and pausing momentarily before giving the answer, creating suspense in a clinical vignette) facilitates information retention and future application.

The principles and practices listed here have been expanded to note the importance of obtaining and maintaining learners' attention. Given that learning is unlikely to occur without the learner attending to the educator, experienced medical educators use strategies such as so-called hooks (a brief story or real-life anecdote that is highly relevant to the learners' clinical practice) to capture the audience's attention and stimulate their need to know.[26] Other techniques, such as regularly switching speakers and providing learning activities that vary in their cognitive demand, can be used to sustain learners' attention. Furthermore, educators have highlighted the importance of enhancing retention by making information relatable and emotionally salient through the use of metaphors, storytelling and narratives, and linking new information to learners' daily needs. Affectively laden stories rooted in the contexts and settings in which learners need to apply their new knowledge and skills can help participants make stronger cognitive and emotional connections to learning content. In turn, this can lead to greater learner buy-in and increased likelihood of learner recall and application of the content in their own work or personal environments.[28]

In addition, consistent with the principles of both adult learning and neuroscience research, Stahl and Davis[26] further emphasize the importance of respecting the limits of learners' working memory. Rather than presenting a great deal of factual information, which can overwhelm working memory and interfere with learning, didactic content should be limited to information that is essential to performing the new behaviors or skills, delivered in small amounts. Educators should use a variety of interactive learning formats (eg, dyadic or small-group discussions, question-and-answer panels, role plays), provide multiple opportunities for behavioral rehearsal and practice with feedback, and guide the learner in creating a behavioral goal and implementation plan. Likewise, educators are more effective if they use a 3-act-play mentality to presenting materials: (1) create a cognitive road map about the learning content before any educational information is delivered, (2) deliver the information, and (3) summarize the information just given to the learner.

There are many adult educational resources and guides available to direct educators in designing effective curricula and learning formats.[25–27,29] However, these effective methods are not sufficiently applied in most CME sessions. Little or no attention is given to content delivery and communication methods for professional providers.

Persuasive communication theory

In our experience, the persuasive manner in which messages (or training content) is communicated is a third key theoretic framework to consider when designing an effective training or behavioral change intervention for PPCPs. Different communication models and theories have been proposed to better understand how information is presented and received.[30–32] Common key factors that strengthen communication effectiveness identified within these theoretic models include (but are not limited to):

1. The source of the information
2. The message being communicated
3. The medium (or channel) by which the message is being delivered
4. The recipient or audience the message is intended to reach
5. The situation/context in which the communication occurs

These 5 factors are useful for understanding the processes by which a message is being presented and received, but are not specific to particular goals of communication (eg, change the listeners' beliefs or behavior). The Yale Attitude Change Approach[33] (YACA) is a communication model for understanding how a persuasive message is accepted by the receiver by describing specific aspects of communication that affect people's attitudes and readiness to change.

The source of the information is the person, or group, who creates the message and delivers it to the receiver or audience. According to communication theory models, including YACA, specific characteristics of the source make that person more persuasive and credible. Expertise and trustworthiness have been identified as the two most important aspects of persuasive sources.[34,35] Specifically, the receiver is more likely to pay attention, retain ideas, and accept a message when its source is respected and trusted. The use of personal anecdotes may help to build a source's trustworthiness because this establishes that the source has similar experiences to the audience. Similarly, having a well-structured message that is conducted in a powerful linguistic style can depict expertise. In our PPCP training experience, a high-impact program must have an educational faculty that includes both professionals with specialty expertise (eg, in mental health, child psychiatrists) and trustworthy peer models (ie, other PPCPs) who can confidently speak to the training content as well as describe their personal experience in delivering and applying the techniques presented within their own practices (eg, diagnostic and treatment procedures for children's mental health). Such personal anecdotes by PPCP trainers can help to build their source trustworthiness because this establishes the idea that they have similar experiences to the audience and are authentic role models.

The message is the information that the source is communicating and the receiver is obtaining. According to the YACA model, messages (or content) may contain characteristics that make them more or less believable. These characteristics are categorized into 2 basic parts: organization (eg, the order in which information is presented, use of 1-sided vs 2-sided arguments, explicit vs implicit conclusions) and content (eg, arguments, evidence, appeals). When the message is presented in a simple, tightly organized format without excessive or extraneous details, receivers are able to comprehend and attend to the message more adequately. Two-sided arguments (eg, presenting the pros and cons of a specific clinical behavior) may also promote acceptance from an audience, more so than 1-sided arguments. Two-sided arguments can be presented by mentioning opposing viewpoints, presenting facts that refute them, and then presenting arguments supporting the favorable viewpoint.[36(p87)] Further, it is ideal to make an explicit assertion in favor of new behavioral performance so the audience reaches the speaker's intended conclusion rather than being left to draw their own.[36(p217)] Explicit conclusions help with comprehension and retention of the information provided. With regard to content, messages are more persuasive and accepted if they contain several strong and high-quality arguments,[37] and include powerful evidence such as findings from large-scale randomized controlled trials. In addition, messages are more persuasive if they contain an urgent need that is serious, could affect them personally, and contains a solution. For example, in a training program on mental health in primary care, PPCPs may be presented with data on the frequency of youth depression and suicidality, how often they are overlooked or underidentified in primary care settings, the positive benefits of screening, and the impact and effectiveness of appropriate PPCP treatment.

The medium, or channel, by which the message is delivered refers to the manner in which the message is being communicated. For PPCPs, this means that passively reading information about behavioral health care strategies in pediatric primary care via 1 channel, like a brochure, published practice guideline, or research article, is not as effective for learning and practice behavior change as conveying this information to them via multiple mediums over an extended period of time. Learners vary in their preferred communication channels, so educational methods that provide content via multiple channels (eg, didactic presentations with slides, visual presentation of slide content in workbooks, Web-based resources, table discussions, expert panels) is more likely to successfully reach individuals.

The recipient (or audience) is the person or persons receiving the information being communicated by the source. Motivation, past experience, knowledge, skills, and expectations can influence a recipient's ability to be persuaded by a message. To better understand these factors and consider them during training, our program has found it vital to assess learners' preexisting knowledge, skills, and expectations coming into the course so training content can then be presented from a starting point appropriate for the audience. To better ascertain the extent to which the program is effectively reaching the learners and facilitating actual practice change, postassessments of specific knowledge, skills, and BI to change their practice behaviors in the future are also conducted.

In addition, the context in which the communication occurs refers to the setting and environmental factors surrounding the source and receiver, such as social, cultural, and physical features. In general, the authors have found the most effective setting or context is one that is highly interactive and interpersonal, allows for substantial give and take between learners and faculty, offers both large and small group discussions, and provides opportunities for learners to seek clarification.

Summary

Current educational efforts to promote the use of evidence-based assessment and treatment approaches for mental health problems in pediatric primary care settings fail to incorporate theory-driven mechanisms of learning and behavior change. Trainings developed to educate providers on evidence-based practices should incorporate research from behavioral decision making, adult learning, and communication to optimize the likelihood that PPCPs will adopt recommended practice behaviors. Next, this article describes how these 3 complementary theoretic approaches have been integrated into a program to train practicing PPCPs to screen, assess, diagnose, and manage common pediatric mental health disorders within primary care settings.

The Application of Theory-based Training Strategies

The Patient-Centered Mental Health in Pediatric Primary Care (PPP) Minifellowship program begins with a 3-day course (the training agenda is shown in **Table 1**) that provides PPCPs with training on up-to-date guidelines and recommendations for assessing, diagnosing, and treating pediatric behavioral health concerns in primary care. Training is delivered by a faculty team that consists of child psychiatrists and PPCPs, all of whom are PPP Fellowship alumni with extensive experience treating child mental health difficulties in their primary care practices. All participants of the PPP Fellowship also receive toolkits with guides, assessment instruments, dosing and side effect charts, medication comparison tables, and handouts for families. After the initial 16 hours of in-person learning, consolidation and application of PPCPs' new skills are facilitated by a series of 12 small-group conference calls delivered over a period of several months.

The face-to-face component of the PPP Fellowship program is designed to inspire PPCPs to engage in the learning process and make long-term changes in their mental health care practices, as well as to provide them with an experience of how integrated behavioral health care might operate in their practice settings. Through course content and educator experiences, PPCPs are taught how integrated care teams that include themselves, mental health professionals, school personnel, and parents collaborating can better help youth and families to manage pediatric mental health problems.

Table 1
Training agenda for the Patient-Centered Mental Health in Pediatric Primary Care minifellowship

Training Topic[a]	Length	Learning Activities
Day 1		
Overview and welcome to day 1	30 min	• Ice-breaker and introductions
Opening remarks: "This is not your Grandma's CME!"	10 min	
Introduction to course: common ground and gaps	35 min	• FD: easy vs hard presenting case in PC • SR: review course road map/overview • IE: identify personal learning goals
Pediatric psychopharmacology overview: categories and agents	45 min	• TE: medication reconciliation • SR: introduce REACH First Principles; summarize major areas to be taught • Orientation to toolkits and medication dosing charts
Understanding why assessment is so important	30 min	• TE: Three goals of assessment; • CP: initial visit for youth with multiple behavior concerns • TE: forming initial diagnostic impressions and differential diagnosis • SR: review mental health toolkit card
Tools to know and love	20 min	• SR: presentation of easy-to-use screening measures • TE: compare/contrast 2 screening measures, pick 1 the group likes best, and explain why
Assessment of anxiety disorders	90 min	• CP: interview with anxious 8-year-old and parent • TE: review patient scores on anxiety scales • SR: overview of anxiety disorder assessment issues • FD: humorous mock celebrity interview with pediatrician/expert • FD: reading patients' nonverbal behavior • PRP: interview patient using mental health toolkit card
Treatment of anxiety disorders	30 min	• SR: evidence for anxiety interventions • GD: identifying appropriate medications for anxiety and titration strategies • PD: pharmacologic treatment of anxiety in youth

(continued on next page)

Table 1
(continued)

Training Topic[a]	Length	Learning Activities
Summary and wrap-up of day 1	10 min	
Total training time (not including breaks)	5 h 00 min	
Dinner with REACH faculty (optional)		
Day 2		
Overview and welcome to day 2	5 min	
Understanding the FDA boxed warning	25 min	• SR: background history of FDA boxed warning
Depressions: short course	50 min	• SR: guidelines for diagnosing adolescent depression • CP: 2 presentations (1 mild, 1 moderate–severe) of adolescent depression • TE: review patient scores on depression scales, give initial diagnostic impressions, discuss possible underlying medical causes
Managing adolescent depression in primary care	60 min	• SR: guidelines for managing adolescent depression • PRP: discuss SSRI boxed warning and safety planning with parent • PD: pharmacologic treatment of pediatric depression
Pediatric bipolar disorder	45 min	• IE: read case notes and give initial diagnosis • SR: essential elements for bipolar diagnosis • SR: pediatric bipolar diagnostic algorithm • PD: assessment and treatment of pediatric bipolar disorder
ADHD: the finer points of assessment	80 min	• SR: ADHD diagnosis, cause, and prognosis • TE: responding to tough questions about ADHD • TE: identify ADHD assessment strategies for special populations • TE: score and interpret ADHD rating scales from multiple informants
Treating ADHD: getting most out of medication part I	40 min	• SR: overview of optimal medication management • CP: initial presenting symptoms and follow-up data for patient, including ADHD scales from multiple informants • SR: medication algorithm for pharmacologic treatment of ADHD

Treating ADHD: getting the most out of medication part II	70 min	• TE: initial case formulation and treatment decisions for teen with ADHD • CP: school-aged boy with behavior problems and harried mother • FD: review of modified motivational interview techniques • PD: pharmacologic treatment of ADHD
Q&A: homework	15 min	• IE: prepare a brief case presentation to present on day 3 for homework
Total training time (not including breaks)	6 h 30 min	
Day 3		
Overview and welcome to day 3	5 min	
Assessment and treatment of aggression in youth	55 min	• CP: assessment of child with significant aggression • SR: practice guidelines for assessing and treating aggression • TE: score rating scales for aggressive child, identify optimal treatment plan
Psychosis	25 min	• SR: common presentations and causes of psychotic symptoms in children and youth • PD: assessment and treatment of psychosis
Adverse effects and monitoring of atypicals	35 min	• SR: side effects management • FD: use of AIMS to screen for adverse side effects
Your training is just beginning	45 min	• PRP: conduct a mock consultation call
Coding for billing	30 min	• SR: billing coding for PC-based mental health services • PD: procedure codes for PC-based child mental health services
Next steps for your practice	60 min	• TE: each participant identifies a goal for incorporating new strategies into practice, obstacle to achieving this goal, and a plan to work around the obstacle; makes a commitment to putting plan into place
Completion of exit paperwork	15 min	
Total training time (not including breaks)	4 h 30 min	

Abbreviations: ADHD, attention-deficit/hyperactivity disorder; AIMS, Abnormal Involuntary Movement Scale; CP, case presentation; FD, faculty demonstration; FDA, US Food and Drug Administration; GD, group discussion; IE, individual exercise; PC, primary care; PD, panel discussion; PRP, participant role play; Q&A, question and answer; SR, slide review/content presentation; TE, table exercise.

[a] Faculty presenters rotate at the start of most training topics.

From The Resource for Advancing Children's Health (REACH) Institute, New York, NY; with permission.

Participants hear PPCP faculty present information and success stories related to challenges such as engaging families, obtaining a psychiatric symptom history, conducting a mental status examination, constructing a differential diagnosis, and implementing appropriate treatment plans; topics that PPCPs may think are outside the scope of standard primary care practice. During the subsequent months of small-group consultation calls, 2 PPP faculty and 10 to 12 PPCP learners work together to problem-solve and apply the learning content to learners' own pediatric patients. The opportunity to receive feedback from peers and instructors in conjunction with multiple learning modalities over an extended period of time creates a foundation of knowledge and trust for PPCPs to practice and refine the behavior change needed.

There are 12 core objectives for the PPP Fellowship course, and each one is pursued with educational elements purposefully designed in accordance with behavioral science principles (a summary is shown in **Table 2**). Three have training elements drawn from all 3 theoretic areas, 6 incorporate principles from 2 different areas (adult learning and either behavior decision or communication theory), and only 3 are informed by only 1 area of behavioral science research. The objective to build a supportive learning network among faculty and PPCPs provides one example of how course elements leverage multiple theoretic principles. Strategies such as seating providers at tables with fellow call group members and engaging them in shared exercises are used to cultivate a supportive network with common social norms related to managing children's mental health problems, because participants may not have colleagues who share this goal within their practices. In addition to group team-building collaboration, table exercises introduce variety in the learning modalities and foster deeper-level learning through critical thinking and problem solving that aligns with adult learning principles. In addition, PPCP and child psychiatry faculty coteach to tap into social norms (as in BDT), as well as to target communication theory principles related to the credibility of the speakers. The child psychiatrists have credibility as experts, but PPP Fellowship participants tend to identify more strongly with PPCP faculty because they are able to speak firsthand about the challenges and successes of implementing the recommended practices with primary care populations. This example shows the degree of intentionality given to designing each element of the PPP Fellowship course.

Another aspect of the PPP Fellowship program worth highlighting is that, before introducing specific learning topics, the faculty orient participants to 4 overarching practice principles, called The REACH First Principles, that apply broadly to children's mental health (**Box 1**). These 4 principles are intended to guide high-quality service delivery, irrespective of a specific diagnostic area. They provide a framework for the course as a whole, and, per adult learning research, are reiterated throughout the course to enhance learning and retention. The principles are rooted in an evidence base that supports the interventions and strategies that PPCPs are taught to use. The REACH First Principles underscore not only that this work is within their scope of practice but also that PPCPs are often in the best position to do pediatric mental health care management.

Support for the Patient-Centered Mental Health in Pediatric Primary Care Fellowship program

Evaluation and survey data from several pediatric health care service networks indicate that long-term, measurable attitude and practice changes occur among PPCPs who participate in the PPP Fellowship program. With regard to provider attitudes and perceptions, PPP Fellowship alumni report increased comfort with prescribing antidepressants, stimulants, mood stabilizers, and atypical antipsychotic medications,

Table 2
Summary of training objectives, course elements, and related theoretic principles for Patient-Centered Mental Health in Pediatric Primary Care minifellowship

Training Phase	Objective	Corresponding PPP Course Elements	Behavior Decision Theory	Adult Learning Methods	Persuasive Communication Theory
Pretraining	Assemble a cohort of motivated learners	• Encourage partnering institutions to allow PPCPs to self-select into the course (rather than mandate attendance) • Clearly describe course aims and training activities in promotional materials to attract participants with compatible learning goals		✓	✓
Pretraining	Develop an effective training team of credible teachers to lead the course	• Have specialists and PPCPs colead the course as peers; recruit PPCP alumni to the faculty • Prospective faculty undergo an initial development process in which they gradually assume increasing levels of training responsibilities • Faculty debrief together at the end of each training day to continually refine teaching skills and ensure high-quality content delivery		✓	✓
Registration/ orientation and core Training	Build a supportive learning network among training faculty and learners	• Program faculty personally greet each participant • Faculty converse with PPCPs 1 on 1 during breaks and lunch • Use ice breakers, group role plays, and humor to foster relationships • Optional dinner with faculty after day 1 to build relationships in a relaxed social setting • Learners are intentionally grouped by tables differently each day • TEs encourage team building and foster group critical thinking and problem solving	✓	✓	✓

(continued on next page)

Table 2
(continued)

Training Phase	Objective	Corresponding PPP Course Elements	Behavior Decision Theory	Adult Learning Methods	Persuasive Communication Theory
Registration/ orientation	Provide a comfortable and effective learning environment	• Begin course on Friday afternoon to reduce impact on practitioners' clinic schedules • Deliver course in a professional, comfortable venue • Serve meals and snacks consistent with learners' dietary preferences • Allow PPCPs to self-select seating on day 1 so they are comfortable to begin their learning journey • Faculty model prioritizing for learning by re-training from using electronic devices or having side conversations during the course • Faculty promptly address any distractions in the environment		✓	
Registration/ orientation and core training	Obtain participant input on impact and effectiveness of program for meeting learning needs	• Administer questionnaires to gather data on PPCPs' precourse and postcourse knowledge and confidence in addressing mental health • Administer evaluations immediately following each learning module • Faculty review unit evaluations daily and make course adjustments as needed to accommodate learners' preferences and requests	✓	✓	✓

Core training	Create a trusting learning climate so participants feel safe to take risks with new skills and behaviors	• Faculty convey respect for PPCPs' existing experiences and education by using collaborative language, validating PPCPs' contributions, and soliciting PPCPs' ideas and solutions before offering their own • Sequence learning topics to present more intimidating topics near the end of training, after trust in faculty is established	✓	✓	✓	✓
Core training	Provide learners with knowledge and tools for practice change	• Provide participants with course book (slides) and practice tools (eg, assessment questionnaires, medication guideline cards) • Structure course to dedicate more training time to less familiar skills (eg, administering and interpreting assessment tools) • Prompt PPCPs to identify their own learning needs and goals	✓	✓		
Core training	Capture and retain the learner's attention	• Stimulate need to know (eg, pose a rhetorical question) before delivering information • Use humorous and/or novel presentation methods • Change presenters and/or format at least once per hour • Introduce modules with emotionally salient anecdotes ("hooks")	✓			

(continued on next page)

Table 2
(continued)

Training Phase	Objective	Corresponding PPP Course Elements	Behavior Decision Theory	Adult Learning Methods	Persuasive Communication Theory
Core training	Enhance information retention and recall	• Present course overview and REACH First Principles early in training to begin building a cognitive roadmap • Focus content on relevant critical skills (rather than facts) • Keep content simple and succinct • Deliver content using multiple teaching methods and modalities • Combine information with emotional content (eg, anecdotes) • Present course content using narrative story-telling techniques • Repeat key information and skills across multiple modules		✓	✓
Core training	Enhance learner comfort and self-efficacy with new practice skills	• Engage PPCPs in individual activities, TEs, and role plays focused on practicing critical skills • Faculty provide immediate coaching and feedback during learning exercises and on consultation calls	✓	✓	

| Core training | Address obstacles to practice change | • Provide PPCPs with information on billing for mental health services
• Guide PPCPs in mental contrasting and implementation intention exercises to enhance commitment to practice change and plan how they will overcome obstacles | ✓ | ✓ | ✓ |
| Posttraining | Provide mechanisms for continued learning and feedback | • Faculty facilitate 12 group conference calls
• All PPCPs present cases and contribute to group discussions
• Faculty reiterate key course content, skills, and resources
• Evaluate learners' changes over time in the key predictors of BIs
• At 6 mo, obtain feedback for course improvement from learners | ✓ | ✓ | ✓ |

From The Resource for Advancing Children's Health (REACH) Institute, New York, NY; with permission.

Box 1
The Resource for Advancing Children's Health First Principles

1. Developmental/contextual assessment
   i. Do a thorough diagnostic and biopsychosocial evaluation
      a. Assess strengths and challenges in the child's networks (eg, family, friends, neighborhood, school)
   ii. Psychiatric medications are only 1 part of an effective treatment plan

2. Team formation, communication, and decision making
   i. Engage in shared decision making with the family and child regarding medication use
      a. Ask about concerns and address them in an ongoing manner
   ii. Treat primary problem (or most urgent or impairing problem) with indicated medication first
   iii. Use rating scales to measure target symptoms at baseline and throughout treatment
   iv. Promote recovery and home by providing patient and caregivers with support, empowerment, and self-management tools
      a. Sustain therapeutic alliance and shared problem solving

3. Do no harm
   i. Understand developmental differences between youth and adults in medication efficacy and side effects
      a. For example, children may require proportionally higher doses because of faster metabolism, kidney clearance, and liver/body-size ratio
   ii. Start a new medication at a low dose, and taper (up or down) slowly
   iii. Use a systematic rating method for monitoring side effects over time

4. Evidence-based prescribing practices
   i. Whenever possible, use medications supported by double-blind randomized controlled trial (RCTs) for this age group, gender, and diagnosis
   ii. Strive for a parsimonious medication regimen
   iii. Use care when changing medication regimen
      a. Make only 1 medication change at a time and monitor results
      b. Consider environmental strategies as an alternative or complement
   iv. Evaluate for iatrogenic effects of multiple medications
      a. When unclear, consider tapering or discontinuing the most worrisome medication or the one with the least RCT evidence first

From The Resource for Advancing Children's Health (REACH) Institute, New York, NY; with permission.

---

beyond the impact reported from traditional CME programs.[38] In addition, PPP-trained providers note increased comfort with assessing, diagnosing, and treating pediatric mental health conditions[39]; persistently high BIs (after 6 and 12 months) to practice changes to deliver guideline-based care as a result of the training[39,40]; fewer perceived barriers to guideline implementation[40]; and high satisfaction with the course itself (ie, rated in the top 10% of medical education trainings).[39] As predicted based on the Behavior Decision Theory framework, interpretable associations in the expected directions are found between participants' BI to implement guideline-based practices and their self-reported expectancy beliefs, perceived social norms, and sense of self-efficacy (Peter S. Jensen, unpublished data, 2017).

More importantly, the PPP Fellowship program is associated with a wide range of concrete changes in practice behaviors. Compared with PPCPs who did not attend the course, or PPCPs' own practice behaviors before the training, PPP alumni have shown increased use of symptom rating scales,[39,40] better adherence to recommended prescribing practices (eg, medication initiation, titration, and less poly-pharmacy),[17] higher rates of appropriate patient follow-up[17,40] and/or mental health specialty referrals,[17] and increased use of psychiatric consultation resources.[38]

Furthermore, changes in PPCPs' attitudes and behaviors following the PPP Fellowship program are associated with improved patient medication compliance and substantial cost savings among patients with Medicaid.[17] In sum, a growing body of evidence indicates that the PPP Fellowship program's theory-driven education methods and training strategies successfully translate into PPCP behavior changes, thereby enhancing access to mental health assessment and treatment of youth in primary care.

DISCUSSION

Successful adoption of integrative mental health care models require PPCPs who are willing and able to screen, diagnose, and treat youth mental health problems in the primary care setting. To facilitate this goal, effective teaching methods designed to reinforce positive BIs and maximize the likelihood of practice behavior change are needed. Behavior science, adult learning, and communication theory are three complementary frameworks that can be used to design medical educational strategies to optimize the likelihood of provider practice change. Specific training methods derived from these theoretic frameworks and applied to the design of a medical education course that trains PPCPs to assess, diagnose, and manage child mental health concerns within their primary care practices are discussed. Evaluation and survey data across multiple systems and hundreds of PPCPs supports the utility of the PPP Fellowship program in effecting change in PPCPs' attitudes and practice behaviors as they relate to pediatric mental health. The course objectives and educational elements described herein are specific to the PPP Fellowship program, but may serve as a model for provider educators in any postgraduate medical education field.

No training course will be successful for everyone. The benefit of a theory-driven training model is that it provides a systematic, structured way to predict, evaluate, and refine the impact of an educational course. When a training program fails to have the intended impact on specific individuals, pretraining/posttraining data should be analyzed to identify why and for whom, and then inform subsequent changes to the teaching methodology. For example, analyzing self-report data for providers who show little behavior change following the in-person training might reveal countervailing forces related to social norms (eg, practice partners disapprove of the new procedures), low self-efficacy (eg, providers lacking confidence in their ability to learn how to interpret all these symptom rating scale scores), or negative outcome expectations (eg, believing that, if an SSRI is prescribed to a teen, the teen is likely to become suicidal). All may have the same outcome (ie, lack of provider behavior change), but, armed with data and the theoretic framework, educators can design tailored solutions that target the underlying obstacles (eg, build a supportive peer network, provide additional opportunities for rehearsal and feedback, or provide information to clarify misconceptions).

Focusing on training methods that resonate with an individual provider is only one aspect of a comprehensive, effective medical education/behavior change program. Other system-level, provider-level, and patient-level factors must be identified and addressed to optimize the likelihood that recommended procedures become the standard of care. Although training existing practitioners is an important and valuable step, it would be more efficient and perhaps effective to expose PPCPs to integrative mental health practice during residency or fellowship so they are prepared to deliver these services after graduation.

Future research on PPCP mental health training strategies should systematically evaluate the effectiveness of theory-driven training programs, compared with traditional CME methods, and explore strategies to make them more cost-effective and widely available. Moreover, computerized or web-based training models might allow the individualized assessment of learners' specific needs, and allow future trainings to be more closely tailored to each individual. Thus, future research should examine whether specific training techniques and content can be matched to learners based on variability in relevant characteristics, such as preferred learning styles; communication strengths and deficits; and individuals' BI factors, such as expected values, perceived norms, and self-efficacy.

REFERENCES

1. Liao Q, Manteuffel B, Paulic C, et al. Describing the population of adolescents served in systems of care. J Emot Behav Disord 2001;9:13–29.
2. Bunik M, Talmi A, Stafford B, et al. Integrating mental health services in primary care continuity clinics: a national CORNET study. Acad Pediatr 2013;13:551–7.
3. American Academy of Child and Adolescent Psychiatry Committee on Health Care Access and Economics Task Force on Mental Health. Improving mental health services in primary care: reducing administrative and financial barriers to access and collaboration. Pediatrics 2009;123(4):1248–51.
4. McMillan JA, Land M Jr, Leslie LK. Pediatric residency education and the behavioral and mental health crisis: a call to action. Pediatrics 2017;139(1):e20162141.
5. Bloom B. Effects of continuing medical education on improving physician clinical care and patient health: a review of systematic reviews. Int J Technol Assess Health Care 2005;21(3):380–5.
6. Mansouri M, Lockyer J. A meta-analysis of continuing medical education effectiveness. J Contin Educ Health Prof 2007;27(1):6–15.
7. Davis D, O'Brien MA, Freemantle N, et al. Impact of formal continuing medical education: do conferences, workshops, rounds, and other traditional continuing education activities change physician behavior or health care outcomes? JAMA 1999;282(9):867–74.
8. Giguere A, Legare F, Grimshaw J, et al. Printed educational materials: effects on professional practice and health care outcomes. Cochrane Database Syst Rev 2013;(4):CD004398.
9. Flodgren G, Parmelli E, Doumit G, et al. Local opinion leaders: effects on professional practice and health care outcomes. Cochrane Database Syst Rev 2011;(8):CD000125.
10. Ivers N, Jamtvedt G, Flottorn S, et al. Audit and feedback: effects on professional practice and healthcare outcomes. Cochrane Database Syst Rev 2012;(7):CD000259.
11. Baker R, Camosso-Stefinovic J, Gillies C, et al. Tailored intervention to address determinants of practice. Cochrane Database Syst Rev 2015;(4):CD005470.
12. O'Brien AM, Rogers S, Jamtvedt G, et al. Educational outreach visits: effects on professional practice and health care outcomes. Cochrane Database Syst Rev 2008;(4):CD000409.
13. Arditi C, Rege-Walther M, Wyatt JC, et al. Computer-generated reminders delivered on paper to healthcare professionals: effects on professional practice and health care outcomes. Cochrane Database Syst Rev 2012;(12):CD001175.
14. Shojania KG, Jennings A, Mayhew A, et al. The effects of on-screen, point of care computer reminders on processes and outcomes of care. Cochrane Database Syst Rev 2001;(1):CD001096.

15. Vaona A, Rigon G, Banzi R, et al. E-learning for health professionals. Cochrane Database Syst Rev 2012;(11):CD011736.

16. Forsetlund L, Bjorndal A, Rashidian A, et al. Continuing education meetings and workshops: effects on professional practice and health care outcomes. Cochrane Database Syst Rev 2012;(11):CD003030.

17. Domino M, Humble C, Wegner L, et al. Changes in ADHD prescribing after psychotropic medication training. Paper presented at the 140th American Public Health Association Meeting. San Francisco, CA, October, 27–31, 2012. Available at: https://apha.confex.com/apha/140am/webprogram/Paper270356.html. Accessed March 31, 2017.

18. Perkins MB, Jensen PS, Jaccard J, et al. Applying theory-driven approaches to understanding and modifying clinicians' behavior: what do we know? Psychiatr Serv 2007;58(3):342–8.

19. Fishbein M, Triandis HC, Kanfer FH, et al. Factors influencing behavior and behavior change. In: Baum A, Revenson TA, Singer JE, editors. Handbook of health psychology. Mahwah (NJ): Lawrence Erlbaum Associates; 2001. p. 3–17.

20. Jaccard J, Dodge T, Dittus P. Parent-adolescent communication about sex and birth control: a conceptual framework. In: Feldman S, Rosenthal DA, editors. Talking sexuality: parent-adolescent communication. San Francisco (CA): Jossey-Bass; 2002. p. 11–41.

21. Jaccard J. The prevention of problem behaviors in adolescents and young adults: perspectives on theory and practice. J Soc Social Work Res 2016;7(4): 585–613.

22. Fishbein M, Ajzen I. Belief, attitude, intention, and behavior: an introduction to theory and research. Reading (MA): Addison-Wesley; 1975.

23. Bandura A. Self-efficacy: toward a unifying theory of behavioral change. Psychol Rev 1977;84(2):191–215.

24. Oettinger G, Gollwitzer PM. Strategies of setting and implementing goals. In: Tangney JP, editor. Social psychological foundations of clinical psychology. New York: The Guilford Press; 2010. p. 114–33.

25. Knowles MS, Holton EF, Swanson RA. The adult learner: the definitive classic in adult education and human resource development. 8th edition. New York: Routledge; 2015.

26. Stahl SM, Davis RL. Best practices for medical educators. Carlsbad (CA): NEI Press; 2009.

27. Taylor K, Marienau C. Facilitating learning with the adult brain in mind: a conceptual and practical guide. San Francisco (CA): Jossey-Bass; 2015.

28. Heath C, Heath D. Made to stick: why some ideas survive and others die. New York: Random House; 2008.

29. Lemov D. Teach like a champion. San Francisco (CA): Jossey-Bas; 2010.

30. Shannon C. A mathematical theory of communication. Bell Sys Tech J 1948;7: 379–423, 623–656.

31. Katz E. The two-step flow of communication. Public Opin Q 1957;21:61–78.

32. Weiner N. Human use of human beings: cybernetics and society. Garden City (NY): Doubleday; 1954.

33. Hovland CI, Janis IL, Kelley HH. Communication and persuasion: psychological studies of opinion change. New Haven (CT): Yale University Press; 1953.

34. McGinnies E, Ward CD. Better liked than right: trustworthiness and expertise as factors in credibility. Pers Soc Psychol Bull 1980;6:467–72.

35. Wiener JL, Mowen JC. Source credibility: on the independent effects of trust and expertise. In: Lutz RJ, editor. Advances in consumer research. Provo (UT): Association for Consumer Research; 1986. p. 306–10.

36. Allen M, Preiss RW. Persuasion: advances through meta-analysis. Cresskill (NJ): Hampton Press; 1998.

37. Andrews JC, Shimp TA. Effects of involvement, argument strength, and source characteristics on central and peripheral processing in advertising. Psychol Market 1990;7:195–214.

38. Hargrave TM, Fremont W, Cogswell A, et al. Helping primary care clinicians give mental health care - What works? Presented at the 61st American Academy of Child and Adolescent Psychiatry Meeting. San Diego, CA, October 20–25, 2014. Available at: https://aacap.confex.com/aacap/2014/webprogram/Paper22076. html. Accessed March 31, 2017.

39. Sharma V, Galanter C, Jensen PS, et al. Pediatricians and primary care physician's knowledge, comfort, and practices about children's mental health before and after a theory-based training. Presented at the 60th American Academy of Child and Adolescent Psychiatry Meeting. Orlando, FL, October 19–27, 2013. Available at: https://aacap.confex.com/aacap/2013/webprogram/Paper20549.html. Accessed March 31, 2017.

40. Humble C, Domino M, Jensen PS, et al. Changes in perceptions of guideline-level care in North Carolina. Paper presented at the 140th American Public Health Association. Available at: https://apha.confex.com/apha/140am/webprogram/Paper270346.html. Accessed March 31, 2017.

UNITED STATES POSTAL SERVICE® Statement of Ownership, Management, and Circulation (All Periodicals Publications Except Requester Publications)

1. Publication Title	2. Publication Number	3. Filing Date
CHILD AND ADOLESCENT PSYCHIATRIC CLINICS OF NORTH AMERICA	011 – 368	9/18/2017

4. Issue Frequency	5. Number of Issues Published Annually	6. Annual Subscription Price
JAN, APR, JUL, OCT	4	$316.00

7. Complete Mailing Address of Known Office of Publication (Not printer) (Street, city, county, state, and ZIP+4®)

ELSEVIER INC.
230 Park Avenue, Suite 800
New York, NY 10169

Contact Person
STEPHEN R. BUSHING
Telephone (Include area code)
215-239-3688

8. Complete Mailing Address of Headquarters or General Business Office of Publisher (Not printer)

ELSEVIER INC.
230 Park Avenue, Suite 800
New York, NY 10169

9. Full Names and Complete Mailing Addresses of Publisher, Editor, and Managing Editor (Do not leave blank)

Publisher (Name and complete mailing address)

ADRIANNE BRIGIDO, ELSEVIER INC.
1600 JOHN F KENNEDY BLVD. SUITE 1800
PHILADELPHIA, PA 19103-2899

Editor (Name and complete mailing address)

LAUREN BOYLE, ELSEVIER INC.
1600 JOHN F KENNEDY BLVD. SUITE 1800
PHILADELPHIA, PA 19103-2899

Managing Editor (Name and complete mailing address)

PATRICK MANLEY, ELSEVIER INC.
1600 JOHN F KENNEDY BLVD. SUITE 1800
PHILADELPHIA, PA 19103-2899

10. Owner (Do not leave blank. If the publication is owned by a corporation, give the name and address of the corporation immediately followed by the names and addresses of all stockholders owning or holding 1 percent or more of the total amount of stock. If not owned by a corporation, give the names and addresses of the individual owners. If owned by a partnership or other unincorporated firm, give its name and address as well as those of each individual owner. If the publication is published by a nonprofit organization, give its name and address.)

Full Name	Complete Mailing Address
WHOLLY OWNED SUBSIDIARY OF REED/ELSEVIER, US HOLDINGS	1600 JOHN F KENNEDY BLVD, SUITE 1800 PHILADELPHIA, PA 19103-2899

11. Known Bondholders, Mortgagees, and Other Security Holders Owning or Holding 1 Percent or More of Total Amount of Bonds, Mortgages, or Other Securities. If none, check box ▶ ☐ None

Full Name	Complete Mailing Address
N/A	

12. Tax Status (For completion by nonprofit organizations authorized to mail at nonprofit rates) (Check one)
The purpose, function, and nonprofit status of this organization and the exempt status for federal income tax purposes:
☒ Has Not Changed During Preceding 12 Months
☐ Has Changed During Preceding 12 Months (Publisher must submit explanation of change with this statement)

13. Publication Title	14. Issue Date for Circulation Data Below
CHILD AND ADOLESCENT PSYCHIATRIC CLINICS OF NORTH AMERICA	JULY 2017

15. Extent and Nature of Circulation		Average No. Copies Each Issue During Preceding 12 Months	No. Copies of Single Issue Published Nearest to Filing Date
a. Total Number of Copies (Net press run)		315	257
b. Paid Circulation (By Mail and Outside the Mail)	(1) Mailed Outside-County Paid Subscriptions Stated on PS Form 3541 (Include paid distribution above nominal rate, advertiser's proof copies, and exchange copies)	152	141
	(2) Mailed In-County Paid Subscriptions Stated on PS Form 3541 (Include paid distribution above nominal rate, advertiser's proof copies, and exchange copies)	0	0
	(3) Paid Distribution Outside the Mails Including Sales Through Dealers and Carriers, Street Vendors, Counter Sales, and Other Paid Distribution Outside USPS®	49	45
	(4) Paid Distribution by Other Classes of Mail Through the USPS (e.g., First-Class Mail®)	0	0
c. Total Paid Distribution (Sum of 15b (1), (2), (3), and (4))		201	186
d. Free or Nominal Rate Distribution (By Mail and Outside the Mail)	(1) Free or Nominal Rate Outside-County Copies included on PS Form 3541	72	71
	(2) Free or Nominal Rate In-County Copies Included on PS Form 3541	0	0
	(3) Free or Nominal Rate Copies Mailed at Other Classes Through the USPS (e.g., First-Class Mail)	0	0
	(4) Free or Nominal Rate Distribution Outside the Mail (Carriers or other means)	0	0
e. Total Free or Nominal Rate Distribution (Sum of 15d (1), (2), (3) and (4))		72	71
f. Total Distribution (Sum of 15c and 15e)		273	257
g. Copies not Distributed (See Instructions to Publishers #4 (page #3))		42	0
h. Total (Sum of 15f and g)		315	257
i. Percent Paid (15c divided by 15f times 100)		73.63%	72.37%

* If you are claiming electronic copies, go to line 16 on page 3. If you are not claiming electronic copies, skip to line 17 on page 3.

16. Electronic Copy Circulation	Average No. Copies Each Issue During Preceding 12 Months	No. Copies of Single Issue Published Nearest to Filing Date
a. Paid Electronic Copies ▶	0	0
b. Total Paid Print Copies (Line 15c) + Paid Electronic Copies (Line 16a) ▶	201	186
c. Total Print Distribution (Line 15f) + Paid Electronic Copies (Line 16a) ▶	273	257
d. Percent Paid (Both Print & Electronic Copies) (16b divided by 16c × 100) ▶	73.63%	72.37%

☒ I certify that 50% of all my distributed copies (electronic and print) are paid above a nominal price.

17. Publication of Statement of Ownership

☒ If the publication is a general publication, publication of this statement is required. Will be printed
in the OCTOBER 2017 issue of this publication.

☐ Publication not required.

18. Signature and Title of Editor, Publisher, Business Manager, or Owner

STEPHEN R. BUSHING - INVENTORY DISTRIBUTION CONTROL MANAGER

Stephen R. Bushing

Date 9/18/2017

I certify that all information furnished on this form is true and complete. I understand that anyone who furnishes false or misleading information on this form or who omits material or information requested on the form may be subject to criminal sanctions (including fines and imprisonment) and/or civil sanctions (including civil penalties).

PS Form **3526**, July 2014 [Page 3 of 4]

PS Form 3526, July 2014 (Page 1 of 4 (see instructions page 4)) PSN: 7530-01-000-9931   PRIVACY NOTICE: See our privacy policy on www.usps.com.

Moving?

Make sure your subscription moves with you!

To notify us of your new address, find your **Clinics Account Number** (located on your mailing label above your name), and contact customer service at:

Email: journalscustomerservice-usa@elsevier.com

800-654-2452 (subscribers in the U.S. & Canada)
314-447-8871 (subscribers outside of the U.S. & Canada)

Fax number: 314-447-8029

Elsevier Health Sciences Division
Subscription Customer Service
3251 Riverport Lane
Maryland Heights, MO 63043

*To ensure uninterrupted delivery of your subscription, please notify us at least 4 weeks in advance of move.

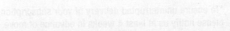

Printed and bound by CPI Group (UK) Ltd, Croydon, CR0 4YY

22/10/2024

01777661-0005